Cardiac Critical Care Made Visual: An Illustrated Guide

Cardiac Critical Care Made Visual: An Illustrated Guide

By Caitlyn Nichols, BSN, RN, CCRN-CMC

JEB Wizard Publishing
Books With Character

Copyright

Cover illustration by David Convissar, MD — a cardiac anesthesiologist & intensivist. He is the creator of Count Backwards from 10, an online multimedia medical education platform for anesthesia and critical care medicine (@countbackwardsfrom10 on Instagram), and Master the Machines — a clinical course in mechanical circulatory support (www.masterthemachines.com).

Medical Disclaimer:

Please note that the information contained within this book is for educational purposes only and is not to be used as medical advice. Readers acknowledge that the author is not engaging in the rendering of legal, financial, medical or professional advice. Although every attempt has been made to provide accurate, up-to-date, and reliable information with the standards generally accepted at the time of publication, the author and publisher are not, under any circumstances, liable for errors or omissions or for any consequences from application of the information in this book and make no warranty, expressed or implied, with respect to the currency, completeness, or accuracy of the contents of the publication. Application of this information in a particular situation remains the professional responsibility of the healthcare professional; the clinical treatments described and recommended may not be considered absolute and universal recommendations. Because medical science is a constantly evolving field, the reader is encouraged to always consult current research and specific institutional policies.

icunursingnotesbycaitlyn

The Story Behind *ICU Nursing Notes by Caitlyn™*, LLC

I started creating my notes in 2021 as a new graduate cardiac ICU nurse. Although I currently work in the cardiac cath lab, I distinctly remember the humbling and challenging experience of being a new grad in a high-acuity environment. The steep learning curve was difficult to navigate and, given the lack of educational resources tailored to visual learners like me, I knew I had to get creative. Determined to succeed and driven by my lifelong passion for art and creativity, I began creating my own study guides to meet my own learning needs. I then organized them into a resource binder for my unit, which I named *ICU Nursing Notes by Caitlyn*. Over time, I refined both the content and format, turning complex topics into visual aids that made concepts easier to understand and remember.

This unique and creative approach to learning helped me grasp difficult material on a deeper level. It encouraged me to ask more questions, think critically, and move beyond surface level learning. As I began to understand the *why*, the how naturally followed. I realized that other nurses likely had similar questions and learning styles, which prompted me to create an Instagram page (@icunursingnotesbycaitlyn) and launch an Etsy shop offering digital downloads. What started as a simple personal study tool has grown into a successful online business and an educational platform that is currently followed by 74,000+ healthcare professionals worldwide. I discovered a unique way to combine my love for art, science, and learning, and *ICU Nursing Notes by Caitlyn* has become my passion project.

This book is the resource that I wish I had as a new grad. It's designed to bridge the gap between nursing school and real-life practice, and it's inspired by my own struggle as a new nurse. Beyond identifying challenging concepts, the broader goal of this book is to make learning meaningful. When you truly understand the *why* behind what you're doing, the *how* becomes intuitive. You'll approach patient care with clarity, purpose, and critical insight and, with a deeper understanding, you'll be better equipped to recognize subtle patterns, see the bigger clinical picture, and anticipate clinical deterioration before it happens.

Starting my career in critical care during an unprecedented time in healthcare was difficult but defining. The unwavering support and mentorship I received from a special group of nurses **(Marie Rahme, Michelle Barbera, Sarah Bailey, Jamil Halaby, Susan Bartos, & Lynn Donatelli)** made all the difference. They shared their knowledge, believed in me, and encouraged me every step of the way. Their lessons continue to guide how I practice and teach. Inspired by their example, I am committed to paying it forward, offering the same support to the next generation of nurses so they can grow, thrive, and believe in themselves as lifelong learners who can make a lasting impact in this ever-evolving profession.

♡ Caitlyn

Table of Contents

1,600+ 5-STAR ETSY REVIEWS!

"5 stars! I really recommend all of her teaching tools. Great graphics with loads of good info. Very useful for my students! Caitlyn always does a fabulous job."
– Brenda M.
(author of *Fast Facts for the Cath Lab Nurse*)

"High quality & very detailed notes! I absolutely love the head-to-toe assessment cheat sheet. As a new grad in the ICU, thorough assessments can be stressful! Keeping this close by helps me double check myself. This one is definitely a must have!"

"All her notes are beautifully done, & very informational and accurate! I'm an experienced ICU nurse, but these are great to refresh and study and help me stay sharp. These would be fantastic for a nurse who is new to ICU."

"Gold mine of incredible information! This is incredibly helpful!"
– Daphne

"I have purchased at least 20 different nursing notes sets. This is HANDS DOWN the best one, especially if you want to work in critical care. They are not cheap, but worth every cent!"
– Tina R.

"I am a cath lab nurse, and I am always trying to learn great ways to explain concepts so that new staff members can understand them. This is such a great tool that shows when/why one device could be chosen over the other."

"I work in CTICU, and these notes are amazing. My coworkers have asked where I got them and I proudly refer them to this little Etsy shop."

– Emmaline A.

"This is an excellent tool to have if you're an ICU or acute care nurse. Explains starting doses, what to monitor, titrations, etc. Completely helpful if you are new to critical drips. Absolutely glad I made this purchase. Caitlyn was very friendly & helpful. Will purchase more very soon. :)"

"As a new grad MICU nurse, I found these so helpful as I've tried to make my own, but these exceeded my expectations and are made so much better than I could have. The time, expertise, and artistry put into these is beyond anything I've seen. Thank you so much, Caitlyn!"

"These notes are so well-made. Worth every penny."

– Claudia R.

"Seasoned ICU nurse, bought as a tool to teach new grads, can absolutely say when I showed them this the pharm finally CLICKED!"

"I have purchased multiple items from this store to show and aid in preceptorship for incoming nurses. This is WAY better than anything I could draw. Highly recommend her documents."

– Sierra J.

"I love this bundle! I went to Staples & had it printed. I've been carrying it around the cath lab & showing everyone. It's very loved, there is so much information that is beautifully displayed. I am a visual learner, & I come from a basic telemetry floor, so the learning curve is huge. I've been feeling much more confident having this to help me."

"Quick visual for when you are trying to figure out what's going on with your patient."

– Shannon S.

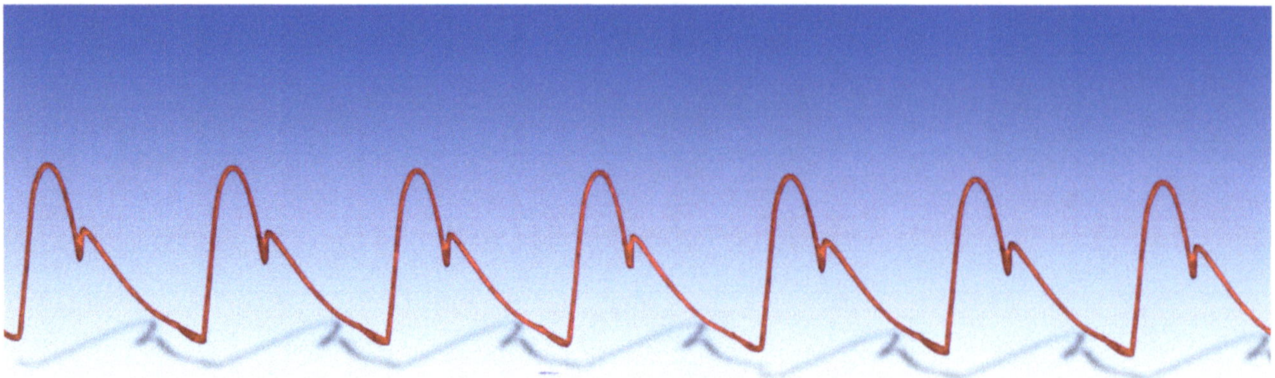

HEMODYNAMICS
hemodynamics

&

CARDIAC CATH LAB
cardiac cath lab

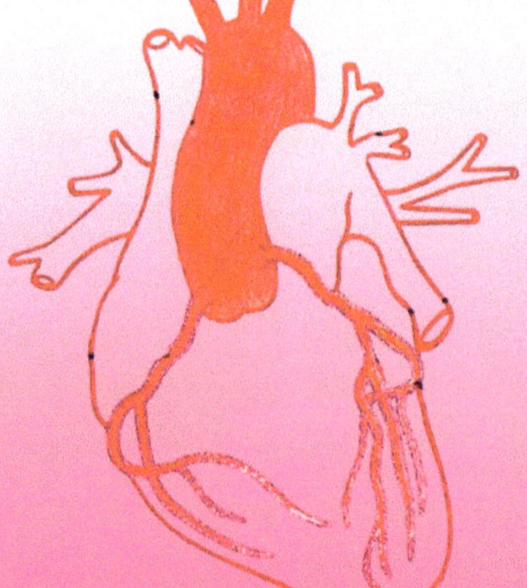

PRESSURE TRANSDUCERS

@ICUnursingnotesbycaitlyn

Indications

Invasive bedside hemodynamic monitoring of intravascular (arterial) and/or intra-cardiac (right atrial and pulmonary artery) pressures.

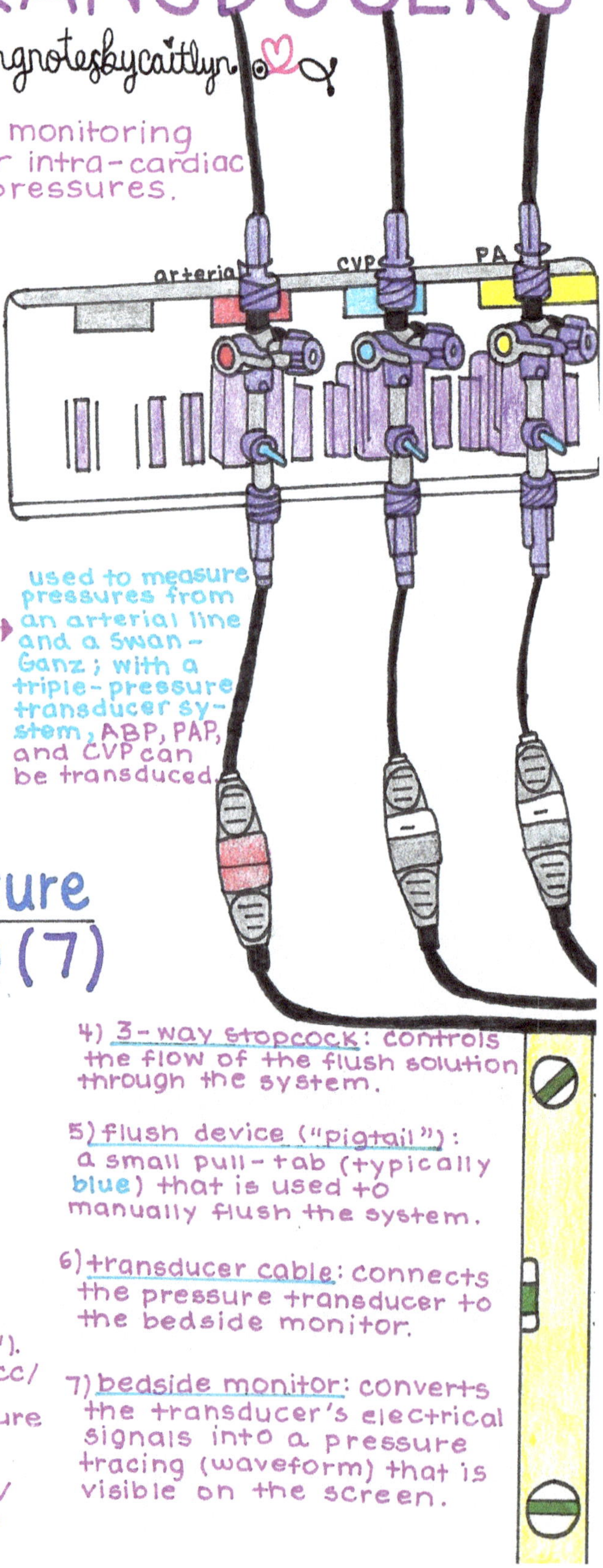

Single, Double, or Triple?

single → used to measure pressure from a single catheter (arterial line or CVC for CVP monitoring).

double → used to measure pressure from two catheters (arterial line and a CVC) or two ports (CVP and PA) on a Swan-Ganz catheter.

triple → used to measure pressures from an arterial line and a Swan-Ganz; with a triple-pressure transducer system, ABP, PAP, and CVP can be transduced.

Components of a Pressure Monitoring System (7)

1) Pressure transducer: detects the pressure waveform generated by ventricular ejection and converts that pressure wave into an electrical signal that is transmitted to the bedside monitor as a CVP/ABP/PAP waveform.

2) Pressure bag c̄ flush solution (NS): a continuous infusion of flush solution, under 300 mmHg of pressure, maintains a constant pressure through the transducer and flush device ("pigtail"). It's kept at a low continuous flow (≈ 3 cc/hr) to maintain patency, prevent blood backflow, and allow for accurate pressure transmissions.

3) Pressure tubing: Rigid and nonpliable IV tubing that connects the catheter in the patient to the transducer system.

4) 3-way stopcock: controls the flow of the flush solution through the system.

5) flush device ("pigtail"): a small pull-tab (typically blue) that is used to manually flush the system.

6) transducer cable: connects the pressure transducer to the bedside monitor.

7) bedside monitor: converts the transducer's electrical signals into a pressure tracing (waveform) that is visible on the screen.

Set Up

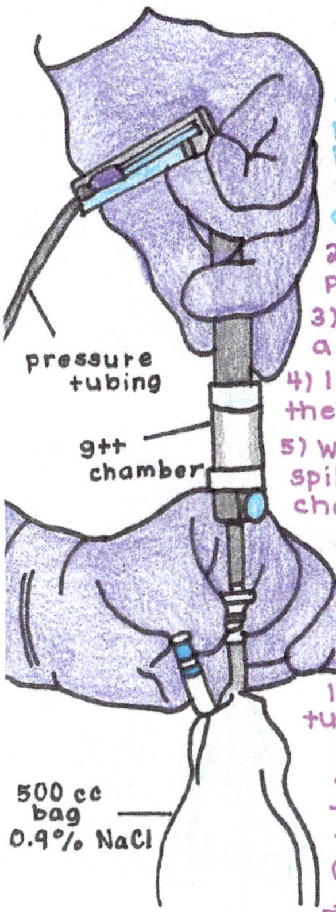

1) Ensure that you have all of the necessary supplies (pressure modules + cables, 500 cc bag NS, pressure bag, pressure transducer kit, dead-end caps, 18G needle, IV pole + transducer mount, labels, carpenter's level).

2) Tighten all connections on the pressure transducer system tubing.

3) Remove air from the NS IV bag c̄ a needle.

4) Insert the 500 cc bag of NS into the pressure bag (wait to inflate).

5) With the spike of the pressure tubing, spike the bag of saline, and fill the gtt chamber.

6) Flush the entire system (including the transducer, stopcocks, and the pressure tubing) by pulling the "pigtail" (fast-flush tab) on the transducer.
   → with the pigtail, flush from the IV bag through the tip of the pressure tubing.
   → turn the stopcock OFF to the patient, and pull the pigtail to flush the stopcock.
   → once the stopcock is primed, replace the vented cap c̄ a sterile nonvented ("dead-end") cap.
   → open the stopcock to the transducer (off to atmosphere, open to the flush solution, open to the patient).

7) Repeat step # 6 if priming a double or triple transducer system (c̄ each of the transducers).

8) Inflate the pressure bag to 300 mmHg.

9) Insert the transducer(s) into the IV pole mount holder.

10) Using sterile technique, connect the end of each transducer to the correct catheter port (i.e. arterial, PA, and/or CVP).

11) Label the tubing.

12) Plug the pressure cable(s) into the correct pressure module(s) on the bedside monitor.

13) Turn parameters on.

14) Level the transducer(s) to the phlebostatic axis (see the "arterial lines" cheat sheet for how to do this).

15) Zero the transducer.

Nursing Care

- Always check that the hemodynamic monitoring alarms and parameters are on and set appropriately.
- Zero and level the system to ensure accuracy.
- Maintain a closed system.
- Check and tighten connections.
- Minimize the use of additional stopcocks and extension tubing for the most accurate waveforms.
- Change the hemodynamic monitoring system per facility protocol.
- Ensure that you remove air from the saline bag on initial set-up and that there are no air bubbles in the tubing.
- Maintain the pressure bag at 300 mmHg.
- Ensure that there are dead-end caps on the end of each stopcock.
- Flush the system and the stopcock after drawing labs to prevent clotting.
- Always use sterile technique.

@sfficunursingnotesbycaitlyn

UNDERSTANDING THE ARTERIAL PRESSURE WAVEFORM

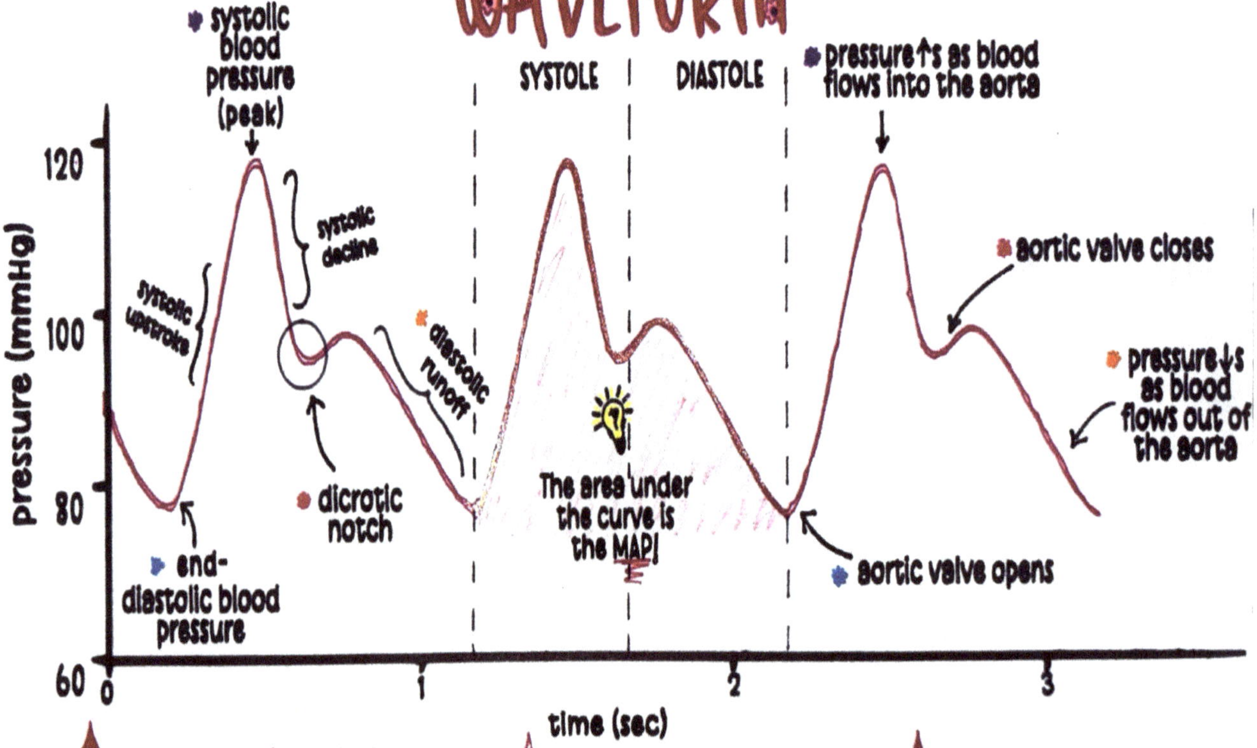

SYSTOLIC UPSTROKE

the rapid ↑ in the arterial blood pressure as the left ventricle ejects blood into the aorta, via the AV valve

SYSTOLIC PEAK

the waveform's highest point; this is the patient's systolic blood pressure.

SYSTOLIC DECLINE

arterial pressure ↓s as blood continues to travel into the peripheral blood vessels.

DICROTIC NOTCH

aortic valve closure & the beginning of diastole.

This is when intra-aortic balloon pump (IABP) inflation occurs!

DIASTOLIC RUNOFF

the decline in arterial pressure as ventricular contraction comes to an end.

END-DIASTOLIC PRESSURE

the lowest pressure during diastole.

@icunursingnotesbycaitlyn

Arterial Line Morphologies!

ARTERIAL WAVEFORMS: CENTRAL TO DISTAL

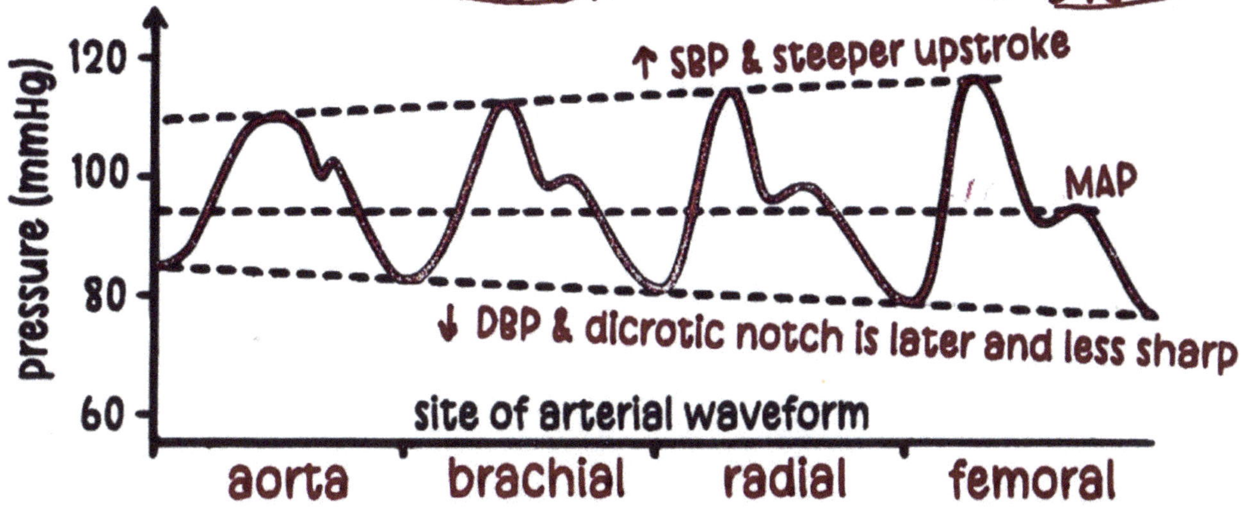

Although the radial artery is the most common site of invasive BP measurement, arterial BP can be measured anywhere along the arterial system (peripherally or centrally)!

CHARACTERISTIC WAVEFORMS:

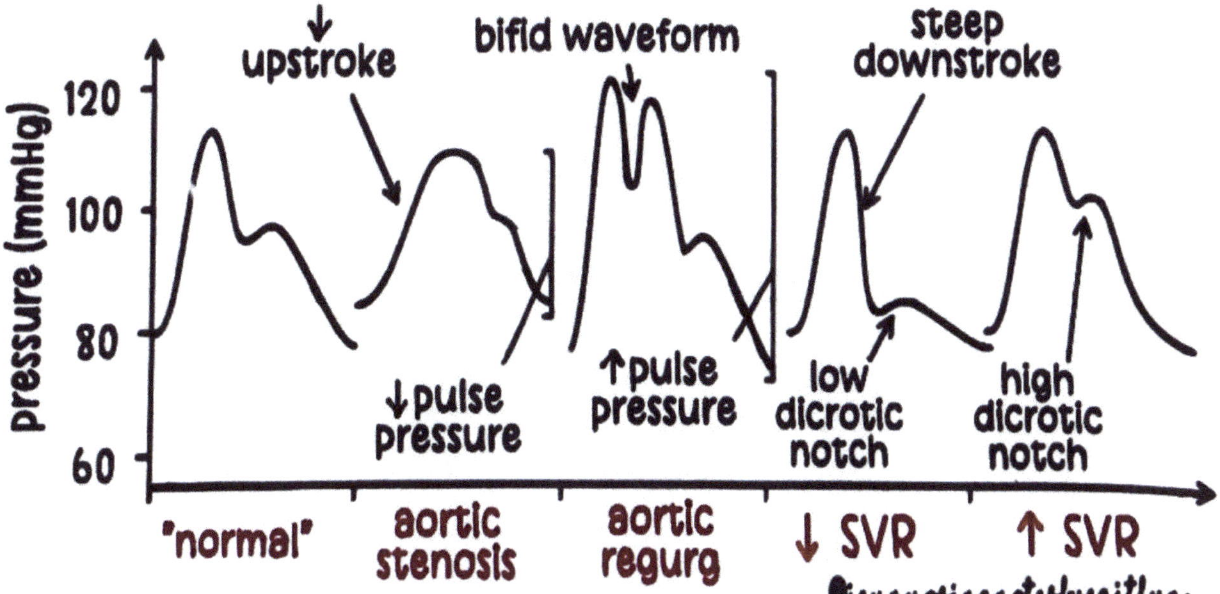

@icunursingnotesbycaitlyn

Cardiac Output

total cardiac output — heart rate — stroke volume

CO = HR x SV

≈4-8 L/min — BPM — mL/beat

mL/beat → preload, afterload, contractility

"How full is the tank?"

PRELOAD

(end-diastole)

the degree to which the ❤ muscle stretches before it contracts.

CVP & EDV are measures of preload!

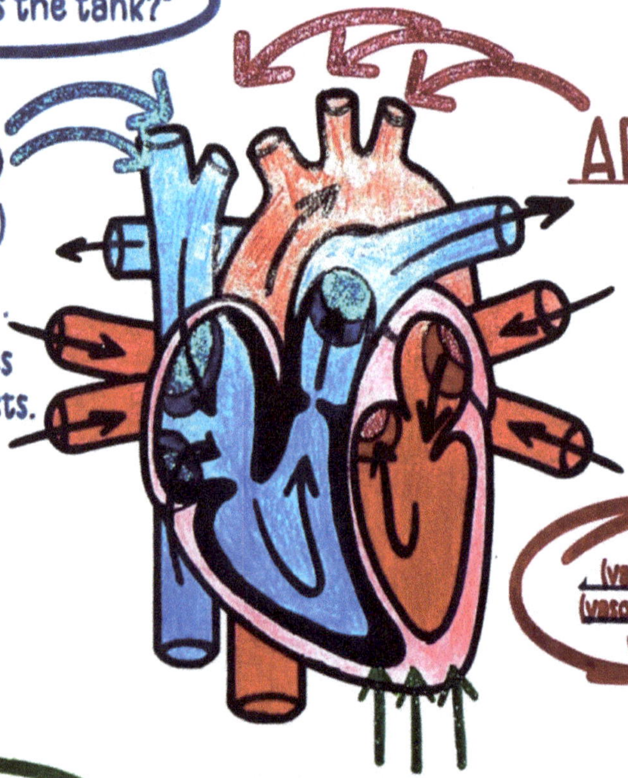

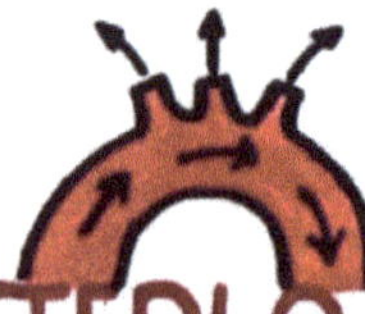

AFTERLOAD

(SVR)

the force that resists contraction.

"How loose (vasodilated)/tight (vasoconstricted) is the vasculature?"

"How is the squeeze?"

CONTRACTILITY

the ability of the ❤ muscle to contract & eject blood into the pulmonary (RV) or systemic vasculature (LV).

The ejection fraction (EF) reflects contractility!

❤ @icunursingnotesbycaitlyn ❤

CORONARY PERFUSION PRESSURE

The pressure gradient between the aortic diastolic pressure (ADP) & the LV end-diastolic pressure (LVEDP) that drives blood flow through the coronary arteries, ensuring oxygen delivery to the heart muscle.

CPP = ADP - LVEDP

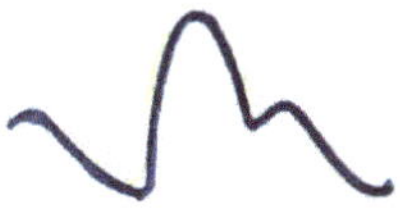

aortic diastolic pressure
(the "driving" force)

left ventricular end-diastolic pressure
(the "opposing" force)

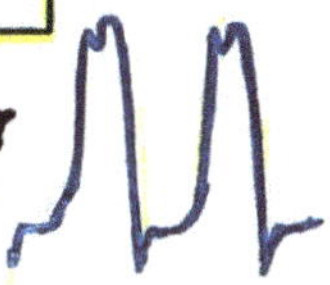

pulmonary wedge pressure can be used as a surrogate for LVEDP!

@icunursingnotesbycaitlyn

PATHOPHYS:

The heart is primarily perfused during diastole when blood comes back towards a closed aortic valve, which diverts blood into the right & left coronary ostia. The diastolic blood pressure meets resistance from the pressure/volume remaining inside the LV at the end of diastole (LVEDP). The difference between these 2 pressures is the CPP.

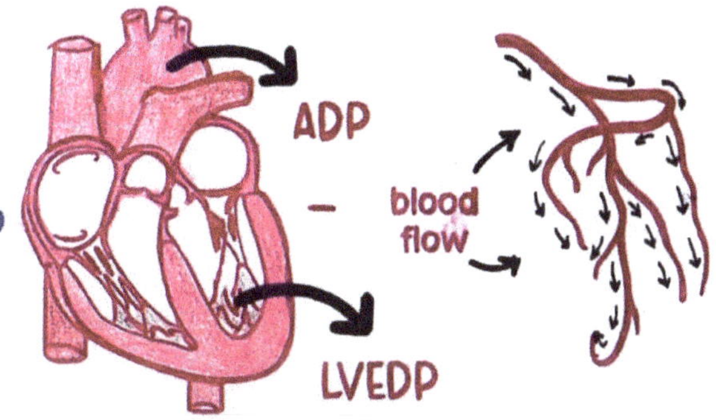

CPP is based on diastolic pressures because most of the blood flow to the myocardium occurs during the diastolic phase (ventricular relaxation) of the cardiac cycle. The left coronary artery is perfused only during diastole, while the right coronary artery is perfused during the entire cardiac cycle (hence why the RV is so sensitive to ischemia!).

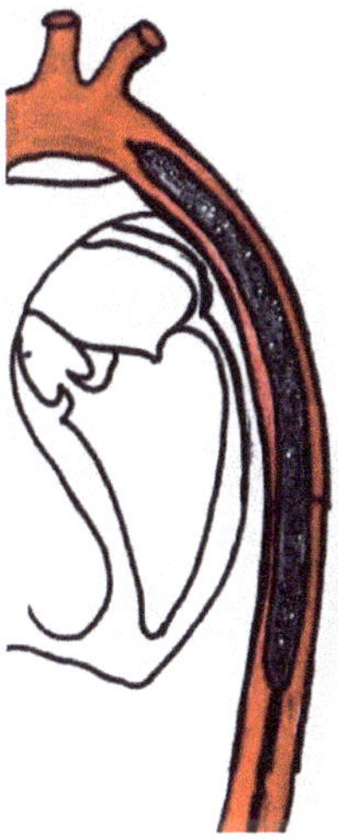

↑ CPP:

- vasopressors & inotropes
- mechanical circulatory support devices (MCS)
- nitroglycerin (↓LVEDP)

Many MCS devices optimize CPP by ↑aortic pressures while ↓ventricular pressures!

↓ CPP:

- systemic hypotension
- cardiogenic shock
- heart failure
- coronary artery disease
- pulmonary hypertension
- aortic & mitral insufficiency
- aortic stenosis
- tachyarrhythmias
- cardiac tamponade
- hypertrophic cardiomyopathy

preload

↑ preload
- hypervolemia
- heart failure
- cardiogenic shock
- cardiac tamponade
- mitral regurgitation
- aortic regurgitation

↓ preload
- hypovolemia
- septic/neurogenic/
- anaphylactic shock
- atrial arrhythmias
- mitral & tricuspid valve stenosis
- tachycardia
- third spacing
- pneumothorax
- ↑ PEEP
- PE

afterload

↑ afterload
- cardiogenic shock
- hypovolemic shock
- cardiac tamponade
- cardiomyopathy
- pulmonary HTN (RV)
- aortic stenosis
- heart failure
- hypothermia
- ↑ PEEP
- HTN

↓ afterload
- anaphylactic shock
- neurogenic shock
- septic shock (early)
- hyperthermia
- vasoplegic syndrome (s/p CABG)

contractility

↑ contractility
- sepsis (early)
- ↑ in HR
- ↑ in afterload (SVR)
- hypercalcemia

↓ contractility
- myocardial infarction
- heart failure
- cardiomyopathy
- valve dysfunction
- acute myocarditis
- cardiac tamponade
- electrolyte imbalances
  → Ca^{++}, Mg^{++}, & K^{+}!
- arrhythmias
- hypoxia
- acidosis
- PE

♡ rate

↑ rate
- ↓ preload
- pyrexia
- anemia
- heart failure
- hyperthyroidism
- hypoxia
- PE

↓ rate
- ↑ vagal tone
- ↑ ICP
- acute MI
- hypoxemia
- hypothermia

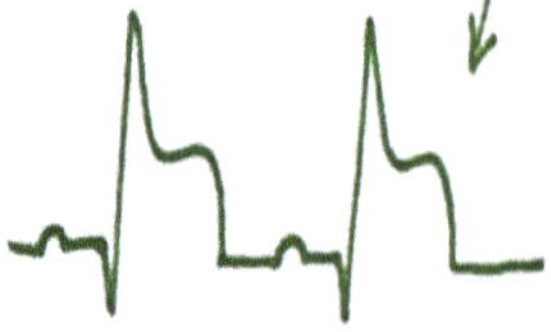

@icunursingnotesbycaitlyn

preload

↑
- fluids
- volume expanders
- blood products

↓
- diuretics
- nitrates
  - *NTG
  - *Isordil
  - *Imdur
- ACE-I & ARBs
- nesiritide (Natrecor)

afterload

↑
- vasopressors
  - *Levo
  - *epi
  - *Neo
  - *vaso
  - *dopamine

↓
- Nipride
- hydralazine
- nesiritide
- nitroglycerin
- beta blockers
- Ca2+ blockers
- ACE-I & ARBs
- inodilators
  - *dobutamine
  - *milrinone
- intra-aortic balloon pump (IABP)

contractility

↑
- dobutamine
- milrinone
- amrinone
- epinephrine
- dopamine
- Digoxin

↓
- negative inotropes
  - *beta blockers
  - *Ca2+ blockers
  - *antiarrhythmics (amiodarone)

@icunursingnotesbycaitlyn

HR

↑
- atropine
- epinephrine
- dopamine
- dobutamine
- Isuprel
- pacing

↓
- beta blockers
- Ca2+ blockers
- antiarrhythmics
- Digoxin
- adenosine

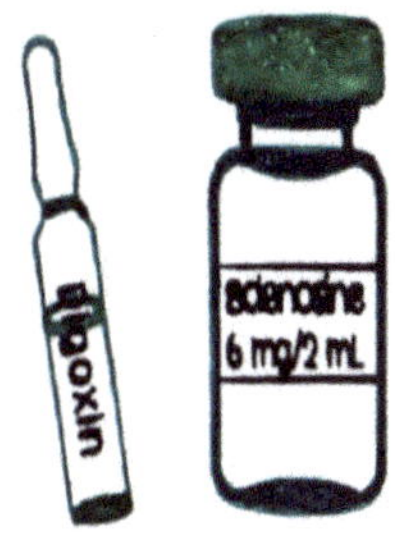

Pulse Pressure

The difference between the systolic & diastolic pressures c̄ a normal value of ≈ 40 mmHg.

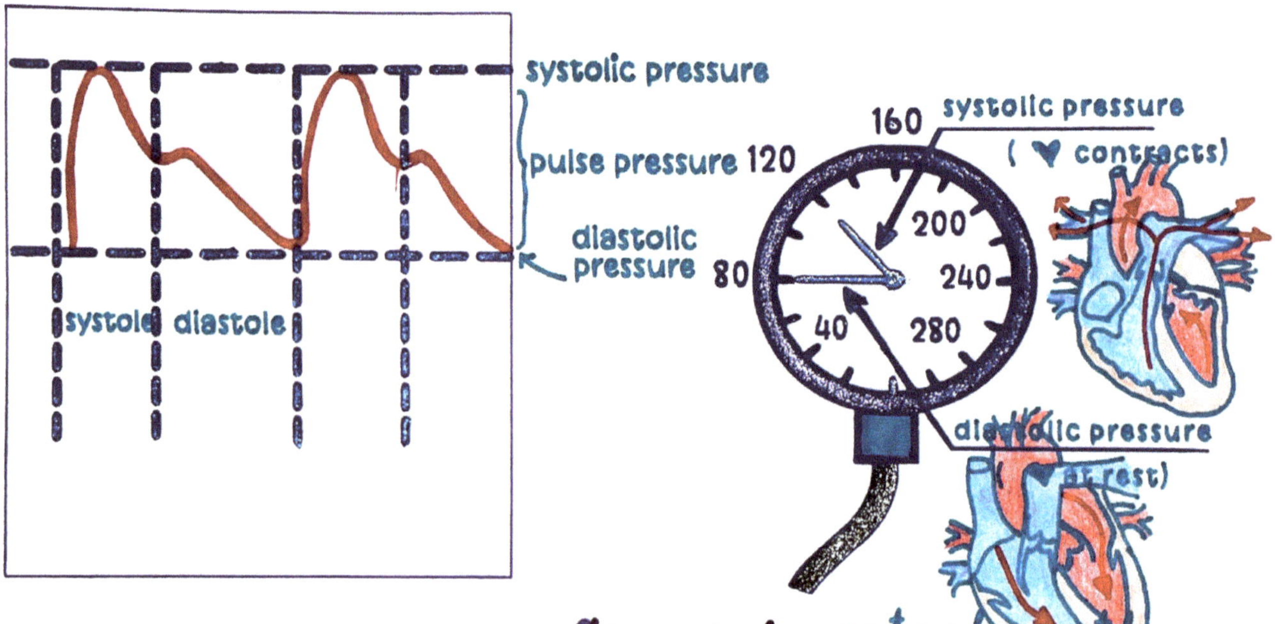

NARROW (LOW) ↓

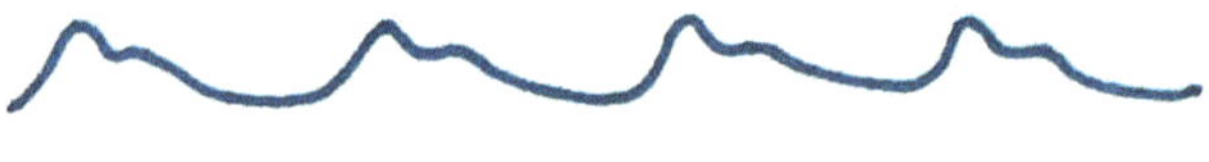

continuous flow LVADs
cardiac tamponade
cardiogenic shock
aortic stenosis (AS)
pneumothorax
hypovolemia
heart failure

WIDE (HIGH) ↑

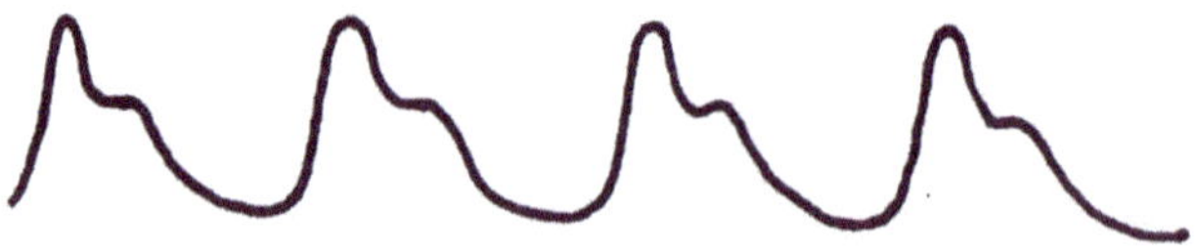

septic shock
aortic regurg
aortic dissection
hyperthyroidism
anemia
↑ ICP

Think high cardiac output states!

RIGHT HEART CATH

A **Swan-Ganz catheter** is used to measure **intra-cardiac pressures**. The catheter is floated through the right atrium & right ventricle, and the balloon at the tip of the catheter wedges into the distal pulmonary artery (PA). Direct measurements obtained during a right ♥ cath: CVP, right-sided intracardiac pressures (RA, RV), PAP, PAWP, CO, & SvO_2. Indirect measurements: SVR, PVR, cardiac index (CI), SVI, LVSWI, RVSWI, DO_2 & VO_2.

@icunursingnotesbycaitlyn

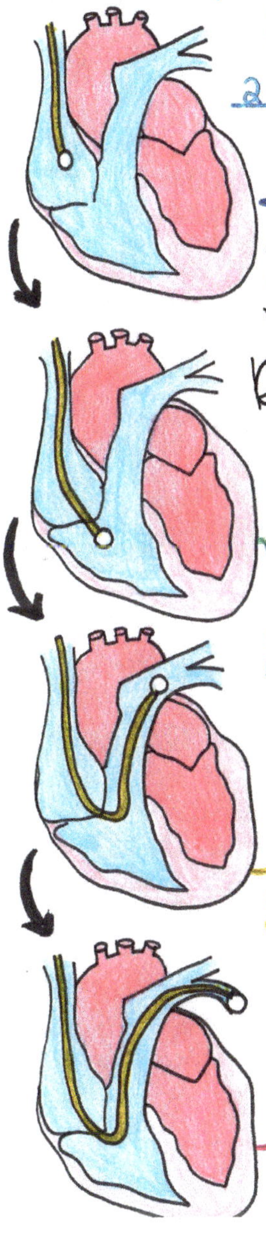

RIGHT ATRIAL/CENTRAL VENOUS PRESSURE (RAP/CVP)

2-6 mmHg

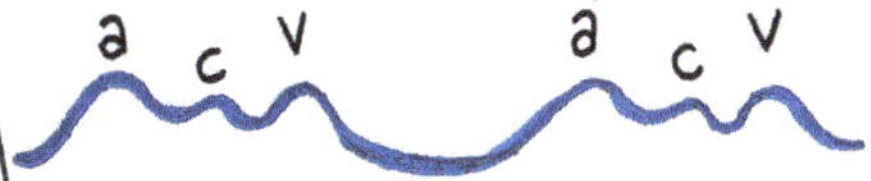

a = atrial systole
c = tricuspid valve closure
v = atrial filling, ventricular systole

- ★ indicator of fluid balance
- ★ ↑ c̄ right-sided HF, volume overload, tricuspid valve stenosis/regurg, constrictive pericarditis, PHTN, cardiac tamponade, & RV infarction.

RIGHT VENTRICULAR PRESSURE (RVSP/RVDP)

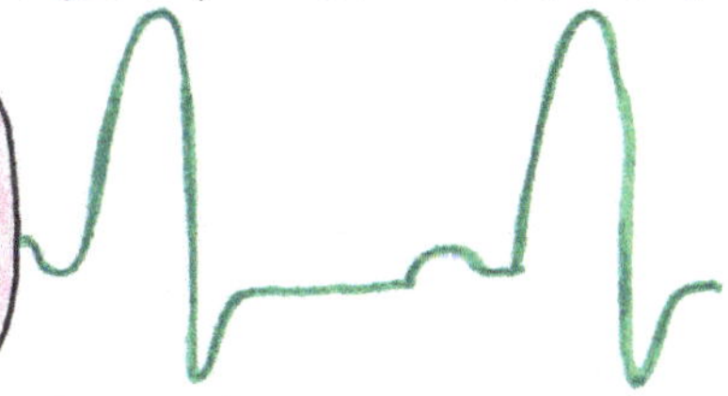

Systolic: 15-30 mmHg
diastolic: 2-8 mmHg

- ★ Distinct pulsatile waveform c̄ systolic (RVSP) and diastolic (RVDP) pressures.
- ★ Common for ventricular ectopy to occur during passage of the catheter through the RV.

PULMONARY ARTERY PRESSURE (PAP)

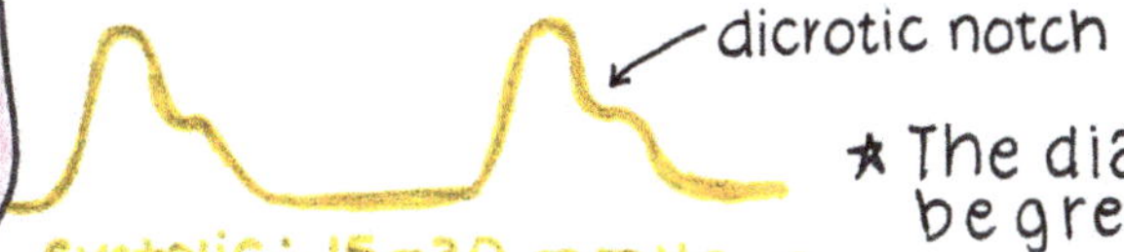

Systolic: 15-30 mmHg
diastolic: 8-15 mmHg } mean PAP: 9-18 mmHg

- ★ The diastolic PAP (PAPD) should be greater than the PCWP.

PULMONARY ARTERY WEDGE PRESSURE (PCWP/PAOP/PAWP)

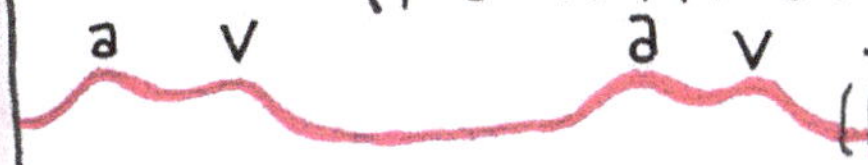

6-12 mmHg

- ★ Reflects left atrial pressure (LAP) and LVEDP; a reliable indicator of LV function.

Pulmonary Wedge Pressure

An indirect measurement of left atrial pressure (LAP) & left ventricular end-diastolic pressure (LVEDP) obtained during a right heart (Swan-Ganz) catheterization.

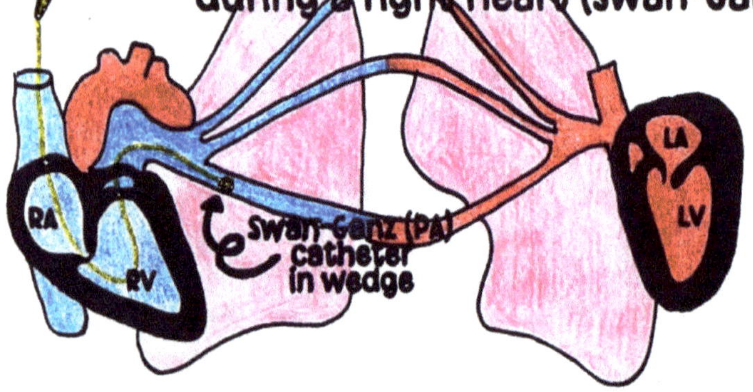

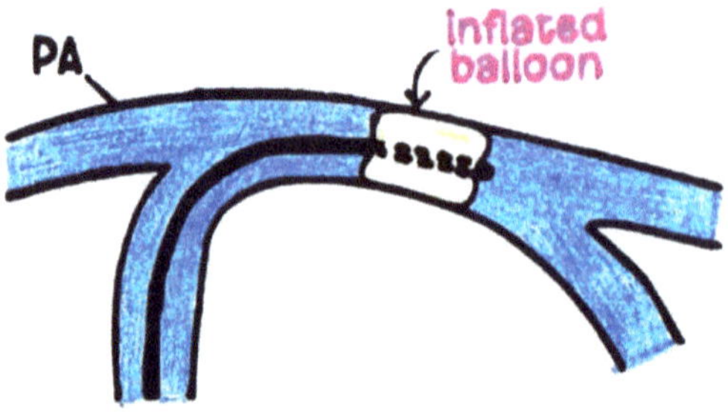

When the balloon is inflated in a branch of the PA ("wedged"), it blocks off all pressures from the right side of the ♥, allowing the pressure sensor at the catheter tip to indirectly "see" left-sided heart pressures (LAP & LVEDP)/left heart preload!

Subtract 2 from the PA diastolic pressure (PADP) to estimate the wedge!

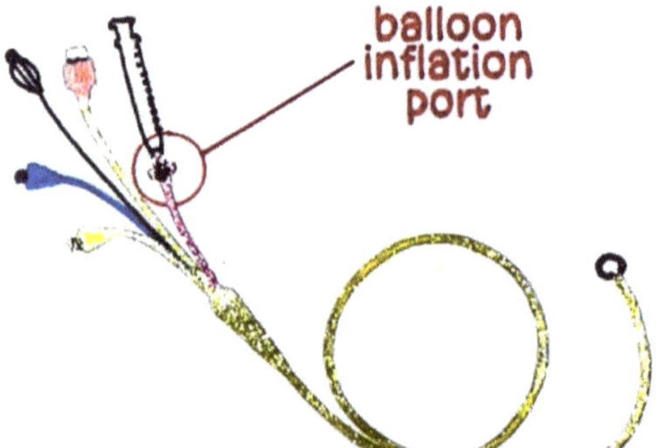

The PAWP Waveform:

The PAWP waveform looks similar to the CVP waveform, but it reflects back pressure from the left side of the heart!

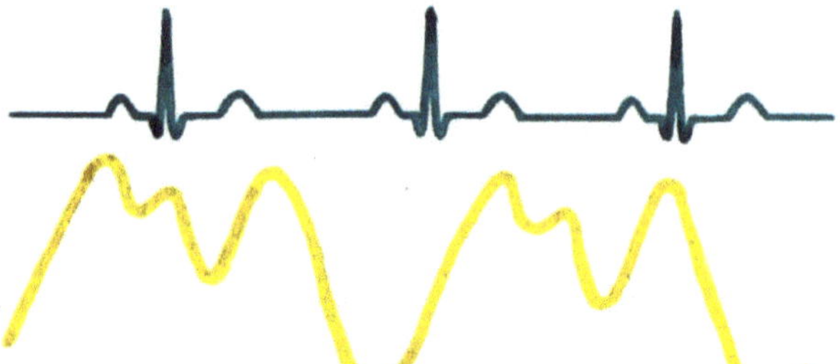

A normal PCWP is 8 to 12 mmHg.

@icunursingnotesbycaitlyn

↑ fluid overload states, LV failure, cardiogenic shock, MI, mitral & aortic stenosis/regurg, & cardiac tamponade.

↓ septic, neurogenic & hypovolemic shock, vasodilation, and hypovolemia.

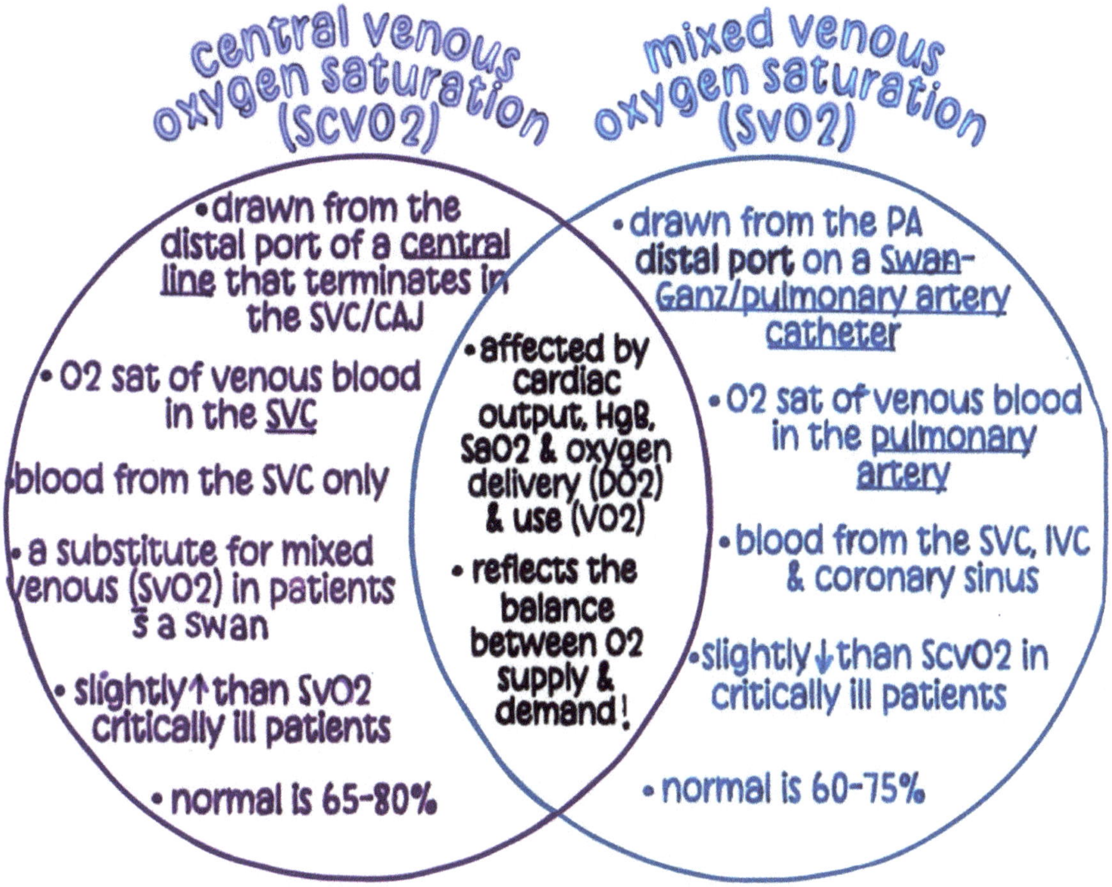

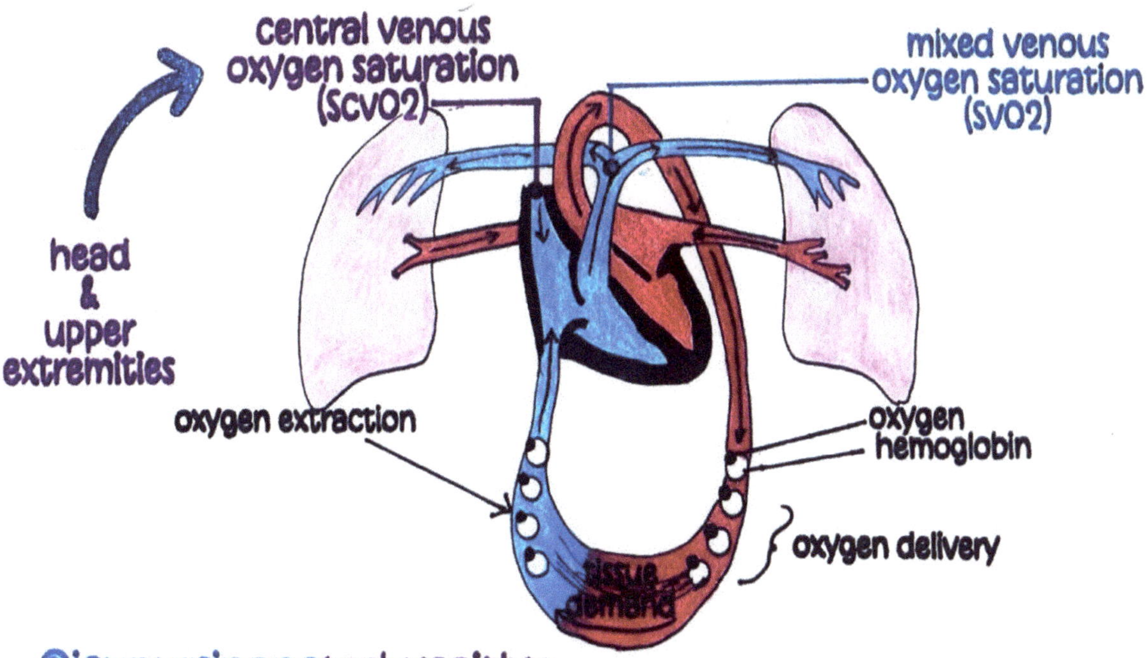

@icunursingnotesbycaitlyn

THE FICK EQUATION

calculating cardiac output

An equation based on the principle that cardiac output can be calculated by looking at the flux of oxygen through the body's peripheral tissues & the arteriovenous difference (the oxygen difference between the arterial & the venous systems).

$$CO = \frac{O_2 \text{ consumption } (VO_2) \times BSA}{[(SaO_2 - SvO_2) \times HgB \times 1.34] \div 10}$$

The SaO_2 is drawn from an arterial line or obtained via an ABG, while the SvO_2 is the mixed venous blood gas that is drawn from the PA distal port on a Swan-Ganz/PA catheter!

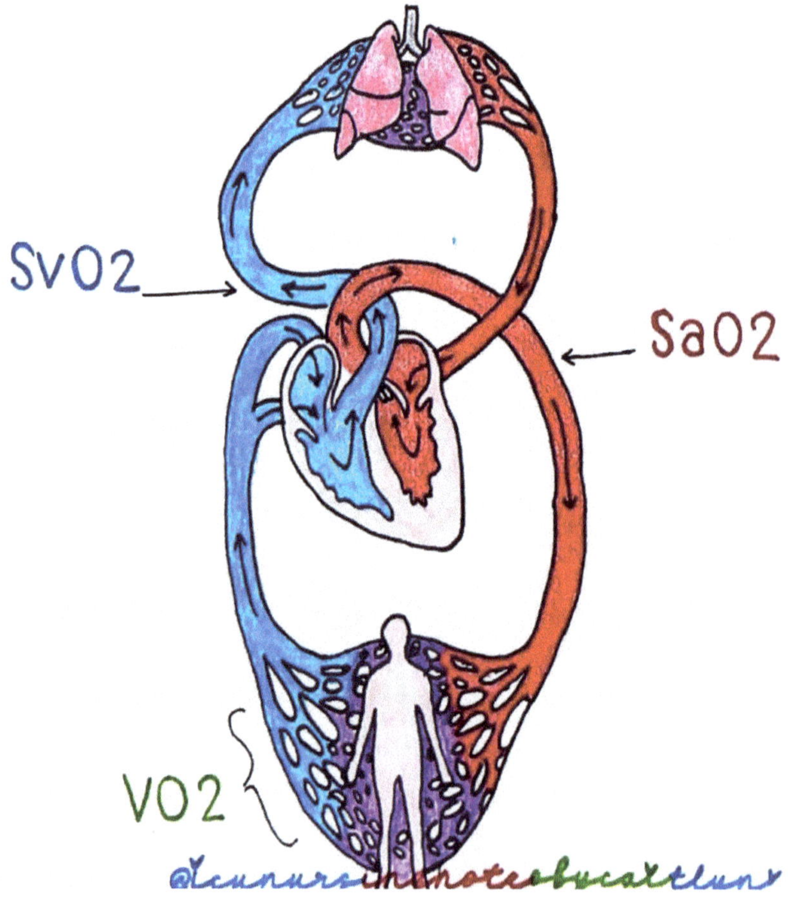

THERMODILUTION

PHYSIOLOGY

Cardiac output (CO) is the amount of blood ejected by the heart per minute & is equal to HR x SV. Monitoring of CO is done to assess the heart's ability to pump oxygenated blood to the tissues & is considered a reliable parameter to determine whether interventions (i.e. inotropes, diuresis, etc) have been successful.

Cardiac output can be measured c̄ the thermodilution method. Using a closed injectate delivery system (see pg. 2), a bolus (10 cc) of room-temp normal saline is injected into the right atrium via the proximal (CVP) port on a Swan-Ganz Catheter, causing a transient ↓ in blood temp as the saline mixes c̄ the blood. The thermistor (in the pulmonary artery) registers this temperature change. The bedside monitor plots the blood temp changes measured by thermodilution as a temperature-time curve. Flow is calculated based on the area under the curve, which is inversely related to cardiac output.

@ icunursingnotesbycaitlyn

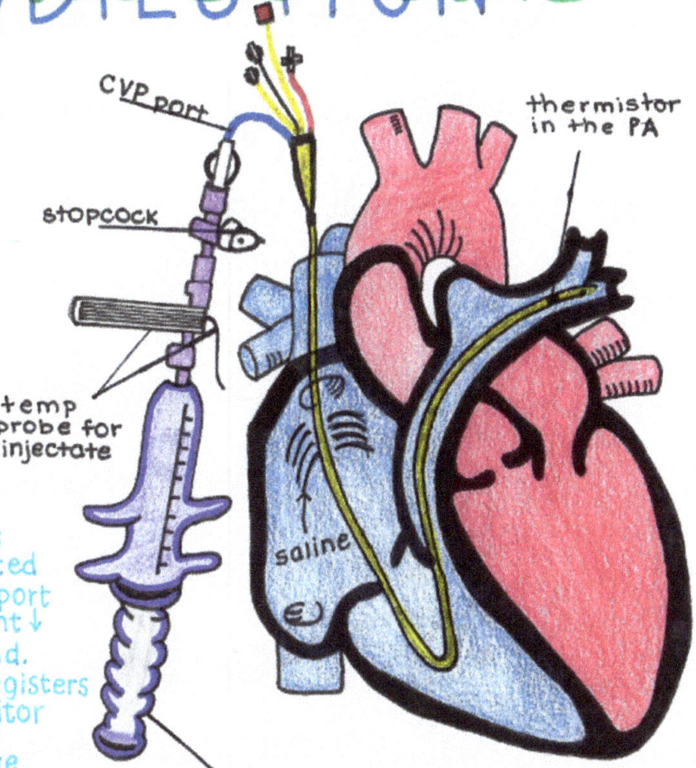

CURVE VARIATIONS

Normal Curve

- rapid, smooth upstroke
- gradual return to baseline

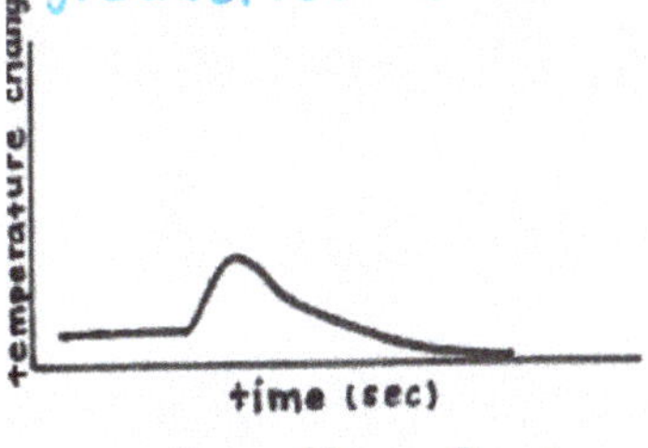

Low Cardiac Output

- rapid, smooth upstroke
- long downstroke
- large area under the curve

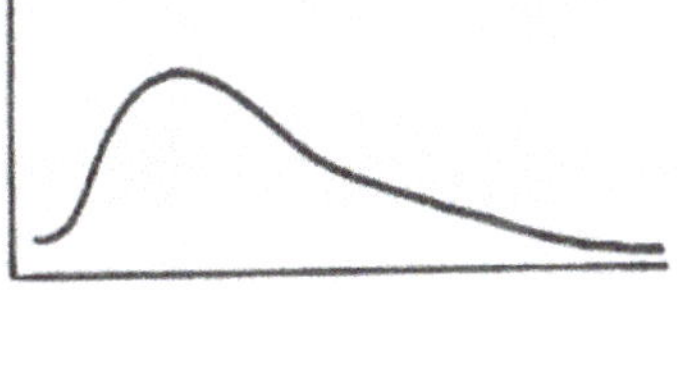

High Cardiac Output

- rapid, smooth upstroke
- rapid return to baseline
- small area under the curve (injectate moves through the ♥ quickly)

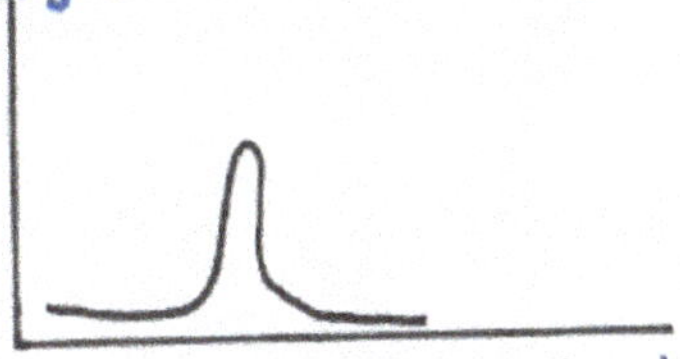

Poor Injection Technique

- uneven + slower than normal upstroke
- large area under the curve

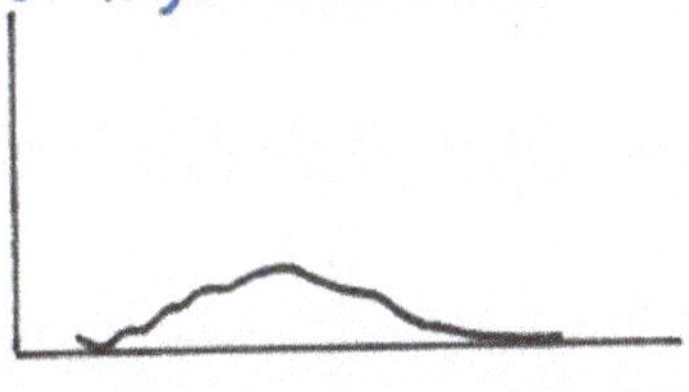

Tricuspid Regurgitation

- prolonged curve
- falsely low thermodilution C.O.

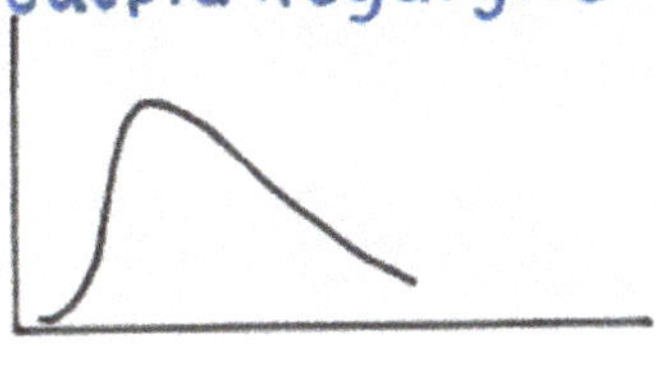

THERMODILUTION STEPS

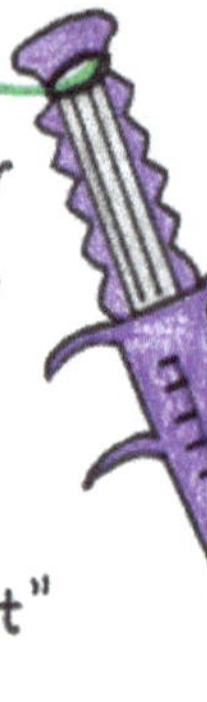
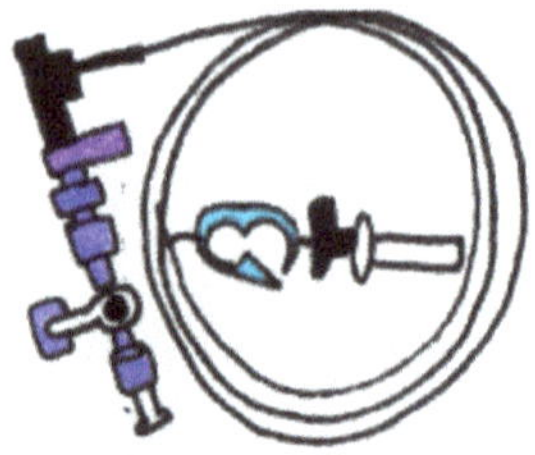

closed injectate delivery system

Supplies: Swan-Ganz catheter, cardiac output module for bedside monitor, cardiac output cable (thermistor/injectate temperature probe & core temperature probe), cardiac output closed injectate set, 500 cc bag of NS

1) Position the patient supine, if tolerated.
2) Level the triple-pressure transducer to the phlebostatic axis.
3) On the bedside monitor, select the "cardiac output" option.
4) Verify the computation constant (typically 0.592).
5) Withdraw 10 cc of saline into the cardiac output syringe.
6) Turn the stopcock on the proximal (CVP) port so that it's closed to the transducer and open to the patient & syringe.
7) When the message "ready for new measurement" is displayed, select "start CO."
8) When the ready tone sounds & the message "inject now!" is shown, depress the plunger on the CO syringe quickly & smoothly (<4 seconds).
9) Assess the CO thermodilution curve & the value on the monitor.
10) When "ready for new measurement" is displayed, repeat steps 3 - 8 until at least 3 satisfactory waveforms are displayed (values within 10% of one another).
11) Select "save co"
12) Turn the stopcock on the proximal /CVP port so that it is open to the transducer & closed to the CO syringe.
13) Perform hemodynamic calculations by pressing the "hemo calc" key.
14) Verify the accuracy of all pre-populated values & manually enter any missing values.
15) Once confirmed, press "perform calc" & press "hemo review" to view the trends in the patient's hemodynamics.

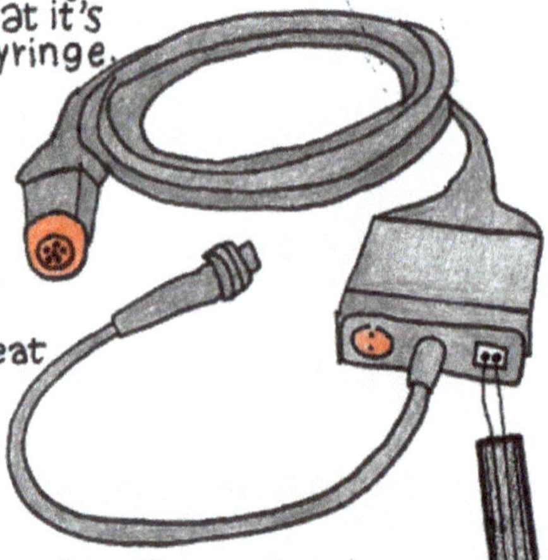

cardiac output cable and injectate thermistor probe

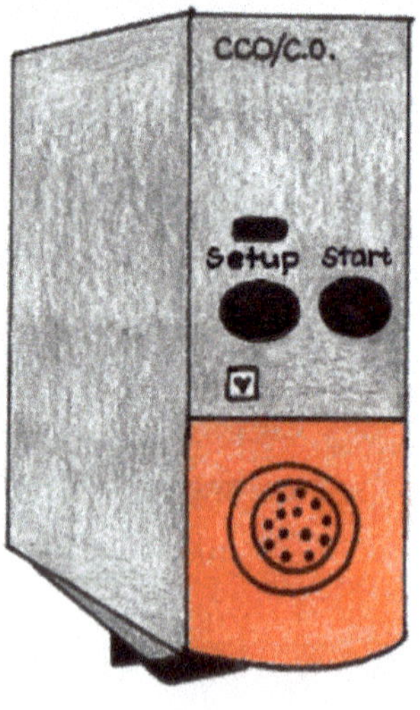

cardiac output module for the bedside monitor

To obtain the most accurate results with thermodilution, inject the saline within 4 seconds at end-expiration to minimize the influence of intrathoracic pressure.

@ icunursingnotesbycaitlyn

2

THE RAMUS INTERMEDIUS

A coronary artery variant resulting from trifurcation of the left main coronary artery (LMCA) that is present in ≈ 20% of the population; it courses between the left anterior descending (LAD) & left circumflex (LCX) coronary arteries.

Illustrations adapted from: Das, D.N. (2023). Clinical examination in cardiology (3rd ed.). Elsevier.

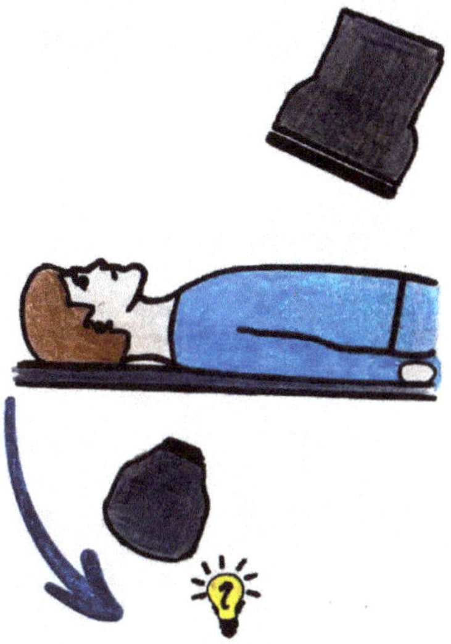

The ramus intermedius (RI) is best visualized in the LAO caudal (spider) view!

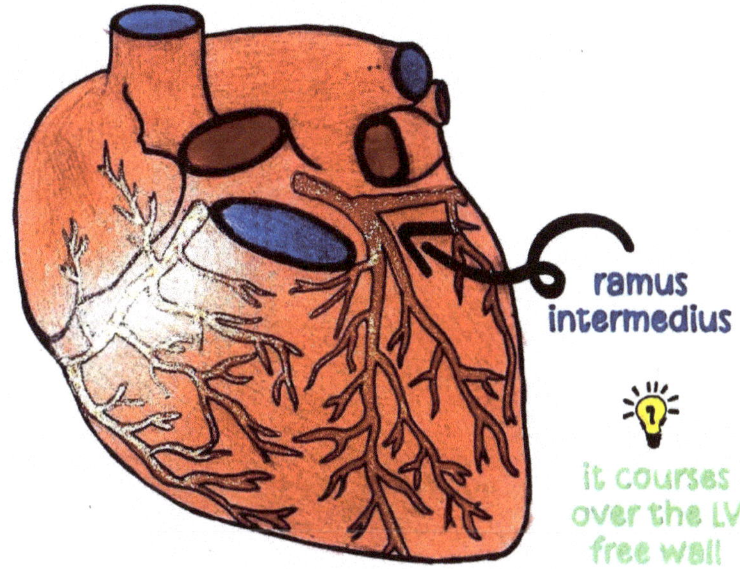

it courses over the LV free wall

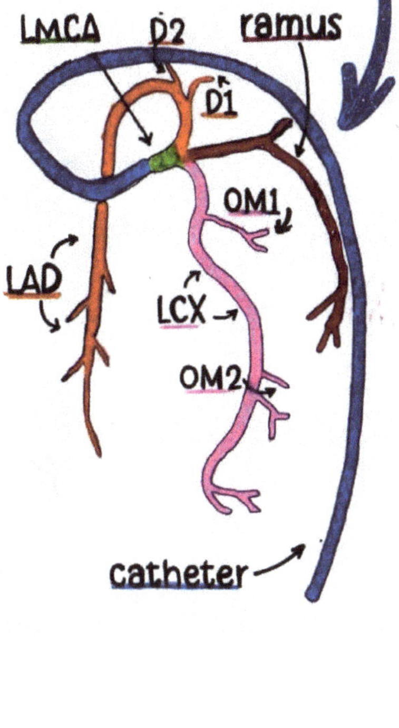

CLINICAL RELEVANCE

The ramus intermedius (RI) can act like an obtuse marginal (OM) or a diagonal branch, depending on whether it supplies the anterior or lateral wall of the LV. Its clinical implications aren't entirely understood: some research suggests that the presence of a RI may be a potential risk factor for ↑atherosclerotic plaque formation in the left main & proximal LAD. Conversely, other sources propose that the RI may contribute to improved survival by providing an additional collateral source of blood supply to the heart muscle (Khachatryan et al., 2024).

@icunursingnotesbycaitlyn

BLAND-WHITE-GARLAND SYNDROME

AKA anomalous left coronary artery from the pulmonary artery (ALCAPA), this is a rare congenital coronary artery anamoly that occurs when the left main coronary artery arises from the pulmonary artery (PA), rather than the aorta.

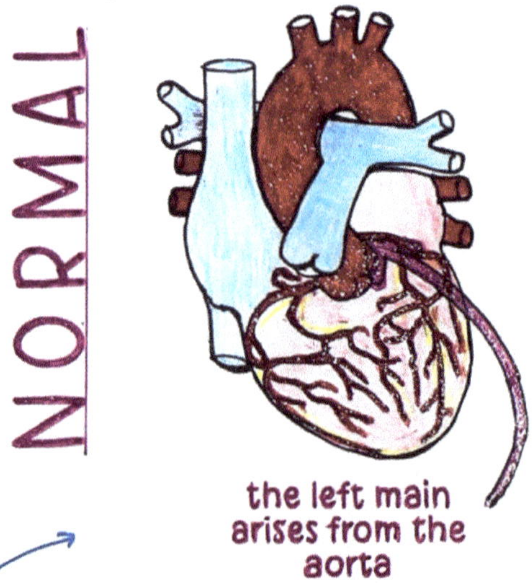

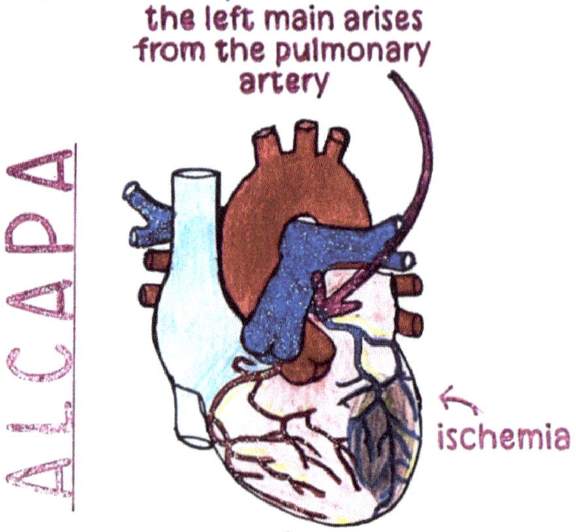

Illustrations adapted from the Children's Hospital of Philadelphia®, @chdidoodles, & @studiesonefortwo!

PATHOPHYS

@icunursingnotesbycaitlyn'

The pathophysiology of BWG Syndrome results from a "coronary-steal phenomenon" that occurs after birth. In utero, pulmonary & aortic (Ao) pressures & O2 saturations are essentially =, & the myocardium is well-perfused by the anamolous artery. Weeks to months after birth, there's a normal physiological ↓ in the pulmonary vascular resistance (PVR), pressure (PAP), & SvO2, so resistance in the coronary arterial system becomes ↑ relative to the pulmonary circulation. Because coronary blood flow will take the path of least resistance, as the LCA pressure falls, blood flows into the low-pressure pulmonary circulation rather than into the high-resistance myocardial circulation, causing a left-to-right shunt (coronary steal phenomenon); s̄ adequate collateral circulation between the RCA & the LCA, myocardial ischemia/infarction, LV dysfunction, & acute MR occur! Survival beyond infancy (10% of cases) is related to the degree of collateral circulation, but chronic hypoperfusion causes subendocardial ischemia that predisposes patients c̄ ALCAPA to a ↑ risk of sudden cardiac death (SCD) in adolescence or adulthood 2/2 ventricular arrhythmias!

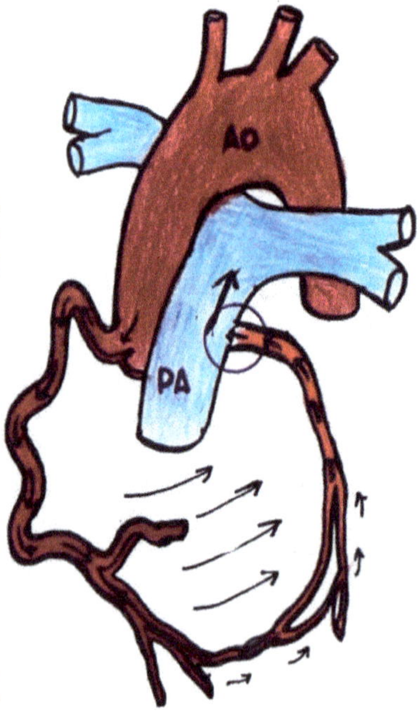

CORONARY DOMINANCE

A term that refers to whether the PDA originates from the RCA (right-dominant), LCx (left-dominant), or both the RCA & LCx (codominant).

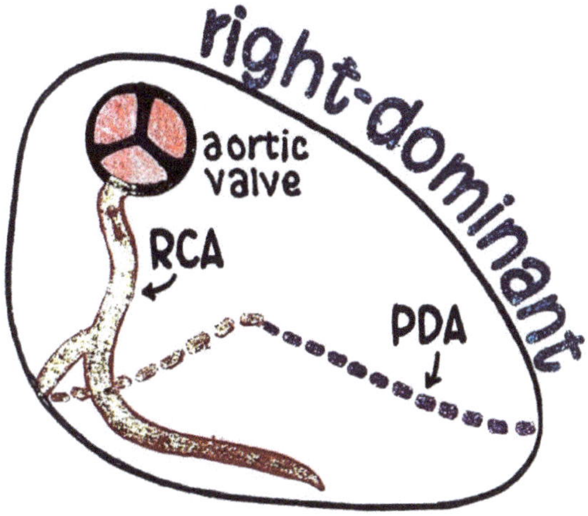

- The RCA supplies the PDA.
- A majority of the population is right-dominant.

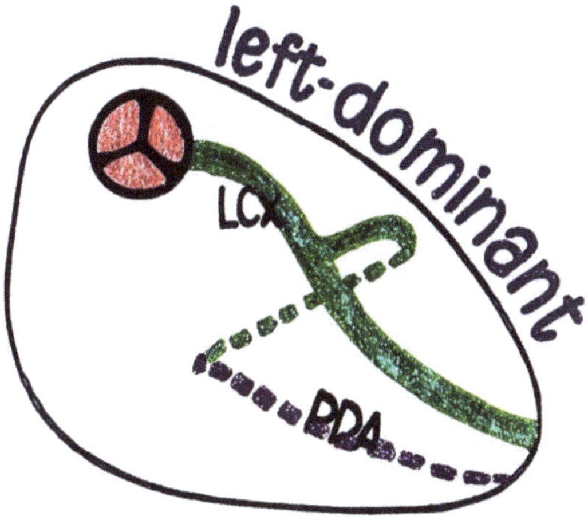

- The LCx supplies the PDA.
- Less common type of coronary dominance (10% of the population).

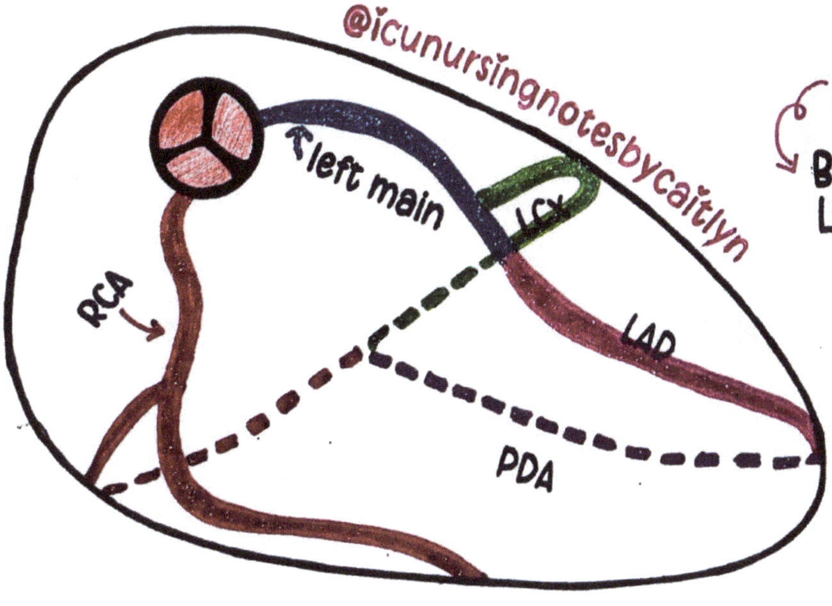

CODOMINANT

Both the RCA & the LCx supply the PDA

Coronary dominance plays an important role in MIs & coronary artery bypass grafting (CABG)!

Basics of Coronary Angiography

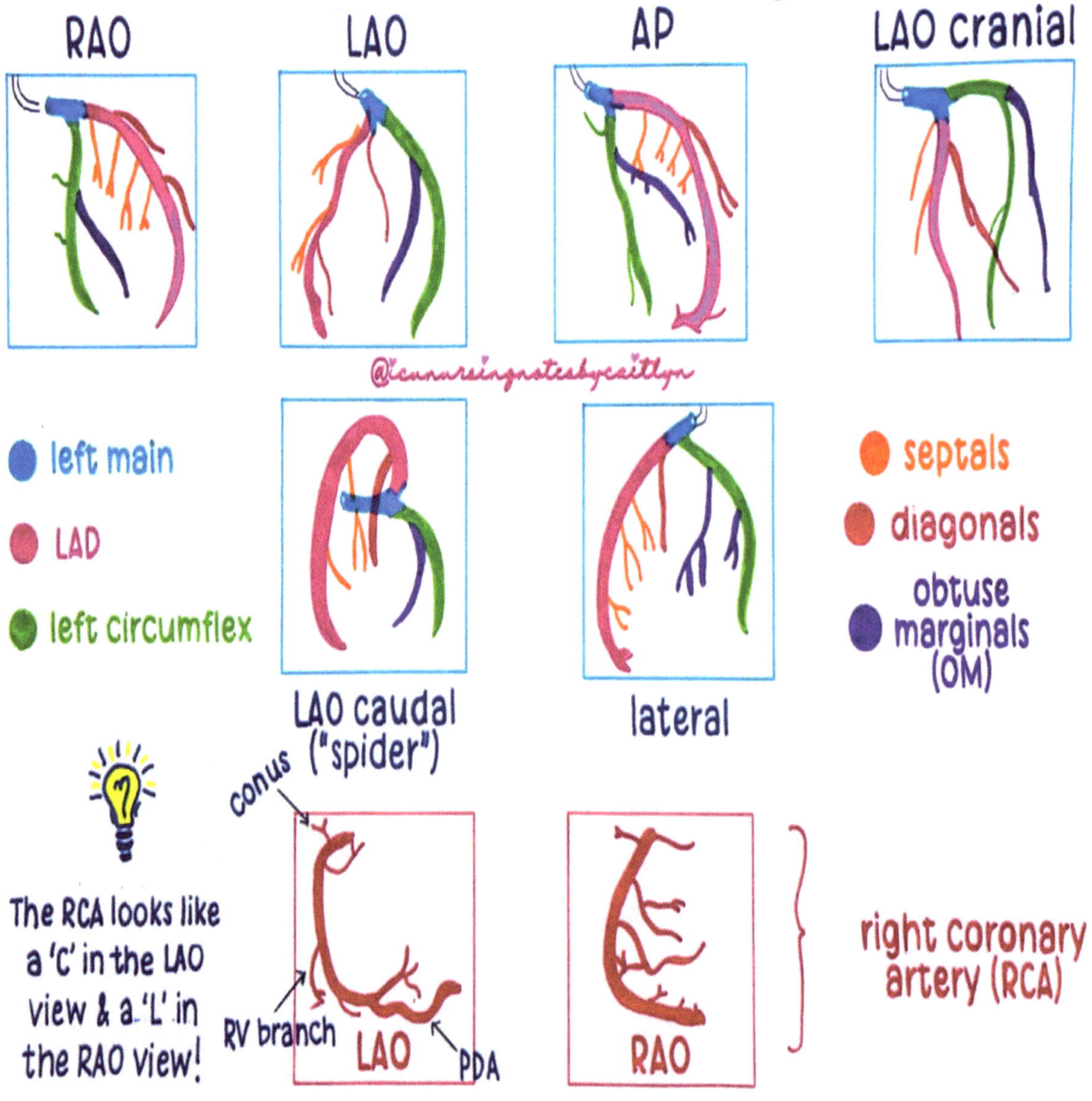

Cardiac Catheterization

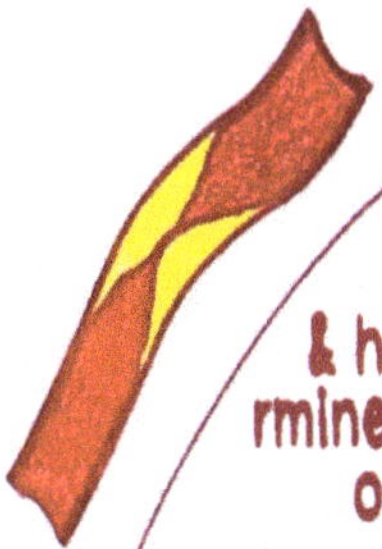

LEFT HEART CATH

- diagnoses coronary artery disease (CAD), evaluates heart valve & heart muscle function, & determines the need for PCI (stenting) or bypass grafting (CABG).
- requires arterial access
- uses a variety of coronary catheters (diagnostic or guides)
- can be non-emergent (elective) or emergent (STEMI)
- can be diagnostic or interventional
- requires fluoroscopy & contrast dye to visualize the coronary arteries
- requires heparin administration for anticoagulation (exception: diagnostic LHC via femoral approach)
- measures aortic (Ao) & LV pressures (systolic & end-diastolic)
- radial cocktail (IA nitro, heparin, & verapamil) is given to prevent radial artery spasm (RAS)

Both

- a sheath is inserted into a blood vessel
- percutaneous approach
- require sterile technique
- can be done via a femoral approach (not ideal)
- pressure measurements are recorded
- assess heart valve function
- can induce arrhythmias
- done under conscious sedation

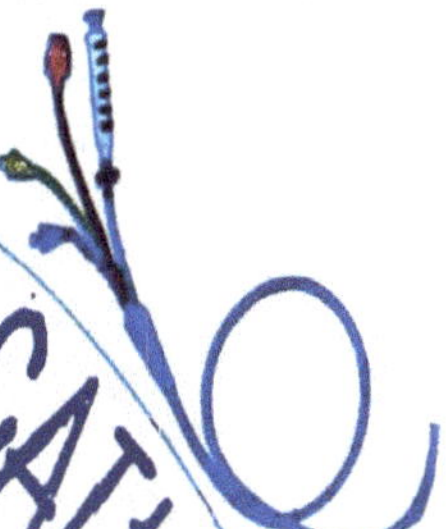

RIGHT HEART CATH

- measures intracardiac pressures (RAP, RVP, PAP, PCWP) on the right side of the ♥.
- requires venous access
- uses a Swan-Ganz/pulmonary artery catheter
- non-emergent & diagnostic only
- can be performed c̄ or s̄ fluoroscopy (can be floated at the bedside or in the cath lab)
- diagnoses intracardiac shunts (oximetry/shunt run)
- estimates cardiac output/index
- doesn't require anticoagulation
- blood is drawn from the pulmonary artery (SvO2) to assess the balance between oxygen supply & demand (useful in shock states)
- a Swan-Ganz catheter can stay in place for continuous hemodynamic monitoring in the ICU.

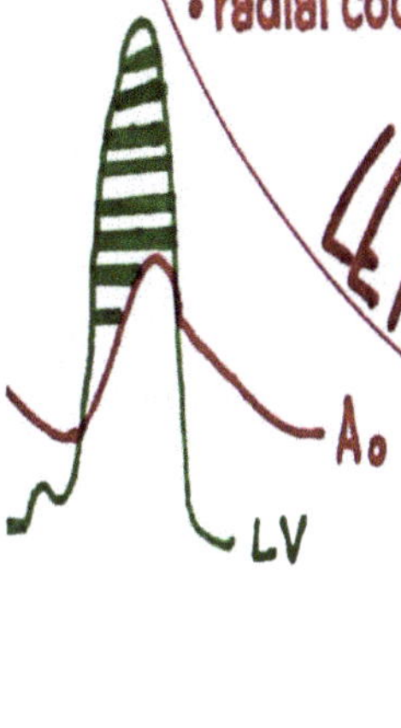

@lannurselaynotesbycaitlyn

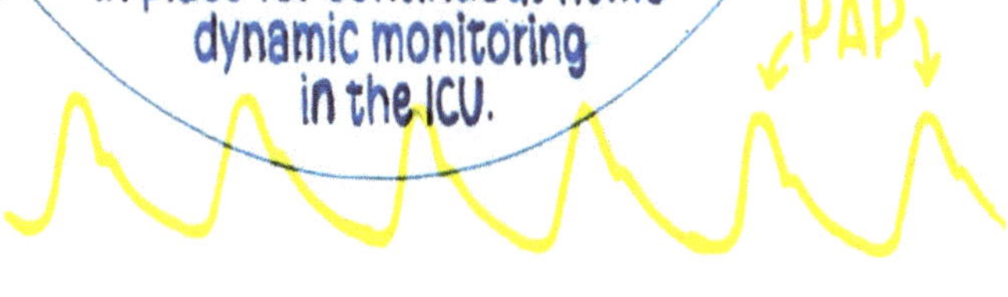

CORONARY COLLATERAL CIRCULATION

THE "BACK UP CIRCULATION" TO THE HEART MUSCLE!

Anastomotic connections between different coronary arteries or between branches of the same artery in response to chronic myocardial ischemia (due to coronary artery disease). When blood flow through a coronary artery is limited, it creates a pressure gradient that stimulates the development of collateral vessels. These small arterial vessels provide an alternative route for blood supply to regions of the heart muscle c̄ ↓ blood flow due to narrowed arteries (atherosclerosis)/in the presence of a chronic total occlusion (CTO)!

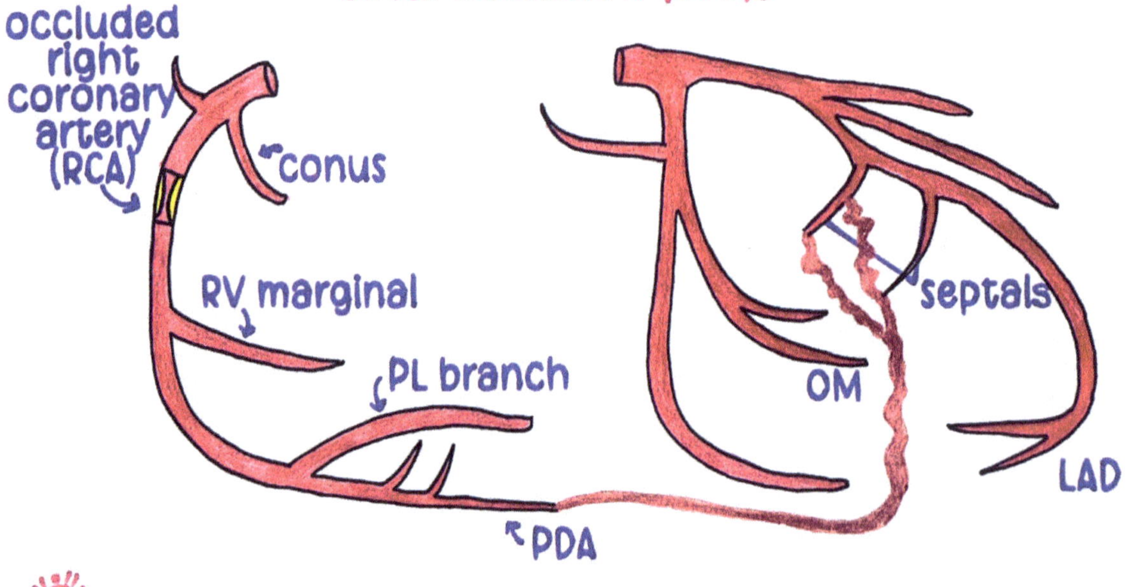

Think of collateral circulation as the body's natural "detour," or bypass, for blocked arteries!

@icunursingnotesbycaitlyn

Competitive Flow

Residual blood flow through a partially stenotic native coronary artery competes c̄ blood flow through an arterial bypass graft, which can lead to graft occlusion & graft failure.

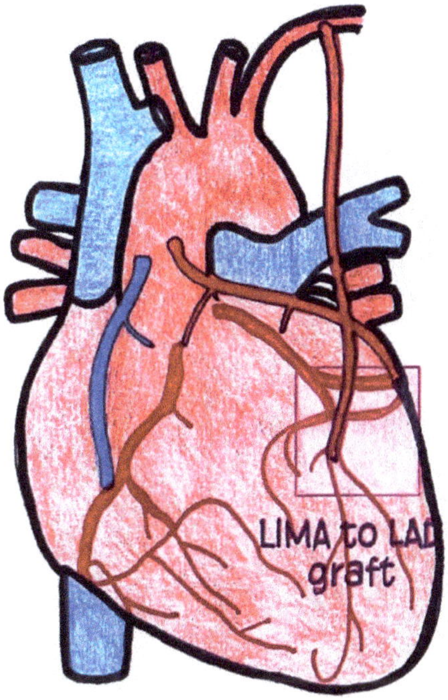

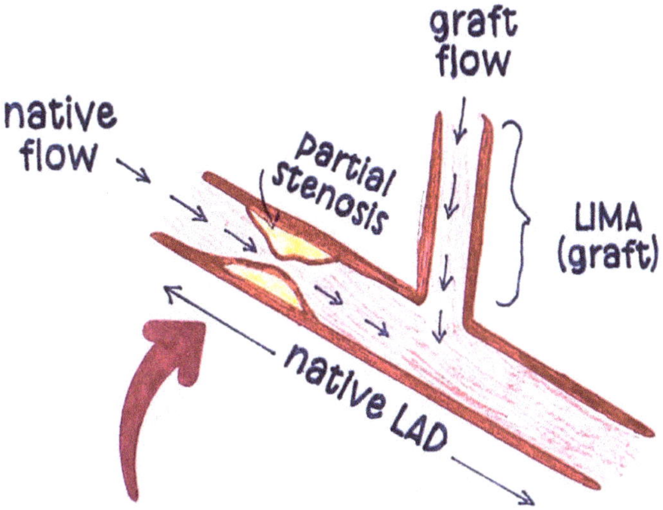

The left anterior descending (LAD) is receiving blood flow from a patent native inflow & a patent left internal mammary artery (LIMA) graft.

↑ Risk of Occlusion, But Why?

Competitive flow can occur after grafting a coronary target that isn't severely stenotic (blocked). Blood flow from the native coronary artery "competes" with blood flow from the bypass graft. In the setting of competitive flow, the native vessel typically wins the competition for flow. Although it indicates a patent (open) bypass graft, it can lead to graft occlusion and, ultimately, graft failure!

Competitive flow isn't limited to bypass grafts; it can also happen in the setting of a chronic total occlusion (CTO) c̄ collateral circulation!

@icunursingnotesbycaitlyn

Myocardial Bridging

The coronary arteries normally run along the outer surface of the heart on the epicardium. Myocardial bridging is a congenital anomaly that occurs when a segment of a coronary artery (most commonly the mid-LAD) is embedded within the myocardium.

@icunursingnotesbycaitlyn

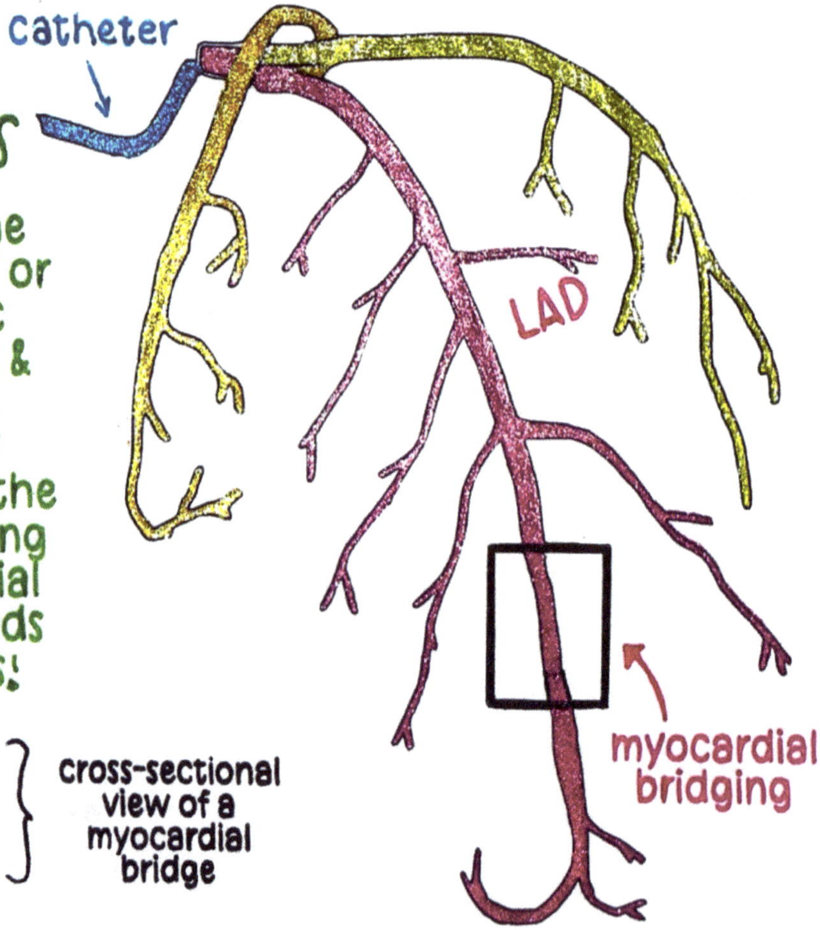

PATHOPHYS

During systole, the overlying "bridge," or band, of cardiac muscle contracts & compresses the coronary artery segment. Because the coronaries fill during diastole, myocardial bridging rarely leads to any symptoms!

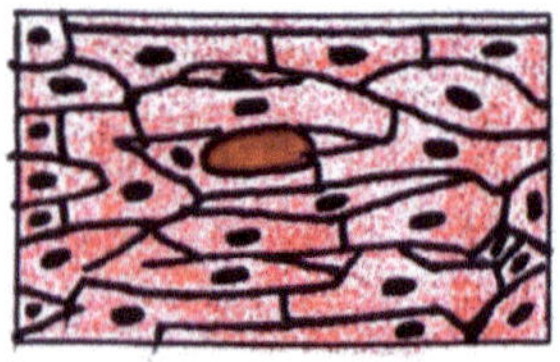

cross-sectional view of a myocardial bridge

Patients c̄ hypertrophic obstructive cardiomyopathy (HOCM) have a higher incidence of myocardial bridging than the general population (Celenk, 2022)!

Fractional Flow Reserve (FFR)

An invasive measurement (FFR) obtained during a cardiac catheterization that is used to evaluate the severity of coronary artery stenosis & to determine the need for revascularization c̄ a PCI (stent).

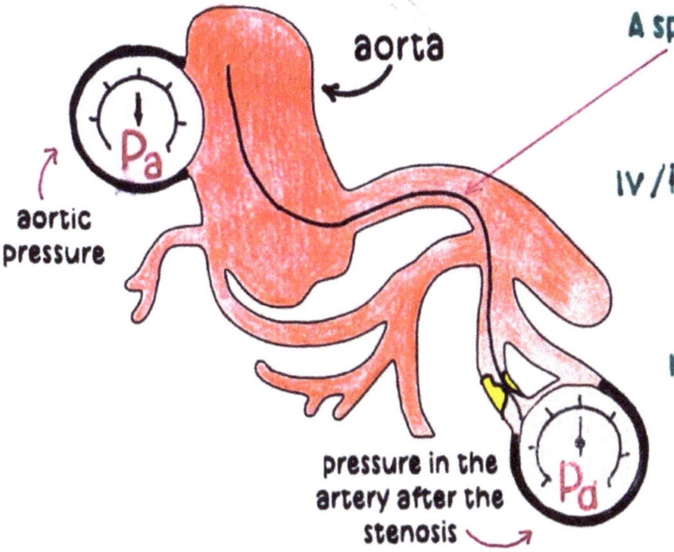

A special pressure-sensor guidewire is advanced past the stenotic coronary lesion.

↓

IV / intracoronary (IC) adenosine is administered to maximize blood flow ("hyperemia").

↓

Intracoronary pressure is measured both proximally (P_a) & distally to the lesion (P_d).

↓

FFR is calculated by dividing P_d by P_a.

To Stent or Not to Stent?

That is the question that FFR answers!

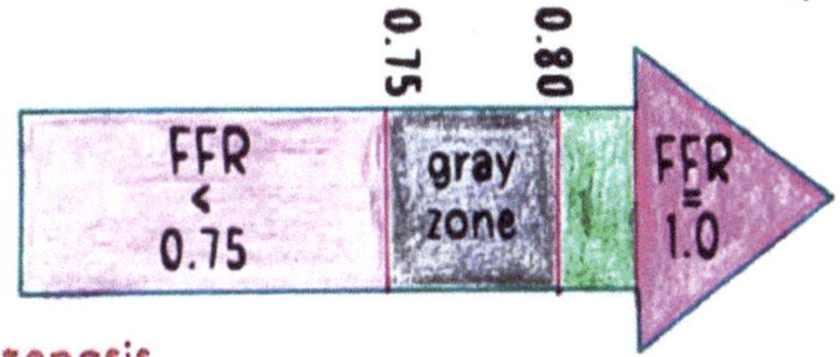

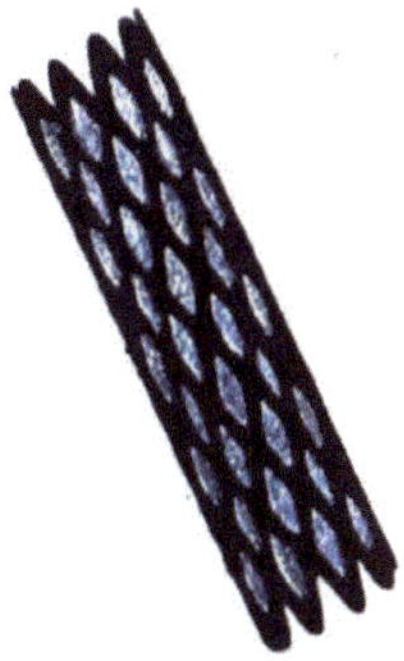

- $FFR = 1$: no obstruction & normal coronary blood flow.
- $0.80 < FFR < 1$: non-ischemia-producing stenosis, medical therapy (medications) is preferred over a PCI ("stenting").
- $0.75 < FFR < 0.80$: the "gray zone" that requires clinical judgement as to whether to perform a PCI or to just treat c̄ medical therapy.
- $FFR < 0.75$: ischemia-producing stenosis that warrants revascularization c̄ a PCI or a CABG.

Remember that not all coronary artery lesions are significant enough to impede oxygen delivery to the ♥ muscle & can be managed c̄ medications (ASA, beta-blocker, statin, & ACE-I or ARB) instead of a PCI!

Acute coronary syndrome

An umbrella term for...

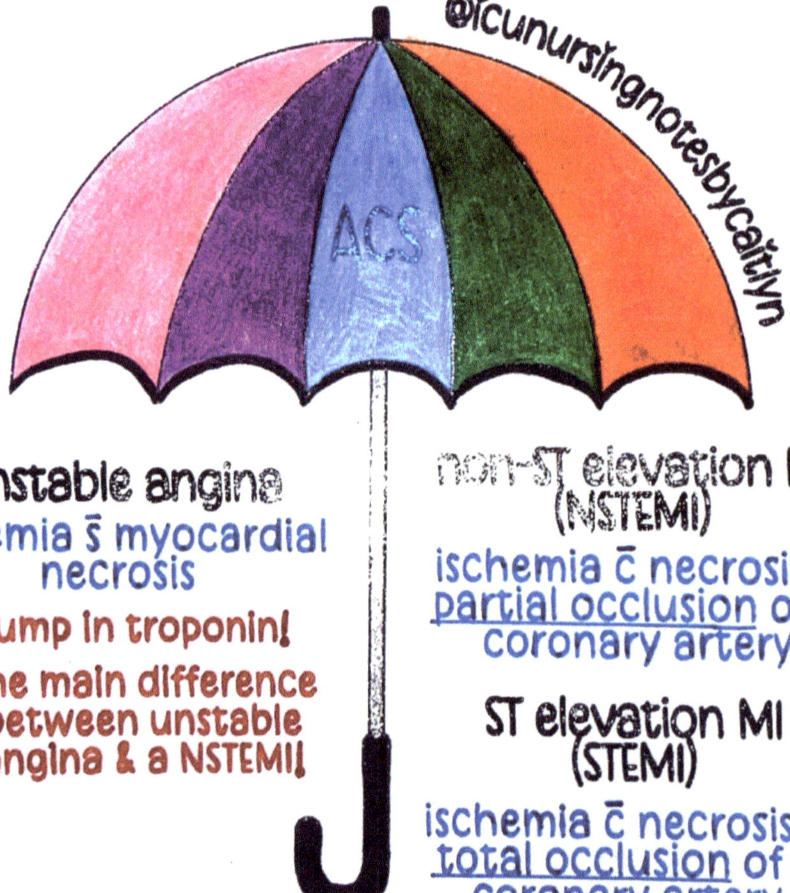

unstable angina

ischemia s̄ myocardial necrosis

NO bump in troponin!

the main difference between unstable angina & a NSTEMI!

non-ST elevation MI (NSTEMI)

ischemia c̄ necrosis & partial occlusion of a coronary artery

ST depression

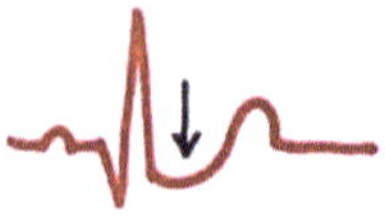

T wave inversion

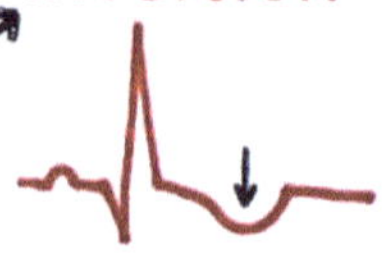

ST elevation MI (STEMI)

ischemia c̄ necrosis & total occlusion of a coronary artery

ST elevation

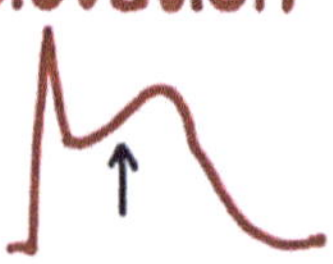

stable angina	unstable angina	NSTEMI	STEMI
- troponin	- troponin possible ST↓/ T wave inversion	+ troponin ST↓ subendocardial infarct	+ troponin ST↑ transmural infarct

12 Lead Territories!

What Supplies What?

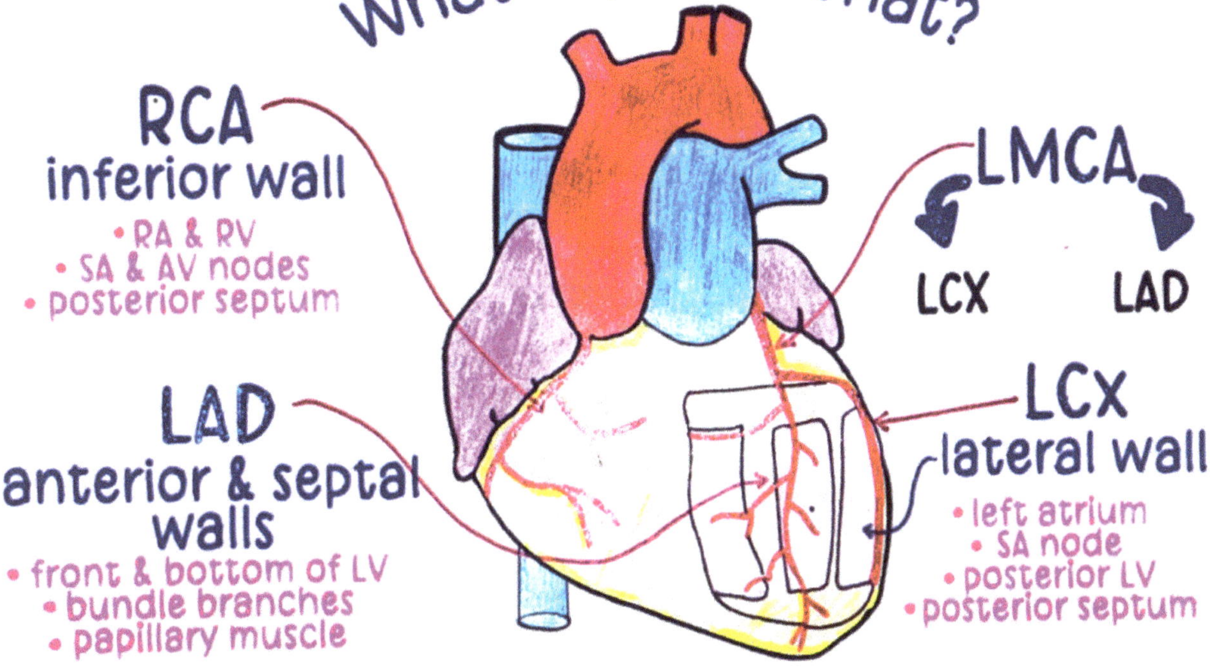

So, Which Artery Is Likely the Culprit?

See page 2 to see this chart in action!

lateral I LCX	aVR	septal V1 LAD	anterior V4 LAD
inferior II RCA	lateral aVL LCX	septal V2 LAD	lateral V5 LCX
inferior III RCA	inferior aVF RCA	anterior V3 LAD	lateral V6 LCX

watch for bradycardia & hypotension c̄ a prox RCA occlusion!!

Coronary Artery Territory Made Visual!

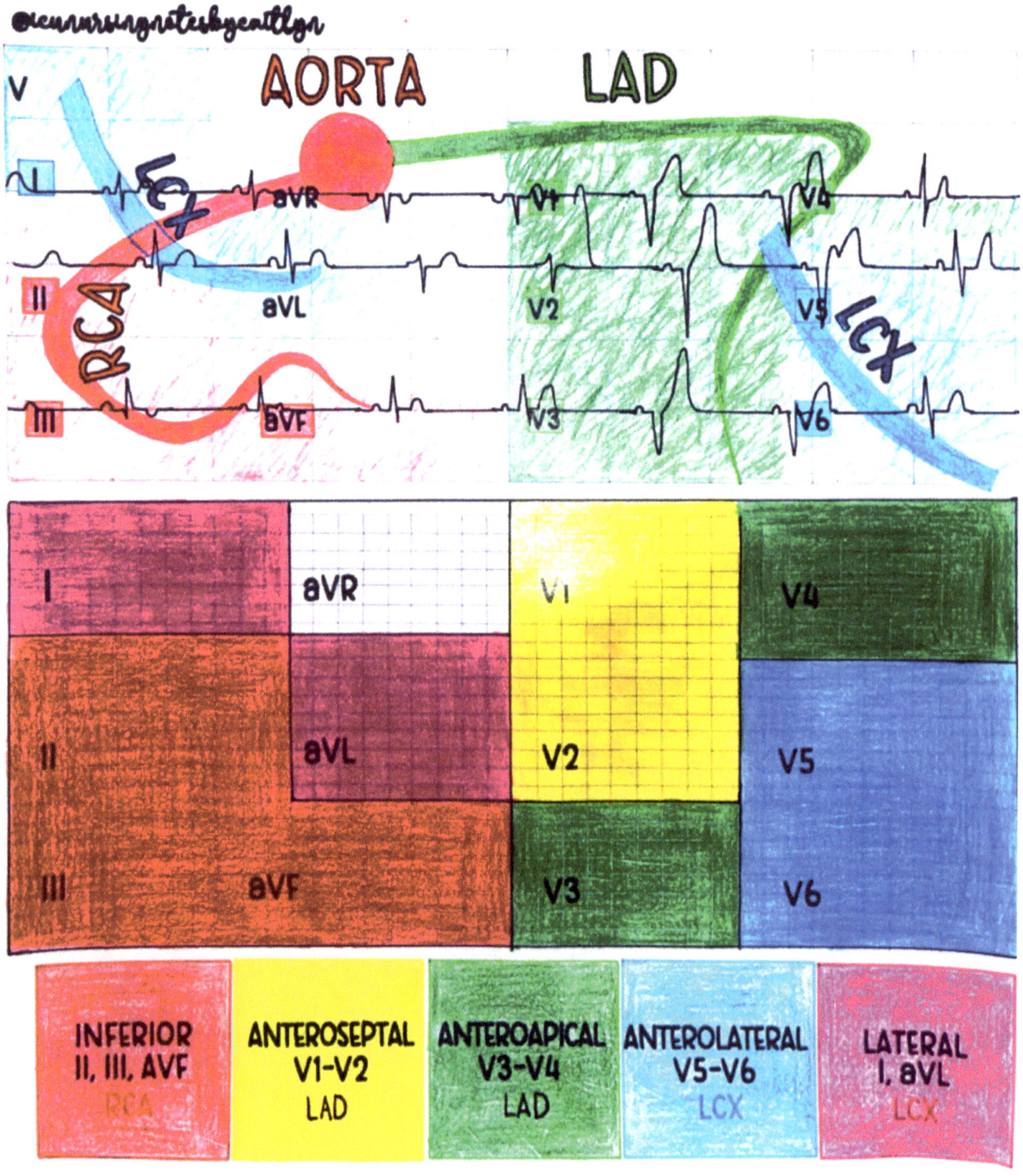

PROGRESSIVE ECG CHANGES DURING AN EVOLVING MI!

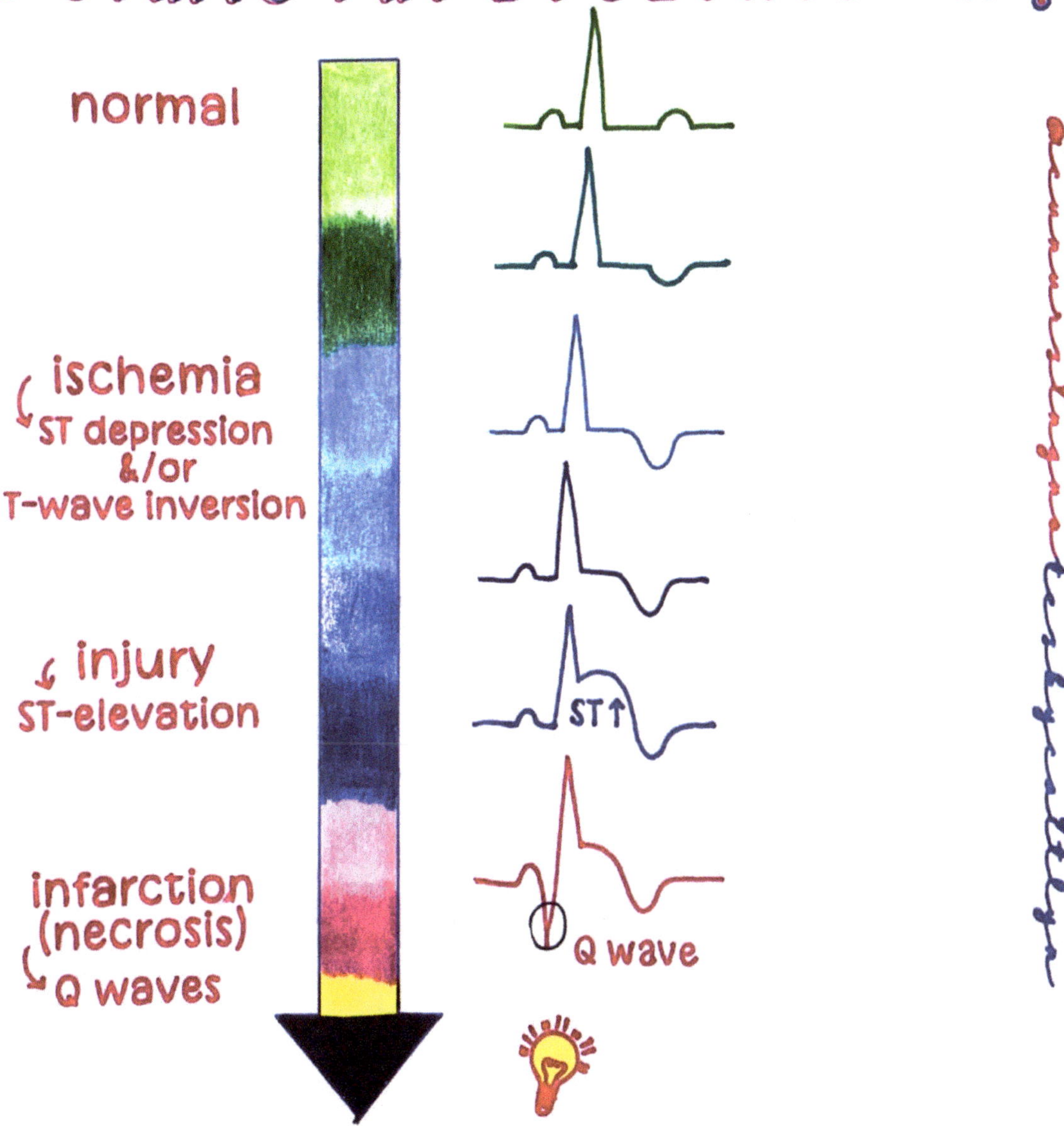

Within days to weeks, the ST segment & T wave return to baseline, but pathological Q waves will persist – these represent scar tissue (remember that dead tissue doesn't conduct impulses – this explains the wide & deep negative deflection!).

PATHOPHYSIOLOGY:

Troponin I & T are two cardiac-specific contractile proteins that are released into the bloodstream by injured cardiac muscle cells. After an acute MI (AMI), troponin levels are typically elevated within <u>3-6 hours</u>, peak within <u>14-20 hours</u>, & return to normal after <u>1-2 weeks</u>.

It's important to remember that <u>a negative troponin doesn't exclude an acute MI</u> (just as a positive troponin doesn't always indicate one)!

troponin

NON-ACS CAUSES OF TROP ELEVATION:

- AFib
- CKD
- PHTN
- HF
- PE
- sepsis
- rhabdo
- myocarditis
- aortic dissection

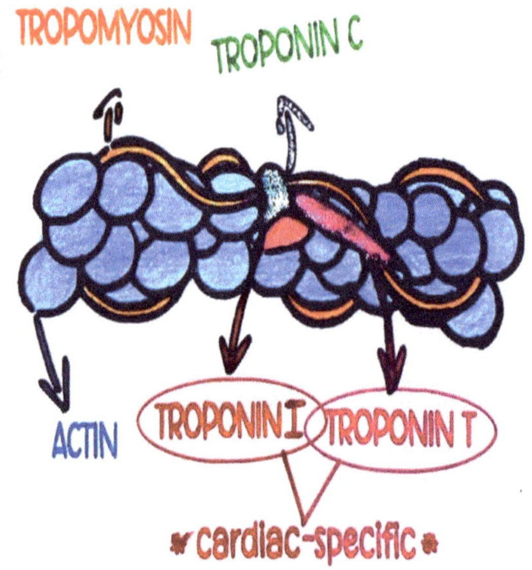

<u>High-sensitivity troponin</u> (hs-cTn) testing is becoming the standard of care in hospitals across the U.S. because it allows for rapid detection of myocardial injury & has ↑ diagnostic accuracy!

ST-Elevation Myocardial Infarction

sudden plaque rupture

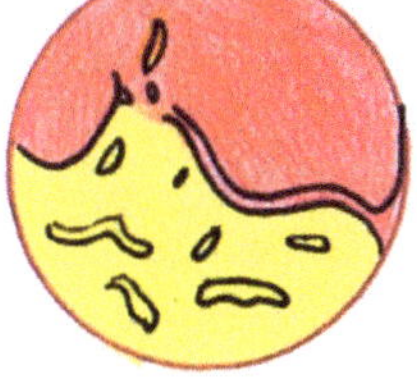

@icunursingnotesbycaitlyn

platelet aggregation & thrombus formation

Priority: Get this patient to the cath lab STAT!

total obstruction of the coronary artery

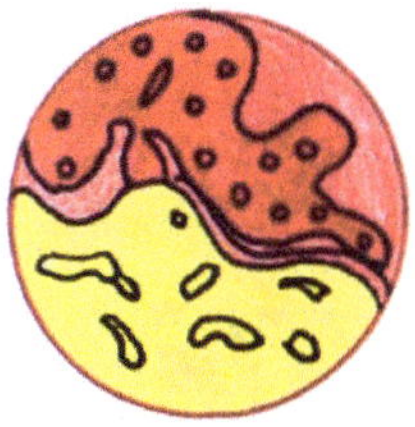

myocardial ischemia & necrosis

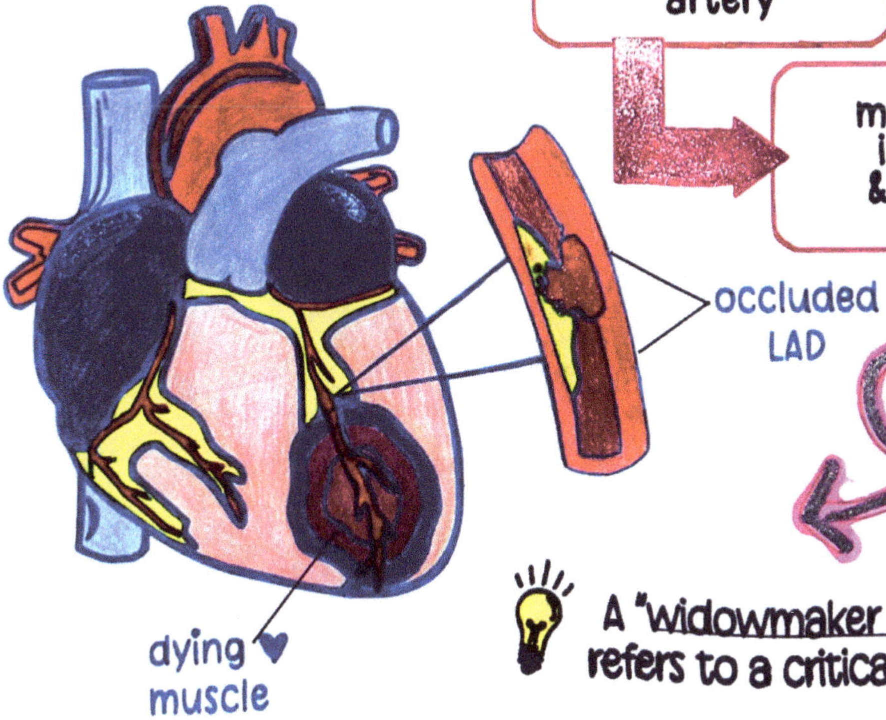

A "widowmaker heart attack" refers to a critical LAD blockage!

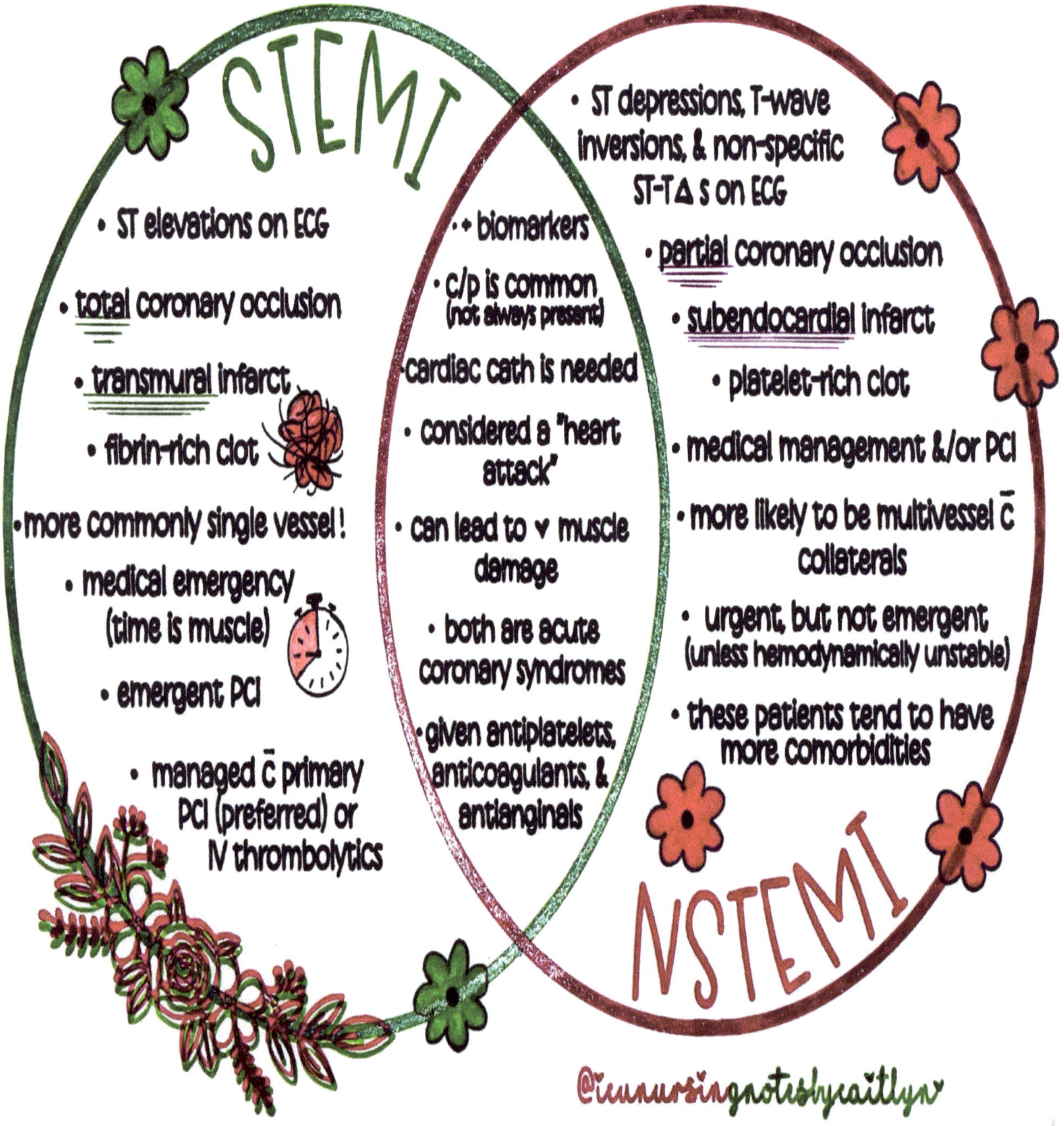
STEMI
• ST elevations on ECG
• total coronary occlusion
• transmural infarct
• fibrin-rich clot
• more commonly single vessel!
• medical emergency (time is muscle)
• emergent PCI
• managed c̄ primary PCI (preferred) or IV thrombolytics
• + biomarkers
• c/p is common (not always present)
• cardiac cath is needed
• considered a "heart attack"
• can lead to ♥ muscle damage
• both are acute coronary syndromes
• given antiplatelets, anticoagulants, & antianginals
• ST depressions, T-wave inversions, & non-specific ST-T Δ s on ECG
• partial coronary occlusion
• subendocardial infarct
• platelet-rich clot
• medical management &/or PCI
• more likely to be multivessel c̄ collaterals
• urgent, but not emergent (unless hemodynamically unstable)
• these patients tend to have more comorbidities
NSTEMI
@icunursingnotesbycaitlyn

CARDIOGENIC SHOCK

A low-cardiac-output state caused by severe impairment in ventricular pump function that leads to inadequate tissue (end-organ) perfusion despite adequate intravascular volume.

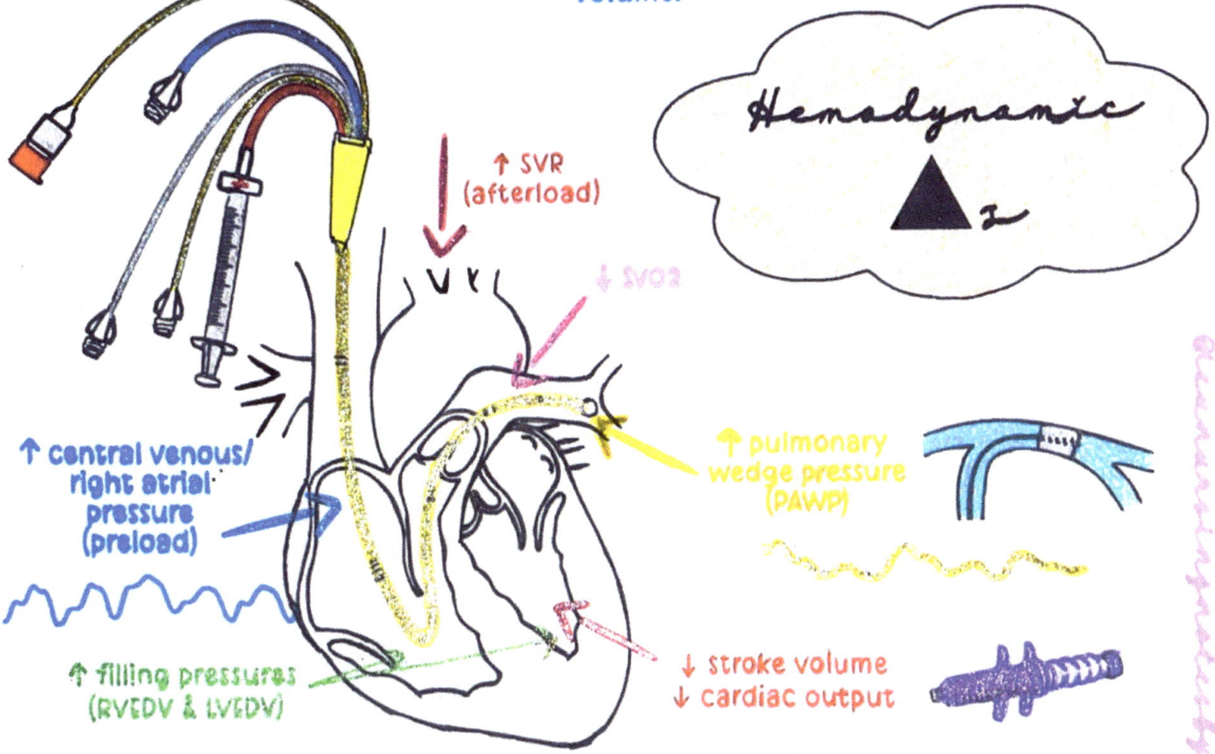

Pathophysiology:

Cardiogenic shock is best understood as a "pump problem." Damage to the heart muscle, most commonly due to an acute MI, impairs its ability to effectively contract & pump enough blood to the rest of the body, resulting in a ↓ stroke volume, ↓ cardiac output, hypotension, & ↓ tissue perfusion. As cardiac output ↓ s & the pumping function of the heart continues to decline, end-diastolic volume (EDV) & intracardiac pressures ↑, which can precipitate pulmonary edema.

The body activates several compensatory mechanisms in an attempt to restore cardiac output & to maintain end-organ perfusion. Activation of the sympathetic nervous system ↑ s heart rate & the force of myocardial contraction. Activation of the renin-angiotensin-aldosterone system ↑ s fluid retention, stimulates vasoconstriction, & ↑ s preload. These compensatory mechanisms further ↑ myocardial oxygen demand & exacerbate myocardial ischemia. Compensatory vasoconstriction, in an attempt to ↑ stroke volume & cardiac output, ↑ s SVR (afterload), which makes an already failing heart work even harder! While initially helpful in the early stages of shock, these mechanisms eventually fail & become maladaptive. ↑ coronary, tissue, & cellular ischemia further perpetuate a vicious downward spiral of cardiac deterioration, hemodynamic instability, & worsening ischemia that will ultimately culminate in end-organ failure & death if not recognized & addressed early.

Cardiogenic shock
part 2

etiology

acute MI, heart failure, mitral & aortic regurgitation, aortic stenosis, cardiomyopathies, cardiac tamponade, cardiac arrhythmias, pulmonary HTN, sepsis-induced cardiac dysfunction, papillary muscle rupture (PMR), myocarditis, & prolonged CPB

assessment

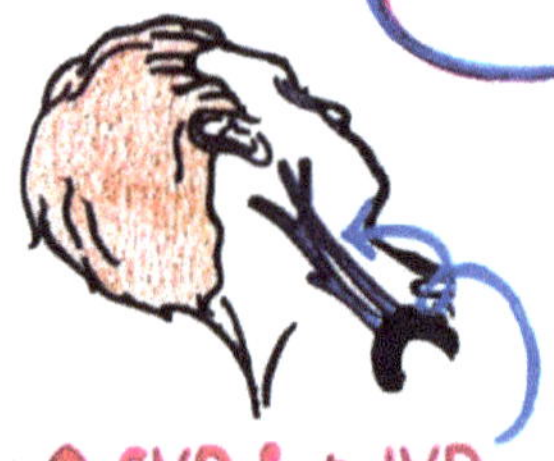

- ↑ CVP & + JVD
- ↑ HR, ↓ BP
- ↓CO/CI
- ↑ PAWP
- ↓ SVO2
- ↑ SVR
- ↑ lactate
- narrow pulse pressure

- pulmonary edema
- cool/clammy skin
- weak peripheral pulses
- AMS 2/2 ↓ cerebral perfusion
- oliguria

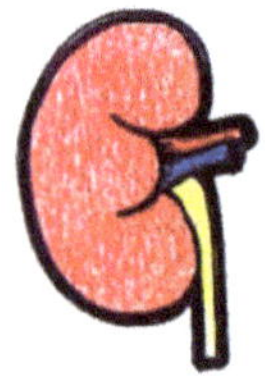

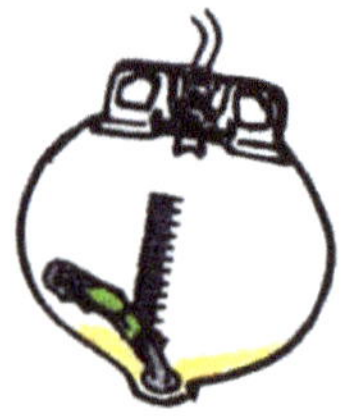

management (acute MI shock)

- **general supportive care:**
  - early revascularization (PCI/CABG)
  - mechanical ventilation (LTVV/↑PEEP)
  - pain control/sedation (↓ MVO2)
- **pharmacological support:**
  - inopressors:
    - -norepinephrine (Levo)
    - -epinephrine
  - inodilators:
    - -dobutamine
    - -milrinone

Remember: lowest possible dose & shortest possible duration. Less is more. Implement MCS early!!

- **optimize fluid status:**
  - be very cautious c̄ fluids
  - IV diuretics (Lasix, Bumex, etc)
  - CRRT

- **mechanical circulatory support (MCS):**
  - intra-aortic balloon pump (IABP)
  - Impella CP/5.5
  - TandemHeart
  - VA-ECMO

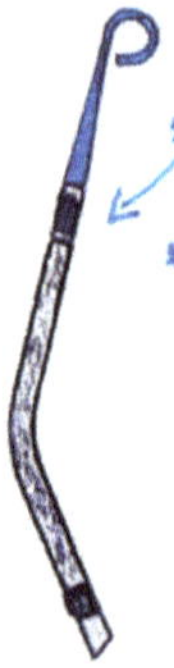

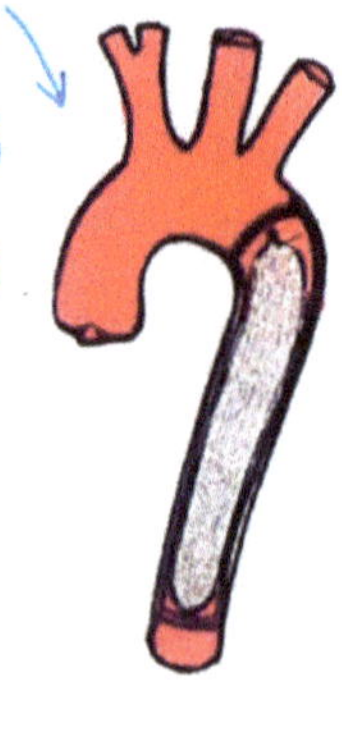

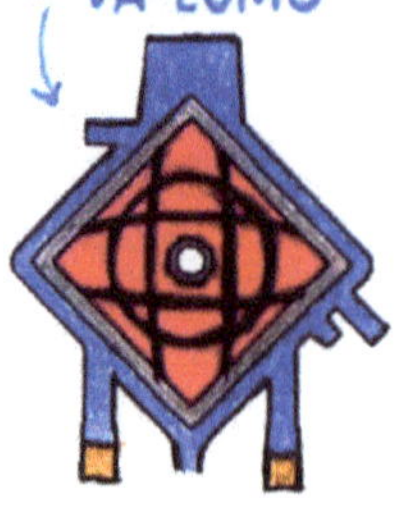

DOOR TO BALLOON TIME

A quality measure in cardiac critical care, specifically in the treatment of a STEMI, that denotes the time that it takes from patient presentation to the ED until balloon inflation (PCI) in the culprit coronary artery.

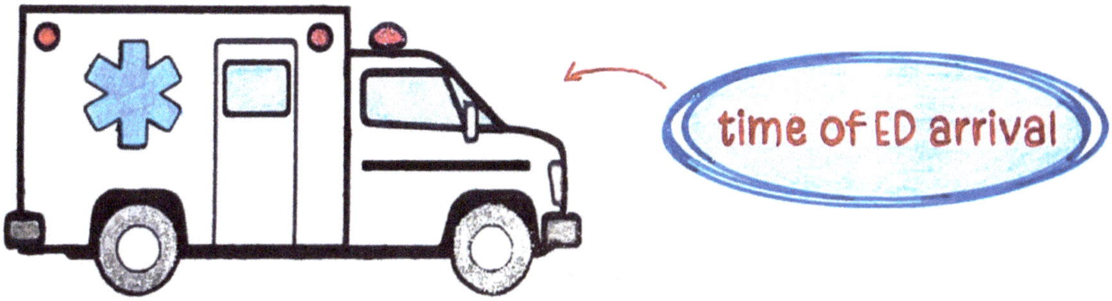

The ideal door-to-balloon time is <90 minutes (American Heart Association)!

If door-to-balloon time is expected to be > 120 min, thrombolytics can be used as a reperfusion strategy (pending that there are no contraindications).

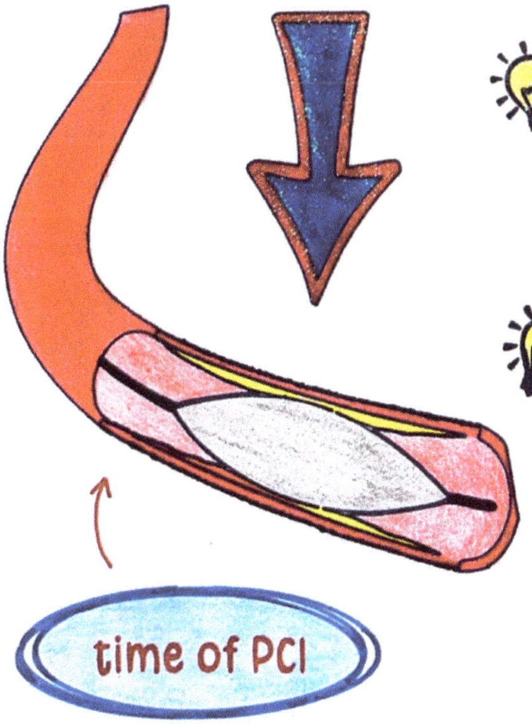

@icunursingnotesbycaitlyn

ACCELERATED IDIOVENTRICULAR RHYTHM (AIVR)

AIVR is a transient reperfusion arrhythmia that can occur during the reperfusion phase of an acute MI when the occluded coronary artery is opened (via PCI or IV thrombolytics), and blood flow is successfully restored to the ♥ muscle.

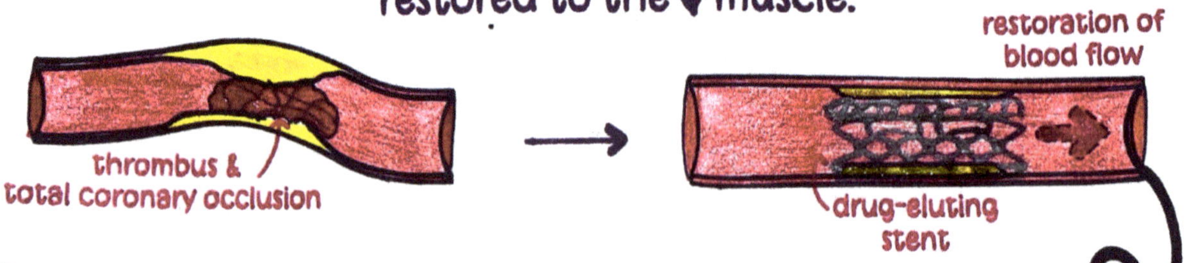

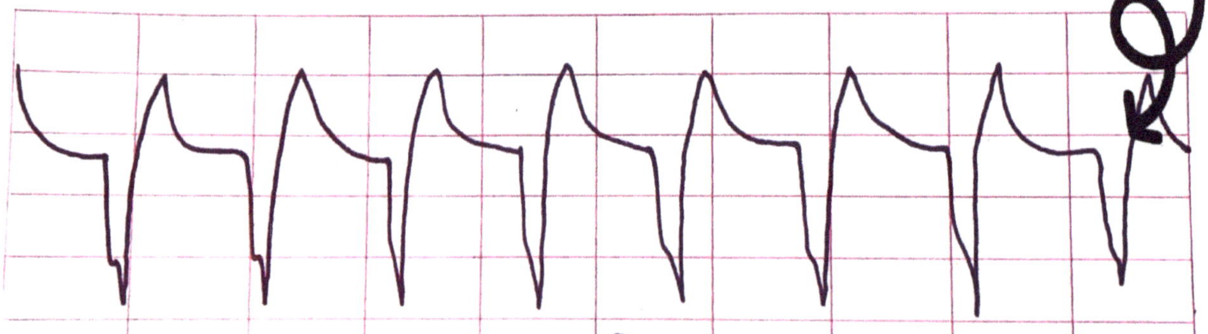

- no P waves
- wide QRS
- origin: ventricular
- rhythm: regular
- rate: 50-100 bpm

OTHER CAUSES OF AIVR:

- drug toxicity
- myocarditis
- cardiomyopathies
- ROSC s/p cardiac arrest
- electrolyte imbalances

@icunursingnotesbycaitlyn

TREATMENT:

In the setting of the reperfusion phase post-MI, AIVR is typically transient, benign, & self-limiting, so it's not typically treated!

NURSING CONSIDERATIONS FOR DIFFERENT MI TYPES

INFERIOR WALL MI

- Associated c̄ a RCA occlusion.
- Look for ST ↑ in II, III, & aVF & ST ↓ in I & aVL.
- Monitor for ↓HR & ↓BP.
- Monitor for S/S of RV infarction & posterior wall involvement.
- ↑risk for high grade AV blocks & conduction delays.
  - sinus bradycardia
  - 1st degree ♥ block
  - Wenckebach
  - complete ♥ block
- Be prepared to externally pace & anticipate possible TVP insertion.
- Remember that atropine will not work for Mobitz II & CHB!

RV INFARCTION

- Associated c ā proximal RCA occlusion/inferior wall MI.
- Monitor for JVD, ↓BP, & tachycardia (the body ↑HR to compensate for the ↓ in stroke volume).
- Severe hypotension is common due to a ↓ in cardiac output.
- Treat hypotension c̄ small boluses of IV fluids (these patients are preload-dependent) & a + inotrope (dobutamine or milrinone)
- Don't give these patients any medications that will ↓ preload! (morphine, nitrates, CCBs, BBs, diuretics).

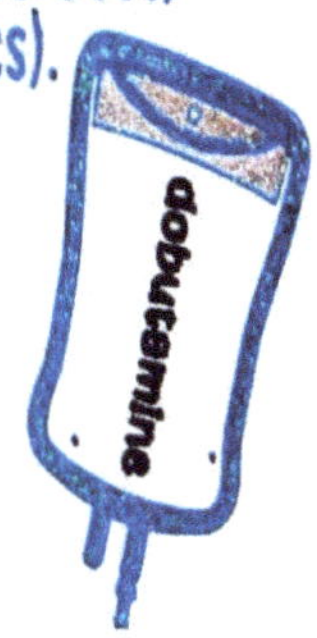

ANTERIOR/SEPTAL WALL MI

- Associated c̄ a LAD/left main occlusion.
- Look for ST ↑ in V1-V4 & ST ↓ in II, III, & aVF.
- Monitor for LV failure, cardiogenic shock, heart block, new BBB, &/or a new murmur (get an echo - could indicate ventricular septal rupture)!
- Monitor for Mobitz II & complete ♥ block.
- ↑risk for V-Fib (especially within the first 48 hrs)!
- Highest mortality rate ("widow maker").

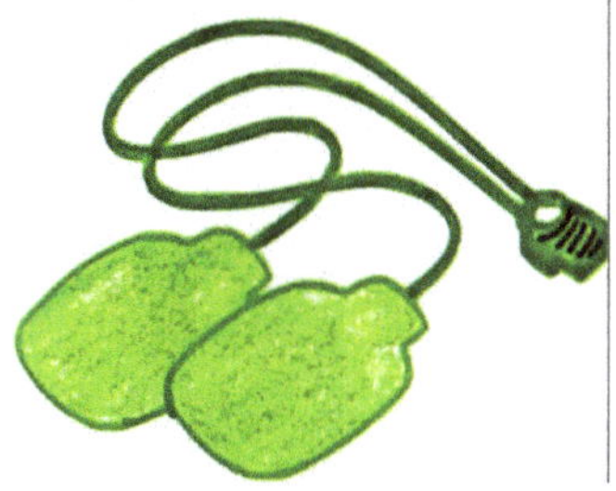

@icunursingnotesbycaitlyn

POSTERIOR WALL MI

- Associated c̄ a RCA (most likely) or LCX occlusion.
- Often accompanied by an inferior &/or lateral wall MI.
- Look for tall, broad R waves & for reciprocal Δs (ST↓) in V1 & V2.
- Monitor for LV dysfunction!!

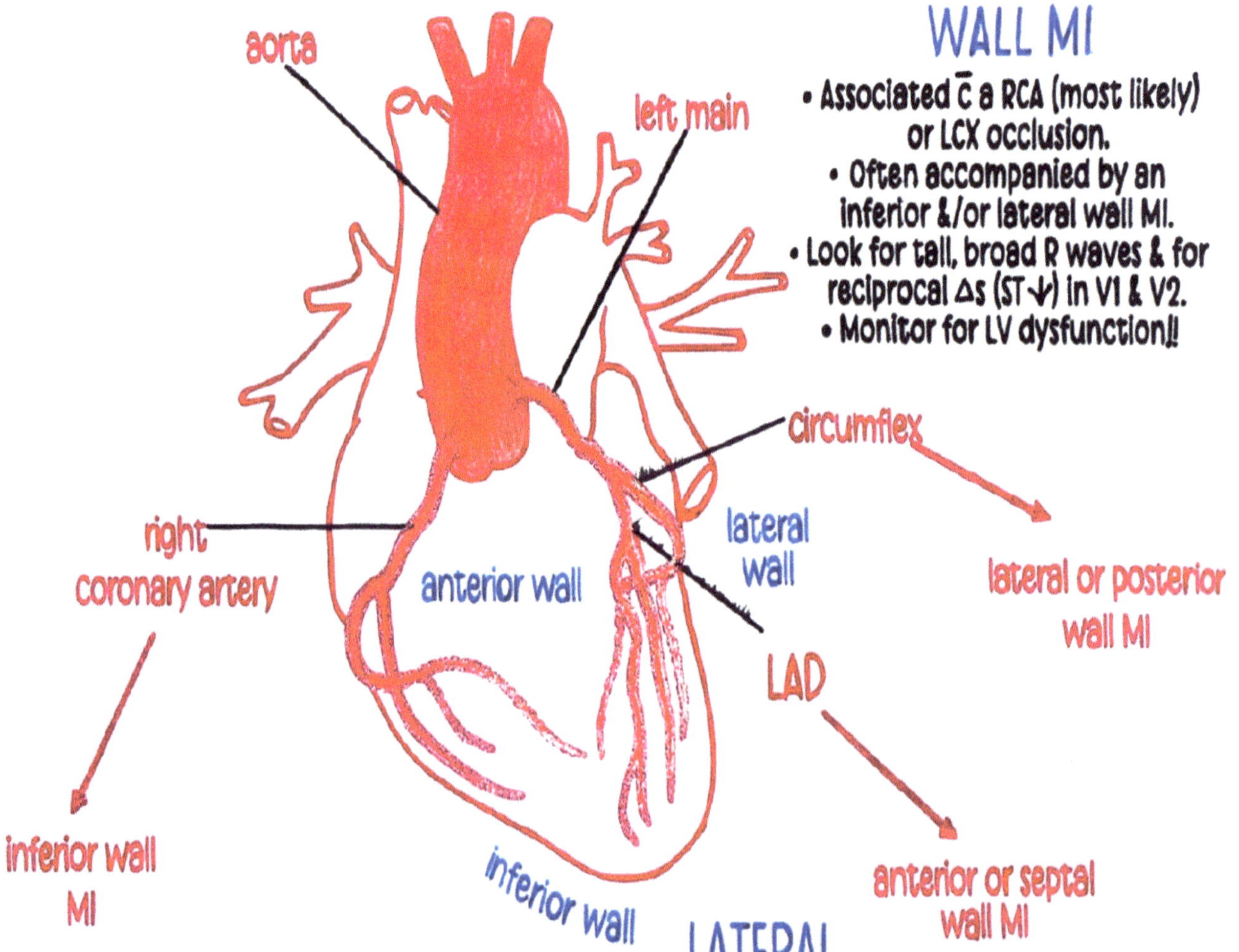

LATERAL WALL MI

- Associated c̄ LCX occlusion.
- Look for STE in I, & aVL, V5 & V6.
- Look for reciprocal Δs in the inferior leads.
- Can be associated c̄ other MI locations (anterior & inferior).

Percutaneous Coronary Intervention

@icunursingnotesbycaitlyn

atherectomy

removing plaque from the lesion (debulking)

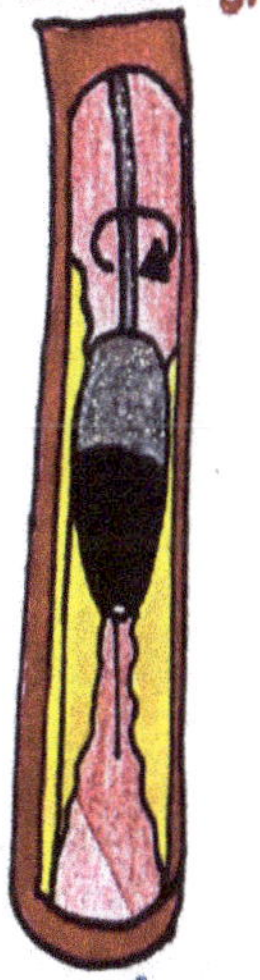

- directional
- rotational
- orbital
- laser

thrombectomy

removing blood clot(s)/ thrombi in the coronaries

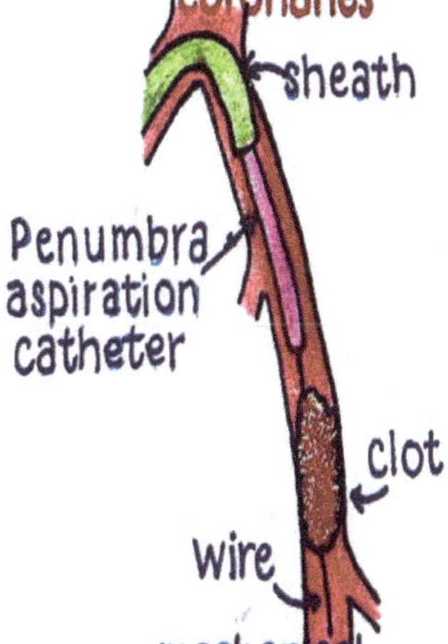

- mechanical (AngioJet & Penumbra)

or

- manual aspiration catheters

PTCA

advancing a balloon-tipped catheter across the lesion & inflating it to compress plaque against the vessel wall

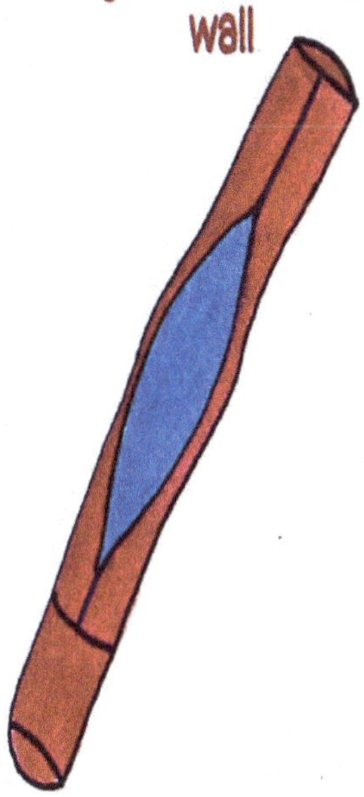

coronary stenting

placing a small mesh tube (stent) in the coronary artery to hold it open after PTCA

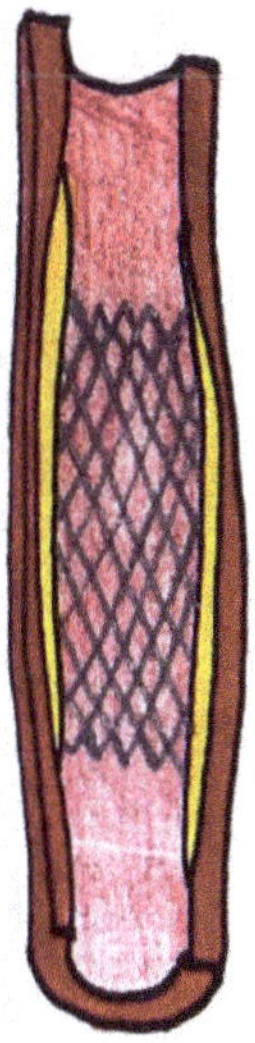

NURSING CARE OF A PATIENT S/P PCI

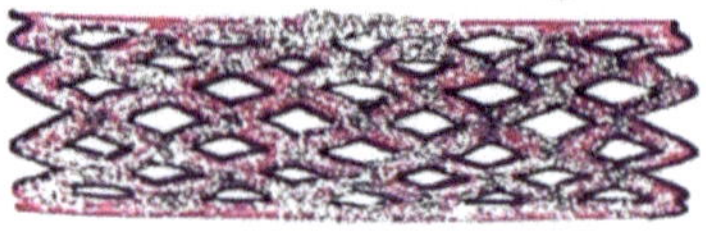

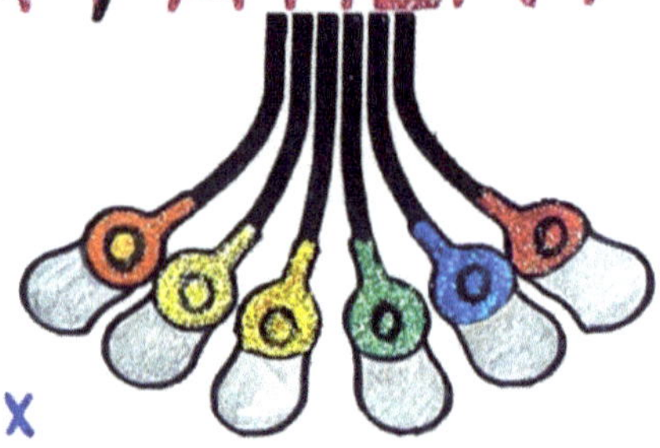

- Check peripheral pulses (radial for radial access & DP/PT for femoral access) & access site c̄ each vital sign check (typically q 15 min x 4, q 30 min x 2, then hourly). Get a 12-lead ECG post-procedure.
- Frequent neurovascular assessments (color, temp, sensation, CRT, etc).
- Monitor for bleeding & for the development of a hematoma at the access site (be on the lookout for S/S of a RP bleed c̄ femoral access).
- For radial access, your patient will have a TR band on (see my TR band cheat sheet to learn more about the nursing care for these)! Put the pulse ox probe on the thumb or index finger & check the SpO2 pleth to confirm perfusion.
- Monitor HR & BP; it's important to keep these under control!
- Give IV fluids as ordered (take your patient's fluid volume status into consideration, of course!) & encourage PO fluids to flush out the contrast dye.
- Monitor for c/p & ST elevations on ECG (can indicate a complication like coronary spasm or acute thrombosis)
- It's not unusual if your patient has a H/A (from the nitro); Tylenol &/ or a simple cool compress usually do the trick!
- If you're pulling a sheath at the bedside, ensure that you have atropine readily available & hold pressure slightly ABOVE (not directly on) the access site.
- Post-PCI patient education is key!
- Ensure that your patient is now on dual antiplatelet platelet therapy (DAPT) & teach your patient about the importance of med compliance!

Venous & Arterial Sheaths!

A sheath is a vascular access device used to introduce wires, balloons, stents, etc during cardiac caths & interventional procedures (PCIs, IABP/Impella insertion, TAVRs, etc).

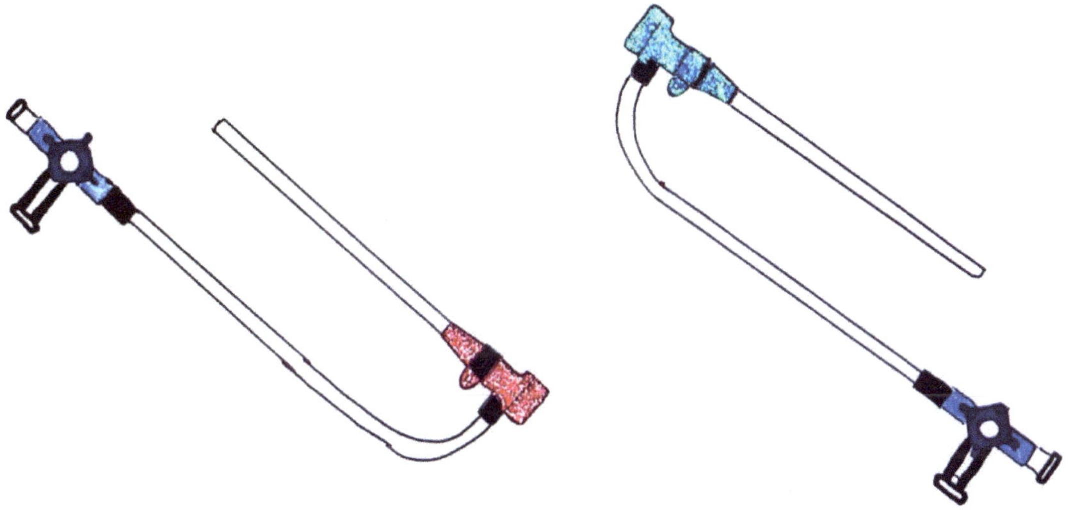

A sheath can be placed in an artery (arterial sheath) and/or a vein (venous sheath).

Sheaths are often removed in the cath lab (i.e. post-cath), but your patient may still have a venous and/or arterial sheath(s) in place post-procedure (i.e. IABP - femoral arterial sheath).

@icunursingnotesbycaitlyn

Nursing Care

*Know your hospital's policy for sheath removal by RNs.

*If your patient has an arterial sheath, ensure it's transduced c̄ an appropriate arterial waveform (although it can be dampened if you're transducing a femoral line). If your patient has a venous sheath, run a KVO through it.

*Frequent peripheral & neurovascular assessments: knowing your patient's baseline is important so that you can compare it c̄ your post-removalassessments. Look for △ s in the strength of pulses (diminished/absent), coolness/pallor, paresthesias, pain, etc. The important thing here is any CHANGE in your assessment: trust your nursing intuition!

*Sheaths are central lines: care & maintenance is imperative! Don't forget about CLABSI prevention!!

*Ensure that you have an order to D/C a venous and/or arterial sheath.

*Know your hospital's policy for VS frequency post-removal: typically, it's q 5 min during removal, then q 15 min x 4, q 30 min x 4, & q 1 hr x 4.

*Check labs ā pulling the sheath(s) - CBC, coags, & ACT.

*If your patient has femoral sheath(s), ensure that the patient is lying flat c̄ legs straight (no bending): educate your patient NOT to raise the HOB (sometimes Reverse Trendelenburg can be helpful).

*Remove the arterial sheath before the the venous sheath.

*Never continue c̄ sheath removal if you meet resistance.

*Be familiar c̄ post-sheath removal complications (bleeding, hematoma, vasovagal response, etc) & assess your patient frequently: before & after removal, make sure that you're checking your patient's PT & DP pulses (femoral access)/radial pulse (radial access) & access site. Mark pulses to save yourself time! ☺

*Remember that the length of time needed to stop the bleeding/achieve hemostasis is going to vary.

*Manual pressure, external compression devices (Fem-Stop), &/or vascular closure devices (Angio-Seal, Perclose) are used to achieve hemostasis.

*Apply sterile gauze & a Tegaderm to the insertion site after removal & monitor it frequently for bleeding & development of a hematoma.

*For radial access, avoid using the affected extremity for blood pressures & blood draws (even after TR Band removal).

TRANSRADIAL (TR) BANDS

transradial tr bands

INDICATIONS

TR Bands are compression devices indicated to assist in hemostasis of the radial artery following a transradial cardiac catheterization or angioplasty.

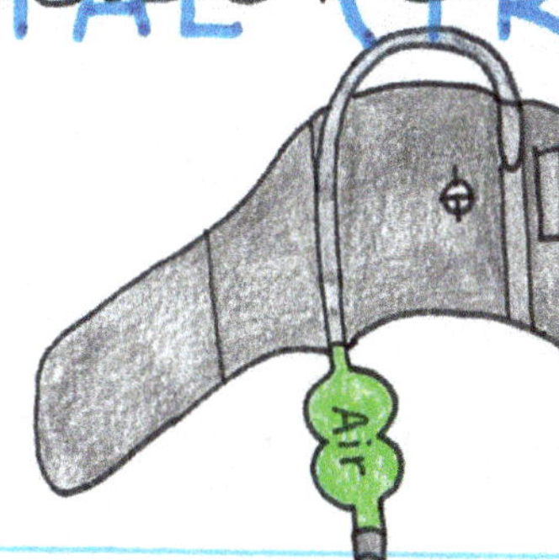

HOW DO THEY WORK?

The TR band is designed to aid in hemostasis of the radial artery after a cardiac cath.

A large balloon compresses the entire puncture site, while a smaller balloon gives it angled direction for point compression. The "dual" compression helps to prevent compression of the nerves and the ulnar artery.

These balloons are inflated using the TR Band Inflator syringe (18 cc) & is designed for air to be slowly injected into the one-way side port. Air is released slowly out of the band upon removal.

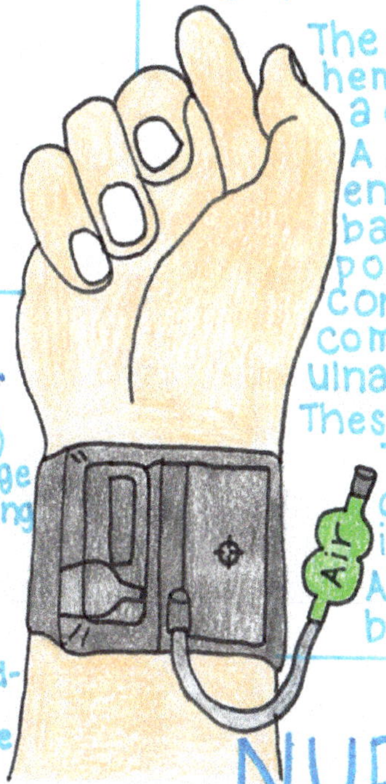

REMOVAL

- Remove 3-5 cc of air q 10-15 minutes (average) using the TR Band syringe
- If bleeding occurs during removal, inflate with enough air to restore hemostasis.
- Once all air has been removed, confirm bleeding has stopped
- Remove the band while stabilizing the access site.
- Apply sterile gauze & a Tegaderm.

NURSING CARE

* Check color, temperature, pulses, sensation, pain & CRT in the affected extremity.
* VS, bleeding & perfusion assessments q 15 minutes x 4, q 30 min x 2, and q 1 hour (general guideline)
* No BPs or venipuncture to the extremity x 24 hours
* Place SpO_2 pulse ox on the thumb of the affected extremity, and monitor the waveform to confirm perfusion.
* Assess for bleeding / hematoma at the access site and above and below the TR band.
* Keep the TR band at the bedside after removal.

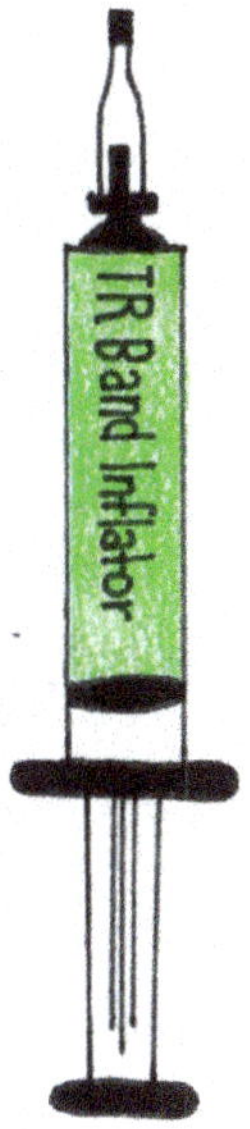

PAPILLARY MUSCLE RUPTURE

papillary muscle rupture

A mechanical complication of an acute MI (typically inferior) that can lead to the development of acute mitral regurgitation (MR) and, subsequently, flash pulmonary edema & cardiogenic shock.

Pathophysiology

When a papillary muscle in the LV ruptures due to ischemia, the mitral valve leaflets don't close completely, resulting in acute mitral regurgitation (MR). Blood from the LV flows backward into the left atrium (LA), abruptly ↑ left atrial pressure (LAP) & forcing blood back into the pulmonary circulation (hence why these patients often present c̄ flash pulmonary edema). Lack of adequate forward flow ↓s cardiac output, leading to hypotension & cardiogenic shock. The body compensates by ↑ the systemic vascular resistance (SVR), but this only exacerbates the MR!

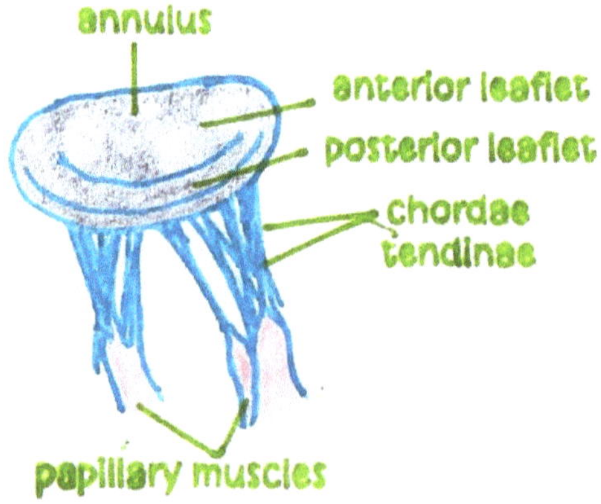

What to Look For

- late-presenting IWMI
- flash pulmonary edema
- c/p, hypotension, & cardiogenic shock
- flail mitral valve leaflet c̄ severe MR on echo
- large V waves on PCWP tracing
- holosystolic murmur radiating to LSB

Don't rely on hearing a murmur - it may be absent 2/2 equalization of pressures (LA & LV) across the mitral valve!

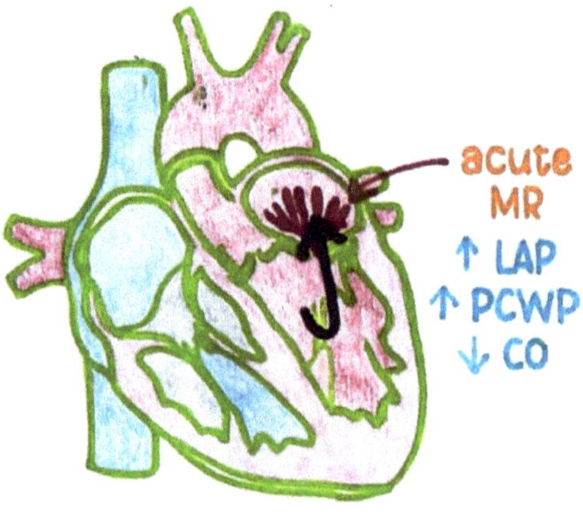

Management

- intra-aortic balloon pump (IABP) as a bridge to surgical intervention
- ↓ afterload c̄ diuretics, vasodilators, & IABP counterpulsation
- mitral valve repair or replacement (once stabilized)

@icunursingnotesbycaitlyn

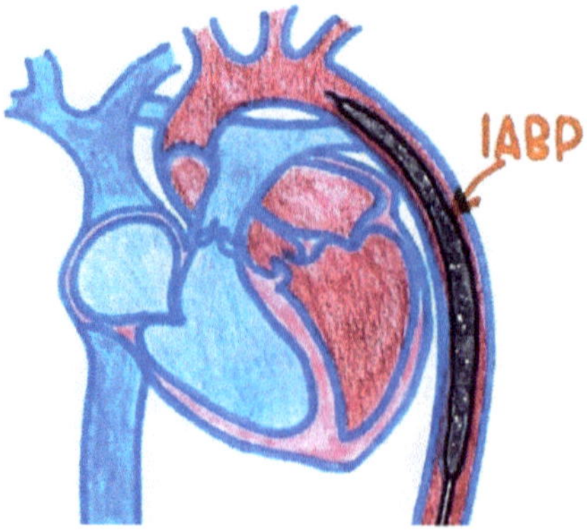

LEFT VENTRICULAR FREE-WALL RUPTURE

A rare & most often fatal complication of an acute myocardial infarction (AMI) in which the left ventricular wall weakens, breaks down & ruptures, leading to hemopericardium & subsequent tamponade c̄ acute hemodynamic deterioration.

delayed STEMI presentation

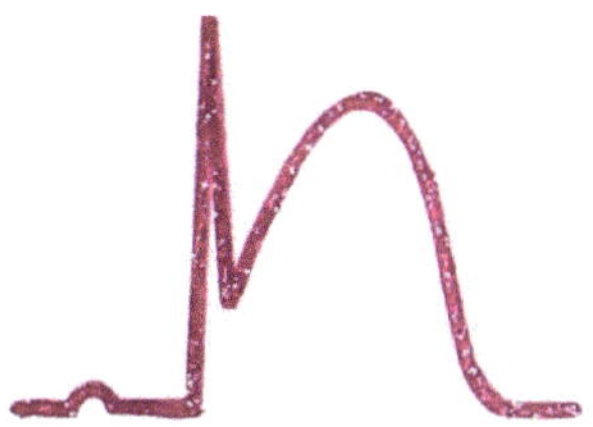

1-4 days post-infarct

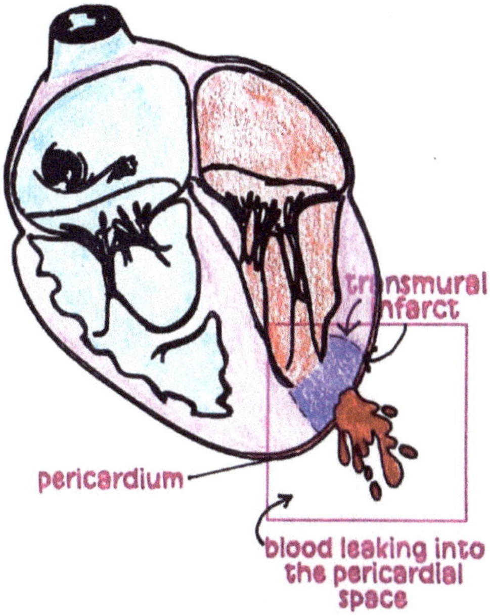

@kcunursingnotesbycaitlyn

PATHOPHYSIOLOGY:

late-presenting transmural MI

↓

necrotic myocardium becomes infiltrated c̄ inflammatory cells 1-3 days s/p infarction

↓

the inflammatory reaction in the infarcted site weakens the myocardial wall

↓

↑ pressure in the LV "blows out" the surrounding necrotic myocardium

↓

blood spills out of the LV & into the pericardial cavity (hemopericardium)

↓

cardiac tamponade & cardiogenic shock c̄ an extremely poor prognosis

RISK FACTORS:

- late-presenting anterior MI
- single-vessel disease
- large transmural infarct
- first MI (poor collateral flow)
- age > 60 years & females
- hypertension

TREATMENT:

- emergent surgical repair
- temporizing measures (IABP, pericardiocentesis, fluids, & inotropes)

Ventricular Septal Defect

An opening in the wall (septum) between the two ventricles allows blood to pass directly from the left ventricle to the right ventricle (left-to-right shunt); in the setting of a large VSD, this can lead to pulmonary hypertension, RV hypertrophy, & heart failure!

Pathophysiology

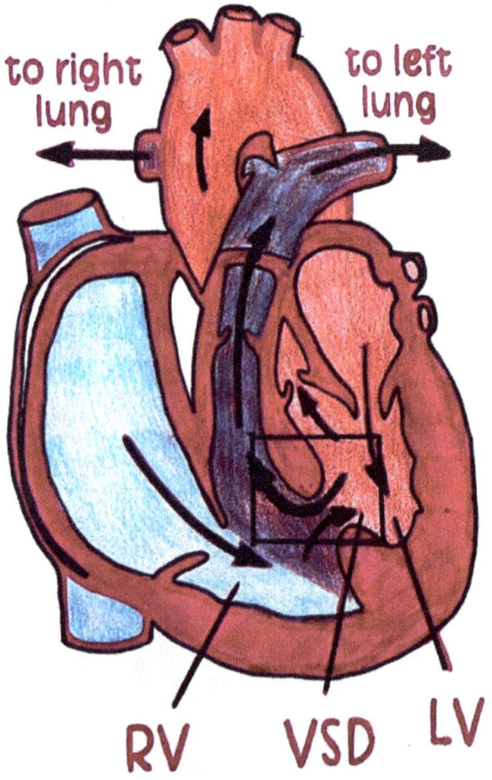

@ycunursingnotesbycaitlyn

A large opening in the interventricular septum allows blood to flow through the septal defect from the left ventricle (LV) to the right ventricle (RV); this is called a "left-to-right shunt." Less blood leaves the left ventricle (↓s stroke volume & cardiac output), & more blood enters the pulmonary circulation.

An untreated VSD can lead to pulmonary hypertension & heart failure. Over time, pulmonary hypertension can cause reversal of the shunt to a right-to-left shunt because of the abnormally high pressure in the RV - this is known as "Eisenmenger syndrome" (Rogers, 2022).

Remember that an intracardiac "shunt" refers to diversion of normal cardiac blood flow to alternate pathways within the ♥!

Post-MI VSD

A rare but often fatal complication of an anterior/septal wall MI. Low forward cardiac output due to a massive left-to-right shunt causes the sudden onset of cardiogenic shock.

NURSING CONSIDERATIONS

A majority of post-MI VSDs occur within 24 hours to one week after an acute MI (Fisher & Reich, 2017).

These patients may present c̄ a new murmur, hemodynamic instability, & cardiogenic shock. (Wing & Schiffman, 2021).

Thermodilution cardiac output (via a Swan-Ganz/PA catheter) will be falsely ↑ in these patients, & the SvO2 (mixed venous blood gas) will be ↑!

Temporizing management until surgical repair include: mechanical circulatory support device, afterload reduction & inotropic support.

Treatment

depends on defect size!

- Smaller congenital VSDs often close during infancy as the heart grows
- percutaneous transcatheter VSD closure
- surgical VSD closure (requires cardiopulmonary bypass)

@icunursingnotesbycaitlyn

Dressler's Syndrome

An immune-mediated form of pericarditis that occurs c̄ or s̄ a pericardial effusion weeks to months after a myocardial infarction (MI) or cardiac surgery.

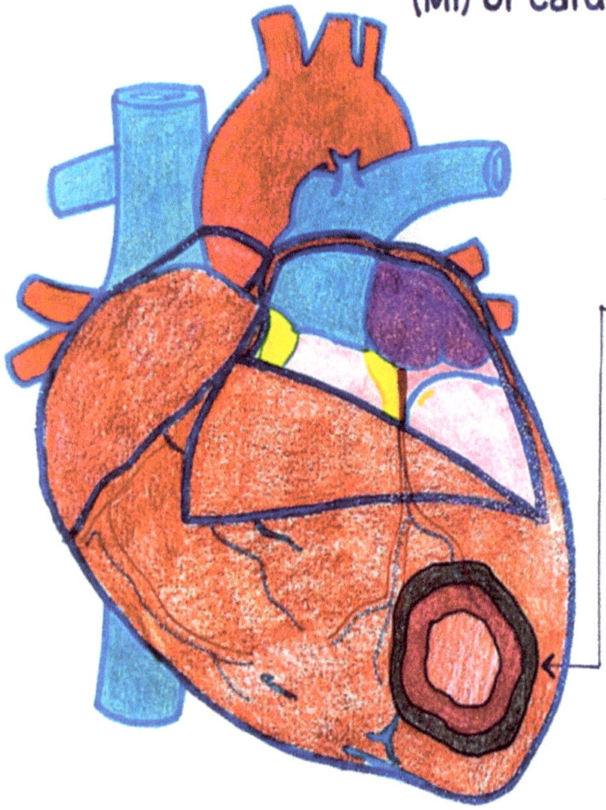

Pathophysiology:

Dressler's syndrome is thought to result from an immune-mediated response to myocardial injury &, specifically, to the pericardial mesothelial cells. The damaged heart muscle releases antigens that form immune complexes c̄ antibodies, producing an inflammatory response that affects the pericardium!

Signs & Symptoms:

- pleuritic chest pain
- tachycardia
- low-grade fever
- pericardial effusion c̄ or s̄ tamponade
- ↑inflammatory markers (ESR & CRP)
- widespread ST-elevations & PR depressions on ECG

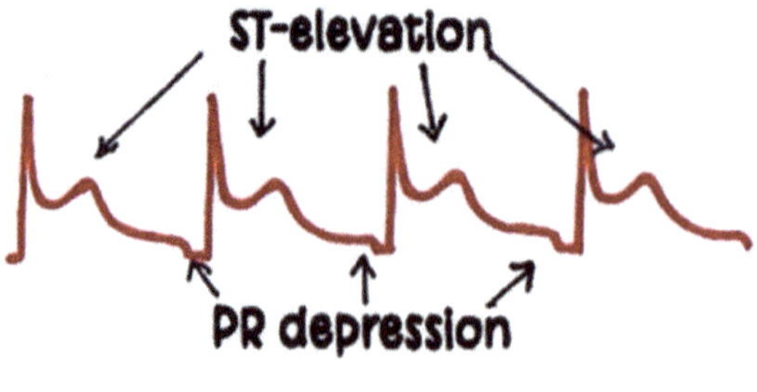

Management:

- high-dose aspirin
- NSAIDs
- colchicine
- corticosteroids
- pericardiocentesis (for large pericardial effusions c̄ tamponade)

WELLENS' SYNDROME

An ECG pattern of biphasic (type A) or deeply inverted (type B) T waves in V2 & V3 that typically indicates critical stenosis of the proximal left anterior descending (LAD) coronary artery.

TYPE A

biphasic T wave inversion

V2

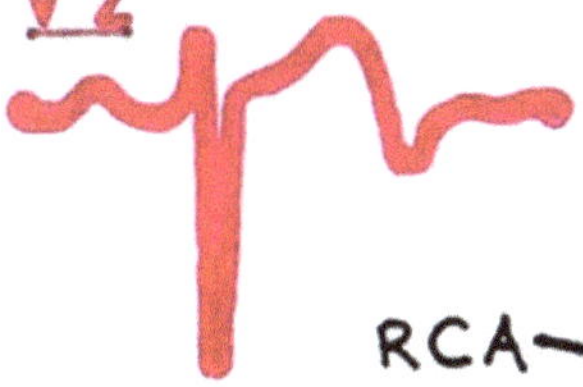

V3

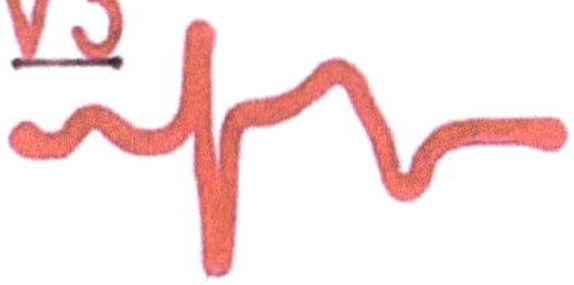

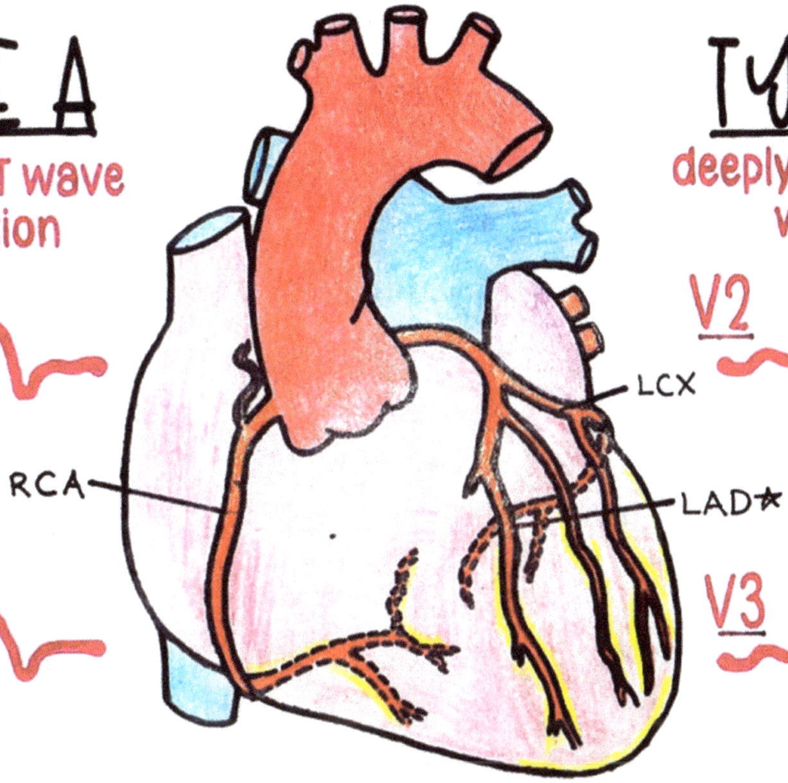

TYPE B

deeply inverted T waves

V2

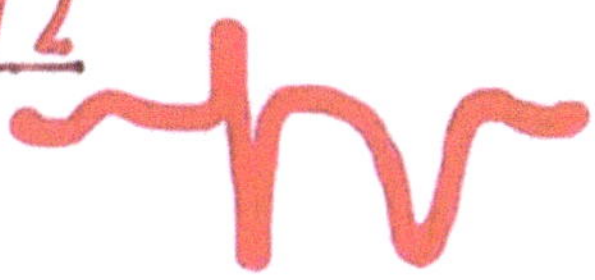

V3

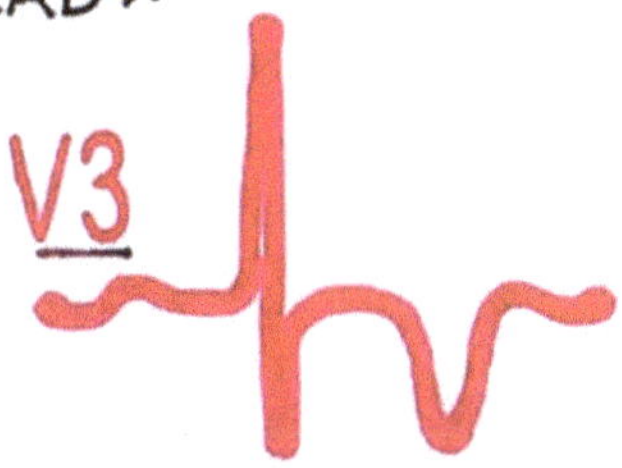

Patients presenting c̄ Wellens' syndrome have a 75% chance of developing an extensive anterior wall MI (AWMI) within days to weeks without coronary intervention (PCI)! (Mead & O'Keefe, 2009).

PATHOPHYSIOLOGY

Wellens' syndrome is thought to involve a transient LAD occlusion that spontaneously resolves. These patients often present c̄ anginal pain that has resolved, & the characteristic ECG findings are seen in a pain-free state. These ECG findings represent coronary reperfusion (similar to what is seen after a successful PCI)!

Aortic Valve Anatomy

@rcunursingnotesbycaitlyn

During systole, the pressure in the LV pressure > aortic pressure, forcing the aortic valve open.

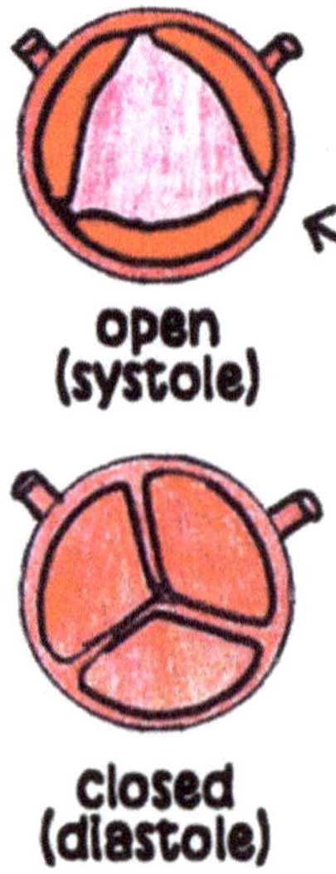

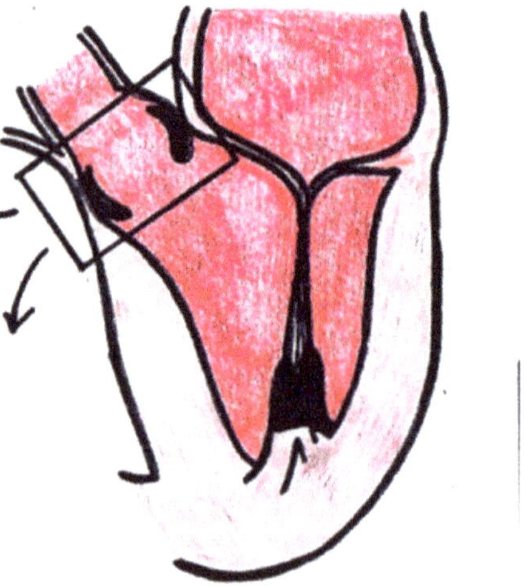

During diastole, the aortic pressure > LV pressure, closing the aortic valve. This is important because it prevents regurgitation & perfuses the coronaries.

The aortic valve is a trileaflet valve that separates the left ventricle from the aorta.

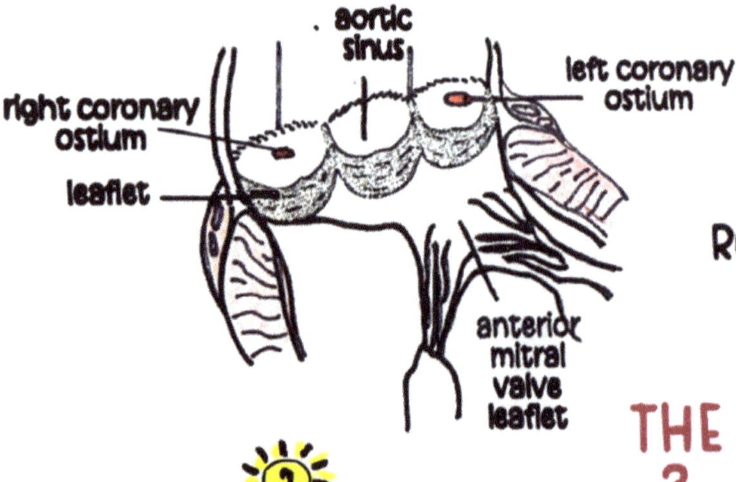

THE 3 CUSPS:

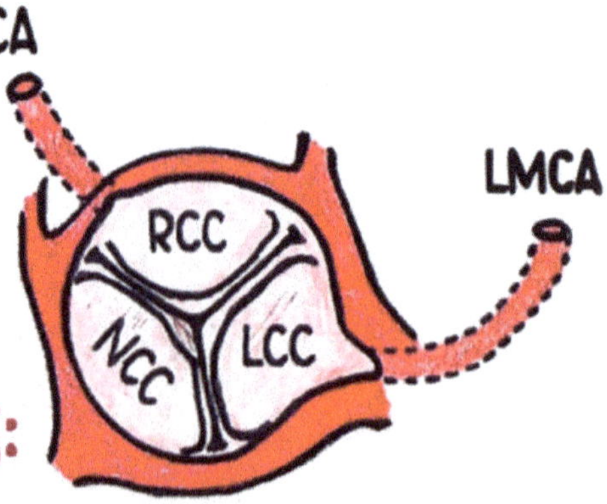

The cusps (leaflets) are named for their association c̄ one of the coronary arteries.

RCC: right coronary cusp
LCC: left coronary cusp
NCC: non-coronary cusp

Aortic Stenosis

ETIOLOGY & RISK FACTORS

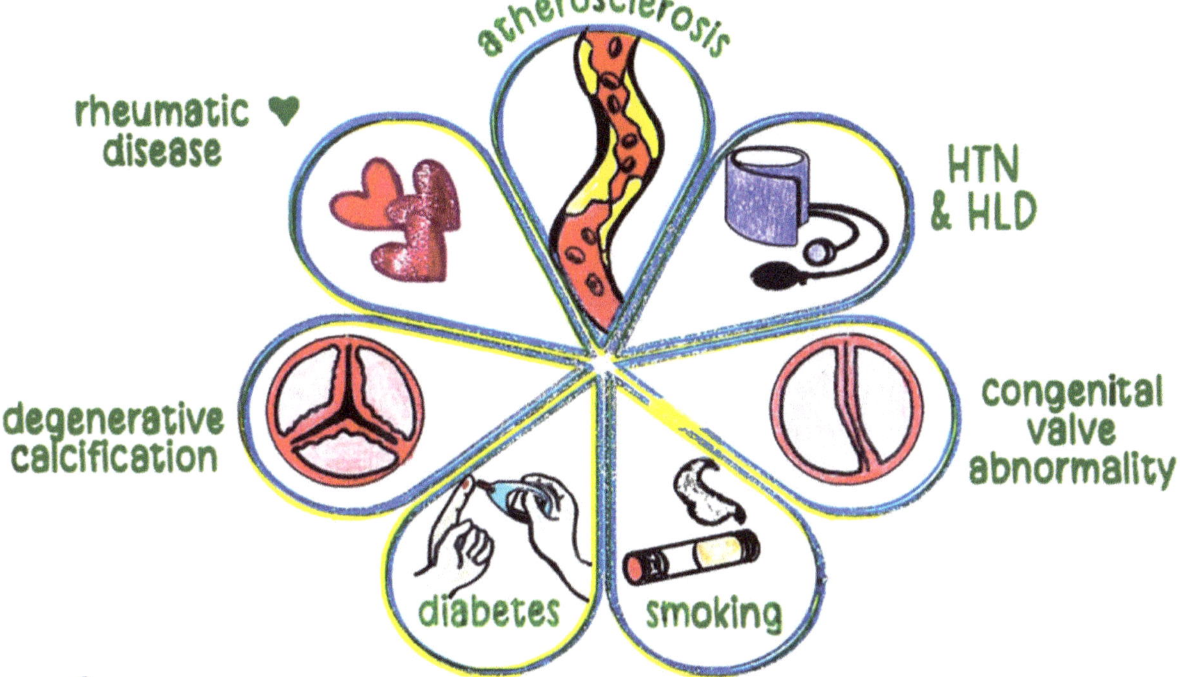
atherosclerosis
rheumatic ♥ disease
HTN & HLD
degenerative calcification
congenital valve abnormality
diabetes
smoking

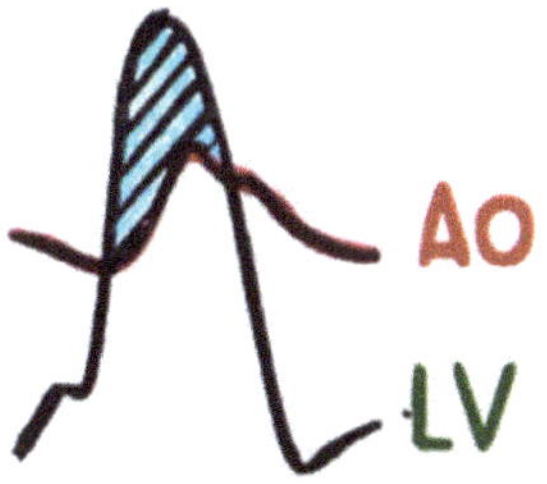
Ao
LV

SEVERITY OF AORTIC STENOSIS

MILD
mean gradient < 25 mmHg

MODERATE
mean gradient > 25 mmHg & < 40 mmHg

SEVERE
mean gradient > 40 mmHg

AORTIC STENOSIS

Signs & Symptoms

- heart failure
- fatigue & weakness
- delayed systolic upstroke
- narrow pulse pressure
- systolic ejection murmur
- ↑filling pressures, ↓SV & ↓CO
- possible LBBB & LVH on ECG
- split S2, S3 (HF) & S4 (LVH)

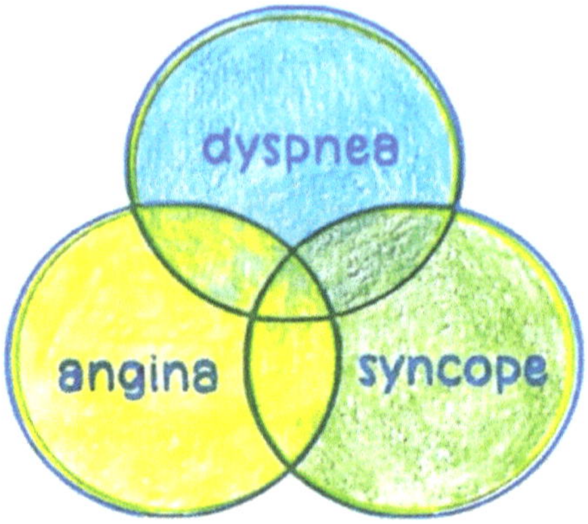

the classic triad of symptoms seen in severe AS

@icunursingnotesbycaitlyn

Treatment

repair the valve!

- surgical aortic valve replacement (SAVR)
- transcatheter aortic valve replacement (TAVR)

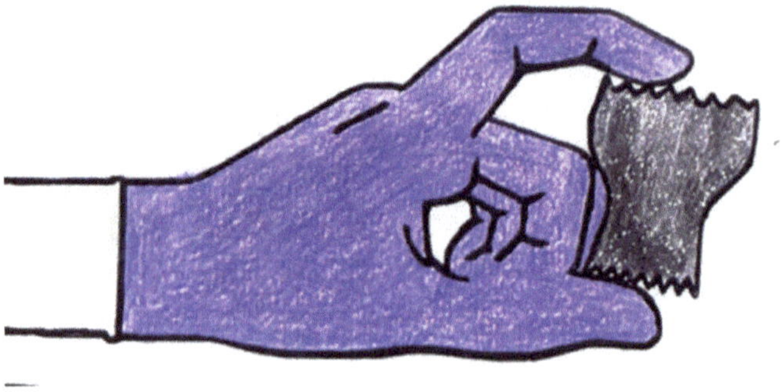

Acute Decompensated AS

- intra-aortic balloon pump
- VA-ECMO
- inotropic support
- vasopressors
- temporizing balloon aortic valvuloplasty (BAV) as a bridge therapy

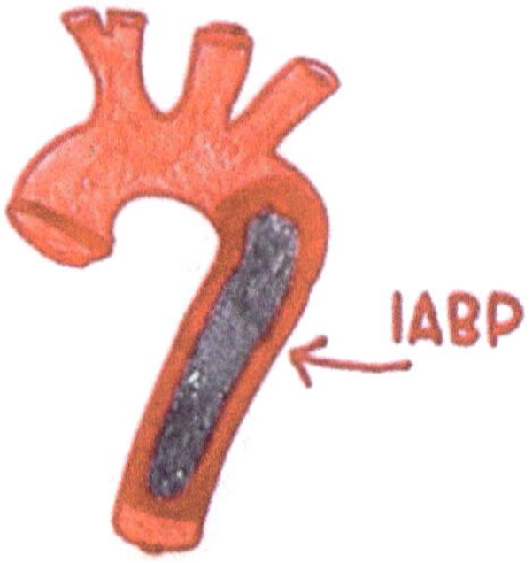

The Langston® Catheter

A dual-lumen pigtail catheter used to obtain simultaneous left ventricular (LV) & aortic (Ao) pressure measurements during a left heart catheterization.

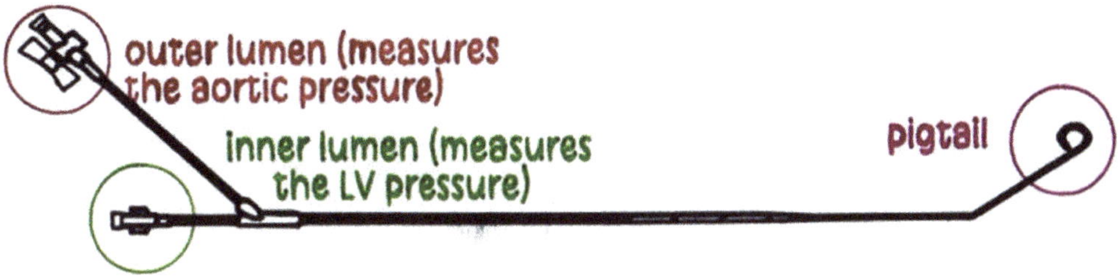

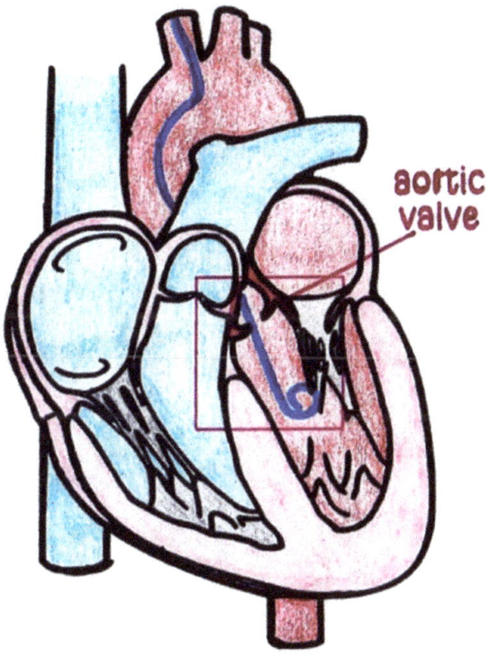

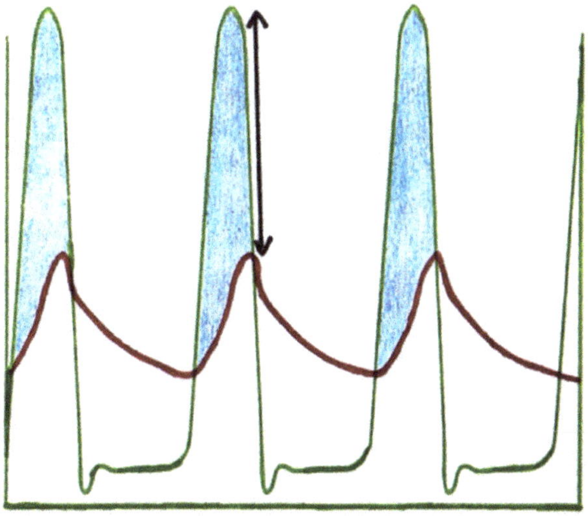

- LV pressure (inner lumen)
- aortic pressure (outer lumen)
- peak-to-peak gradient

The Langston catheter is useful in determining the severity of aortic stenosis (AS). In a patient c̄ AS, the aortic valve is narrowed, altering flow & causing a pressure difference (gradient) between the aortic (Ao) & the LV pressure!

@icunursingnotesbycaitlyn

AORTIC VALVE GRADIENT

aortic valve gradient

Simultaneous aortic & LV systolic pressures are recorded to assess for aortic stenosis.

@zcunursingnotesbycaitlyn

NORMAL

- identical LV & aortic (Ao) systolic pressure tracings
- systolic aortic pressure = systolic LV pressure

"Pressure gradient" refers to the difference in pressure on each side of the valve!

AORTIC STENOSIS

- significant pressure gradient between the systolic Ao & LV pressure tracings
- systolic LV pressure > systolic Ao pressure
- delayed systolic upstroke of the aortic tracing compared to the LV tracing

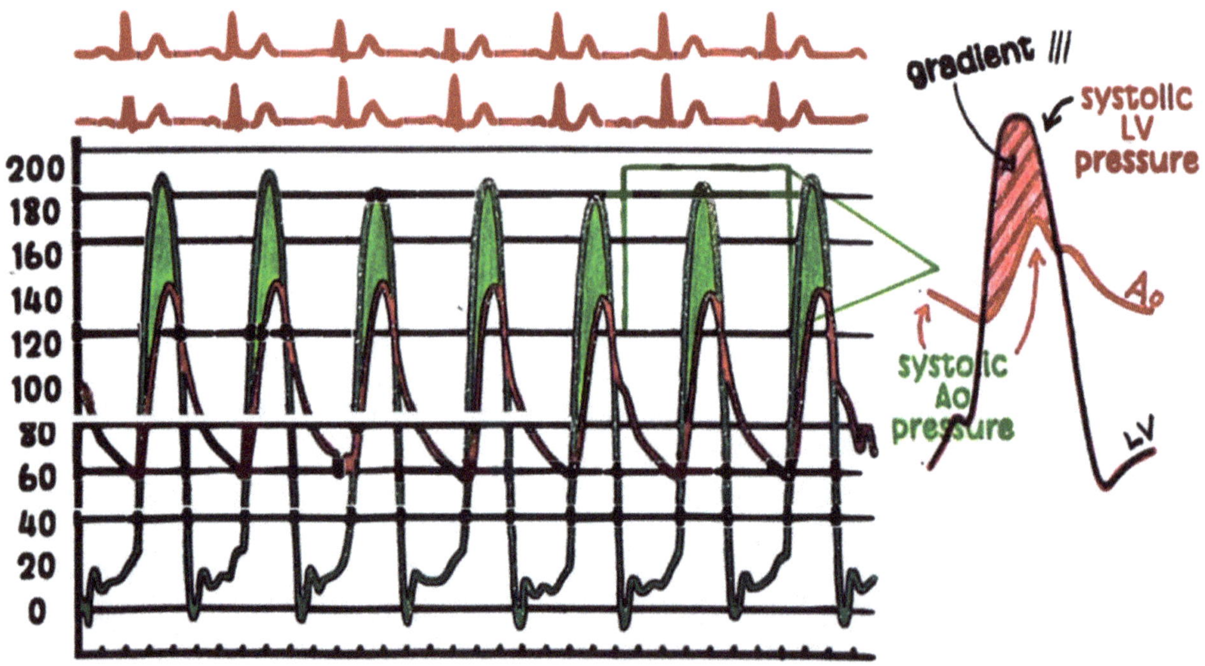

The shaded area is the aortic valve gradient that is characteristic of critical AS!

HEMODYNAMIC CONSIDERATIONS FOR CRITICAL AORTIC STENOSIS

@icunursingnotesbycaitlyn

RHYTHM: SINUS!

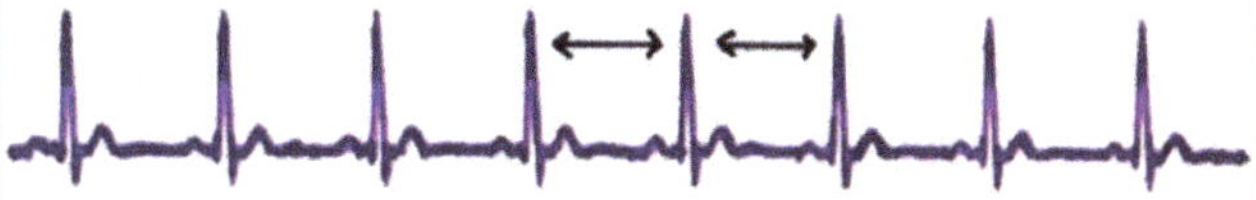

The LV requires the "atrial kick" of sinus rhythm to fill in diastole. Maintaining sinus rhythm ensures AV synchrony which, in turn, optimizes LV filling & the best possible stroke volume!

PRELOAD: ↑

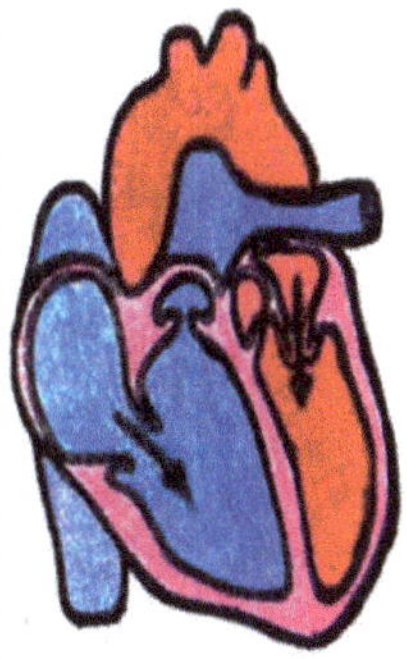

A stiff, hypertrophied LV requires ↑ filling pressures to fill in diastole. These patients depend on preload to maintain cardiac output.

HEART RATE: ↓

Because it takes longer to eject blood through a narrowed valve, a slower HR is important. A ↑ HR promotes ischemia & ↑ s myocardial oxygen demand.

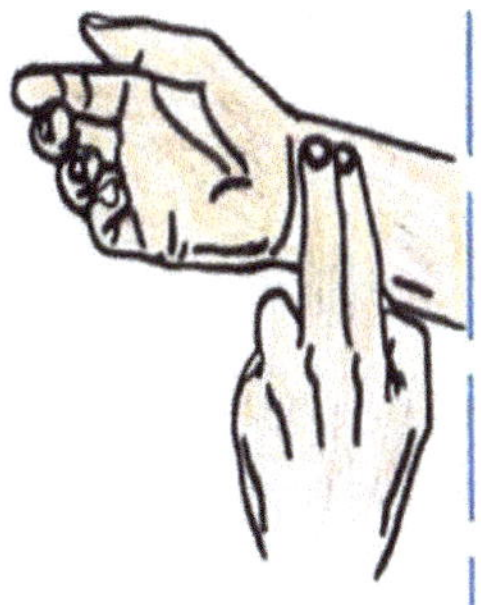

AFTERLOAD: ↑

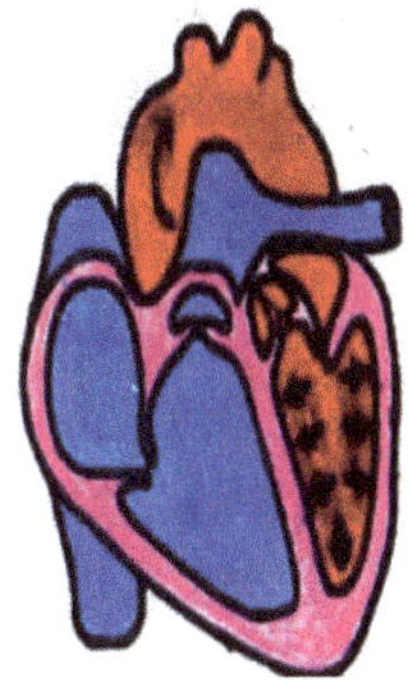

Although afterload is essentially fixed in AS, a ↑ afterload is ideal because of the heart's inability to augment BP by way of stroke volume.

TRANSCATHETER AORTIC VALVE REPLACEMENT (TAVR)

A minimally invasive, catheter-based procedure & alternative to a surgical aortic valve replacement (SAVR) for patients c̄ severe aortic stenosis who are not surgical candidates.

In the transfemoral approach (through the groin), a delivery catheter is threaded up the femoral artery via an introducer sheath & is guided into position under echo and fluoroscopy. Once in place, the new valve is deployed against the orifice of the native valve (the native valve is not removed).

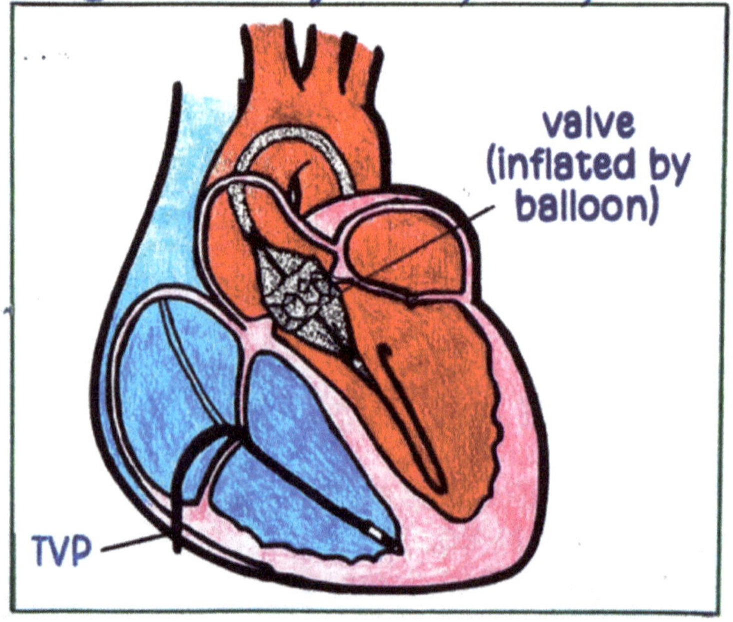

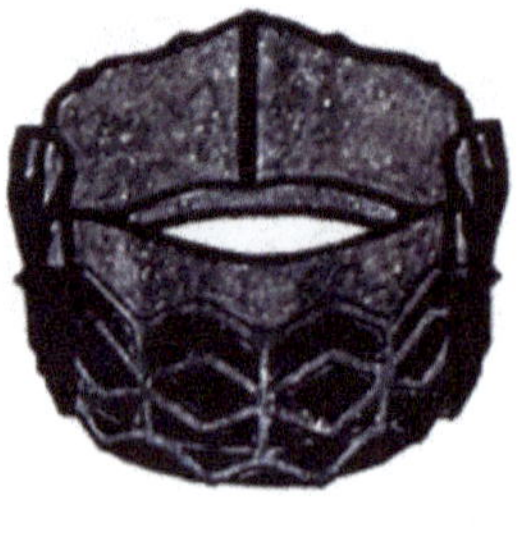

During a TAVR, a temporary transvenous pacemaker (TVP) is typically inserted for rapid ventricular pacing (RVP). During replacement valve depolyment, RVP is used to temporarily ↓ cardiac output to ↓ the risk of valve dislodgement. These patients are also at risk for heart block!

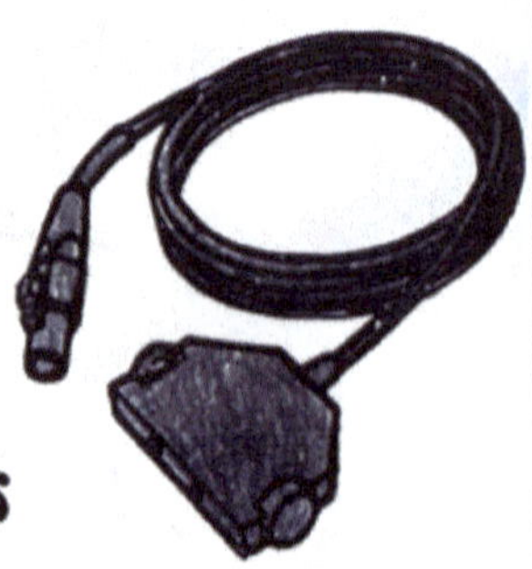

RAPID VENTRICULAR PACING

Rapid VVI pacing of the right ventricle (180-200 bpm) to transiently ↓ cardiac output in patients undergoing a TAVR or a BAV in order to facilitate native valve ballooning (BAV & TAVR) & replacement valve deployment (TAVR only).

Rapid ventricular pacing (RVP) decreases the cardiac output & reduces blood flow pulsatility. Without RVP, the TAVR valve can be ejected out of the aortic valve annulus because of the force of LV systolic contraction.

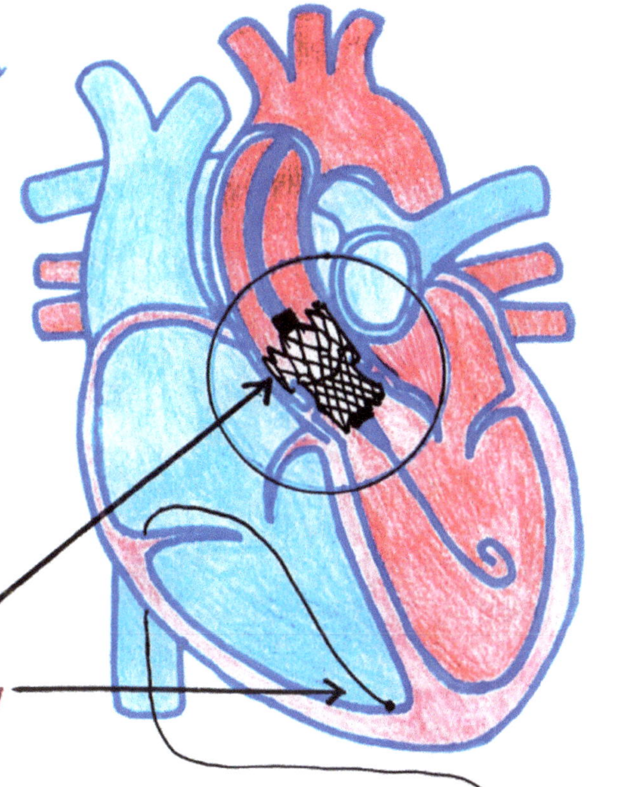

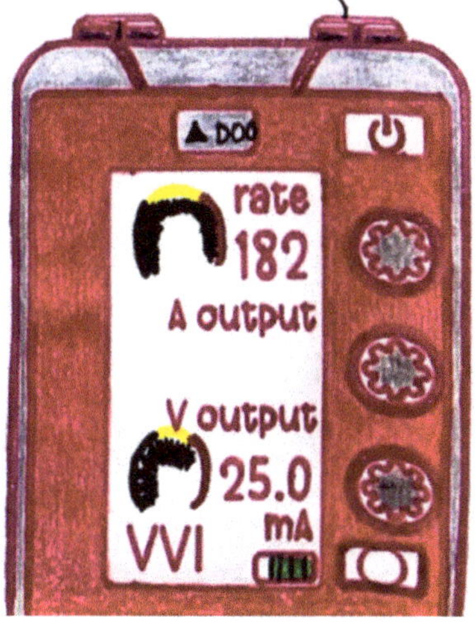

Because of the aortic valve's close proximity to the conduction system, heart block is a TAVR-related complication that requires leaving the transvenous pacemaker (TVP) in place. Patients c̄ pre-existing conduction defects (RBBB, LBBB, & 1st or 2nd degree AVB) are at highest risk)!

POST TAVR NURSING CARE

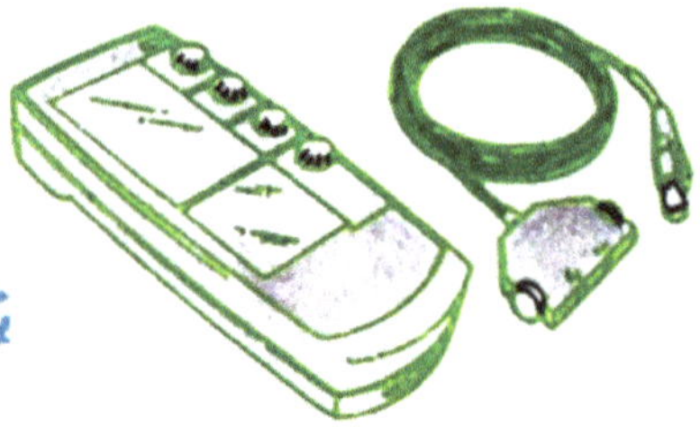

- Frequent neuro checks (post-TAVR patients are at a ↑ risk for stroke).
- Frequent neurovascular assessments of the RLE & LLE (color, temperature, pulse, sensation, etc) for transfemoral access.
- Monitor HR & rhythm (specifically for new-onset A-Fib or heart block).
- If the patient has a transvenous pacemaker (TVP) 2/2 complete heart block (CHB), verify that the settings match those ordered & that it's capturing & sensing properly.

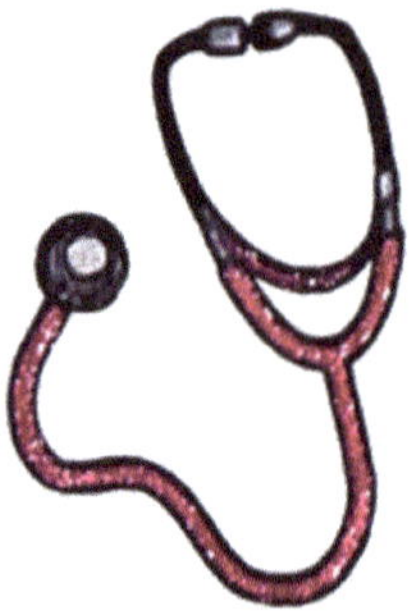

- Monitor for tolerance & recovery from sedation (these patients are typically given MAC or conscious sedation).
- Monitor for vascular complications (hematoma, RP bleed, arterial occlusion, etc).
- Assess for changes in heart sounds & for the development of a new murmur, as this can indicate a paravalvular leak.

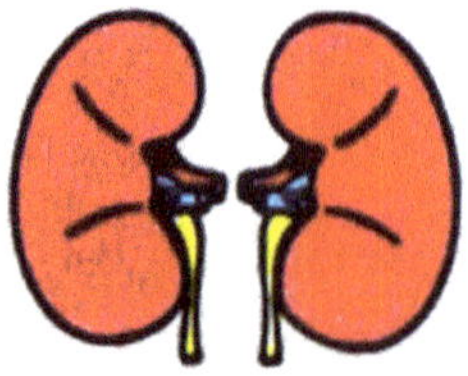

- Keep the patient on bedrest for 4-6 hours (varies per facility policy) c̄ the HOB <30 to minimize access site bleeding.
- Monitor I&O & renal function.
- Monitor for changes in vital signs.
- Remove access site dressings 24-48 hours post-procedure.
- Educate your patient that he or she will be sent home on a dual antiplatelet therapy (DAPT) regimen x 6 months to prevent thrombus formation of the newly placed valve.

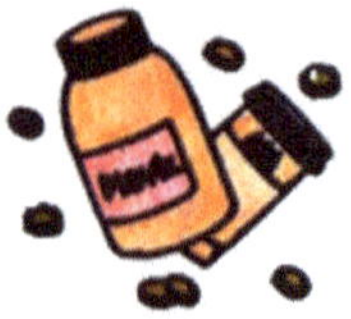

@icunursingnotesbycaitlyn

"SUICIDE LEFT VENTRICLE" S/P TAVR

Acute hemodynamic decompensation that can occur following a transcatheter aortic valve replacement (TAVR) 2/2 a sudden reduction in left ventricular afterload.

PATHOPHYSIOLOGY

Over time, a chronically high afterload from aortic stenosis leads to compensatory LV hypertrophy & diastolic dysfunction. After a TAVR, the new valve alleviates the fixed obstruction & offloads the LV. This sudden ↓ in LV afterload can result in LV cavity obliteration during systole as a hypertrophied ventricle contracts against a significantly reduced afterload; when this compromises cardiac output & causes cardiovascular collapse, it's termed "suicide left ventricle."

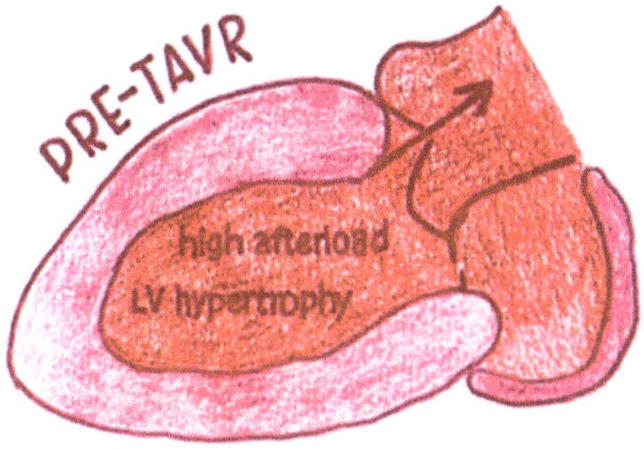

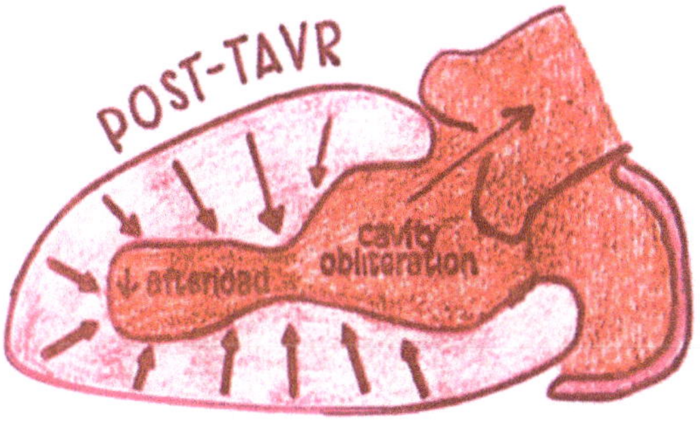

MANAGEMENT

ALLEVIATE THE OUTFLOW OBSTRUCTION!

- Maintain preload (IV fluids)
- Avoid excessive vasodilation & positive inotropes
- Alpha-1 agonist like phenylephrine ("Neo") to ↑ afterload, ↑ BP, & ↓ the intraventricular gradient
- Beta blockers to ↓ inotropy & ↑ diastolic filling time (in the absence of hypotension)

This condition is treated like hypertrophic obstructive cardiomyopathy (HOCM)!

RISK FACTORS

1) small left ventricular outflow tract (LVOT) & LV size
2) preserved/high ejection fraction (EF)
3) high interventricular septum-to-posterior-wall thickness ratio

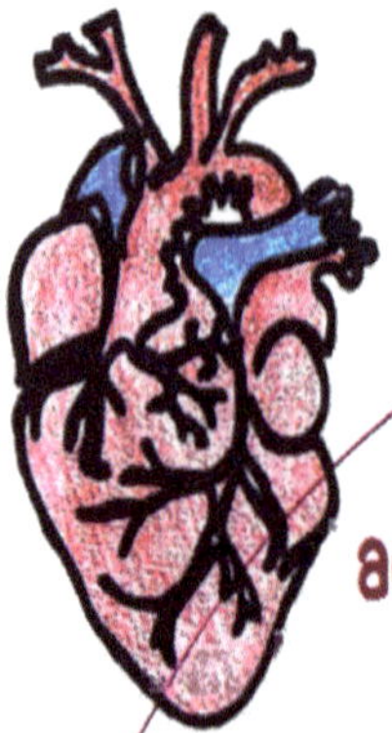

SAVR

- requires cross-clamping of the aorta & cardiopulmonary bypass (CPB)
- the diseased native valve is removed & is replaced c̄ a biologic (tissue) or prosthetic (synthetic) valve
- ideal for lower risk patients c̄ fewer comorbidities
- performed under general anesthesia
- lifelong anticoagulation is required for mechanical valves
- the gold standard & most definitive treatment option for severe AS

SAVR & TAVR

- treatment options for critical aortic stenosis (AS)
- both increase the patient's life expectancy
- both require lifelong low-dose aspirin (ASA)

TAVR

- a minimally invasive, catheter-based procedure that does not require CPB
- a new valve is deployed within the native valve; the native valve is not removed
- ideal for high risk patients who are not surgical candidates
- shorter recovery time
- requires short-term dual antiplatelet therapy (DAPT)
- typically performed under MAC rather than general anesthesia
- ↑ risk of stroke & heart block

@icunursingnotesbycaitlyn

Cardiac Tamponade

...when the heart is under pressure!

A condition in which fluid accumulates in the pericardial space & compresses the heart leading to inadequate ventricular filling & hemodynamic instability 2/2 a decrease in cardiac output.

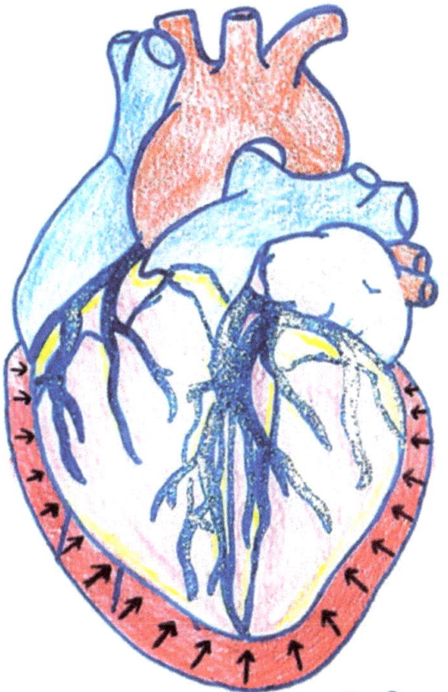

etiology

type A aortic dissection, s/p ablation & PPM insertion, coronary dissection/perforation, LV free wall rupture, s/p CABG, s/p AMI, cancer, infection, trauma, pericarditis, kidney failure, & autoimmune diseases.

@icunursingnotesbycaitlyn

The difference between a pericardial effusion & cardiac tamponade is **the patient's hemodynamic status!**

pathophysiology

The pericardial space typically holds ≈ 50 cc of fluid that protects the heart by preventing friction & wear and tear as the heart contracts. Cardiac tamponade occurs when intrapericardial pressure becomes equal to or greater than the intracardiac pressures because of fluid or blood accumulation within the pericardial space. This compression prevents the heart from stretching & filling during diastole, thereby ↓ venous return to the right side of the heart (preload) which, in turn, ↓s left ventricular filling, too. A ↓ preload (decreased filling) & ↓ stroke volume (decreased blood pumped out) leads to a subsequent ↓ in cardiac output that can lead to cardiogenic & obstructive shock. These patients are often tachycardic because the body attempts to compensate for the low cardiac output by ↑ the heart rate.

CARDIAC TAMPONADE

signs & symptoms

★ jugular venous distention

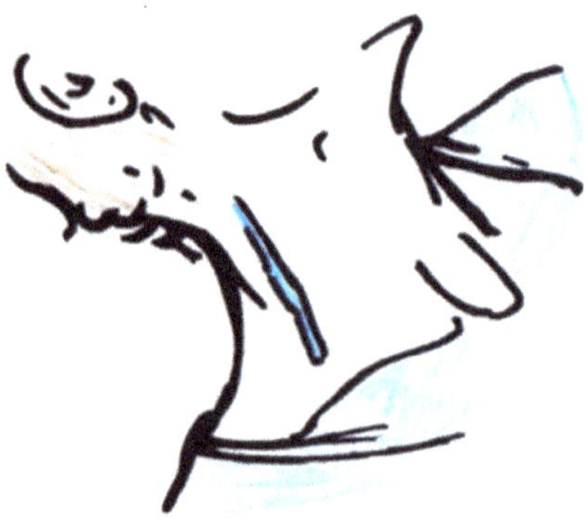

★ distant (muffled) heart sounds

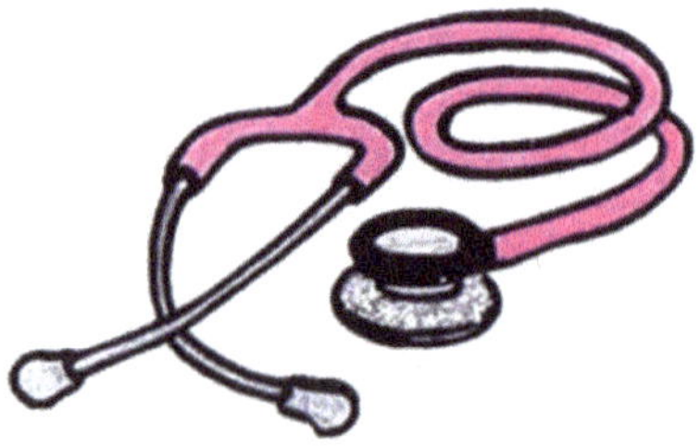

sinus tachycardia

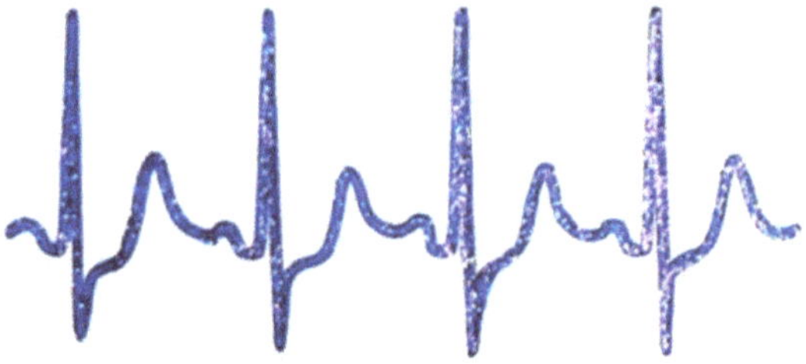

★ hypotension, pulsus paradoxus, &/or narrow pulse pressure

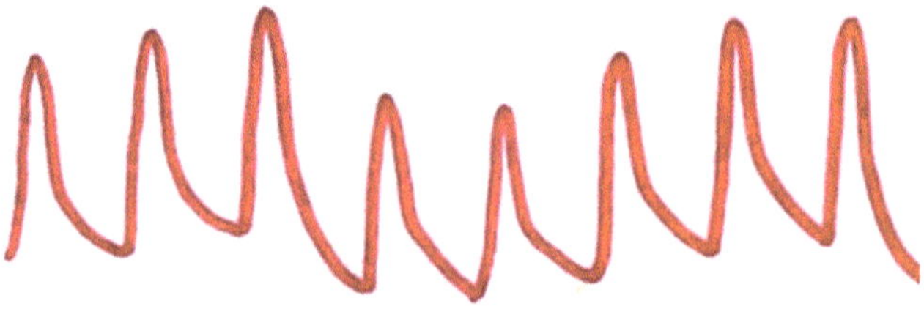

dyspnea

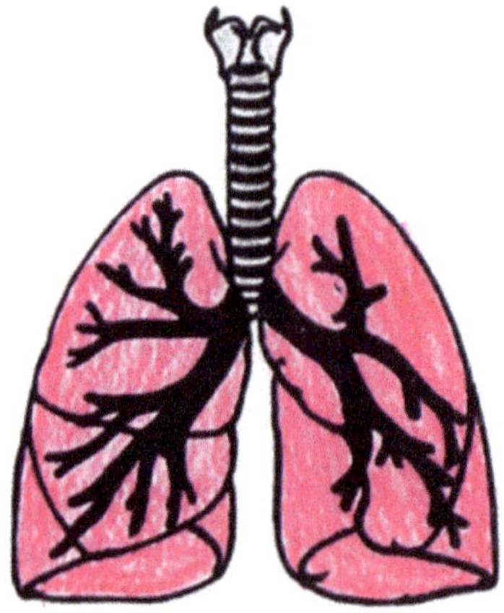

equalization of diastolic pressures

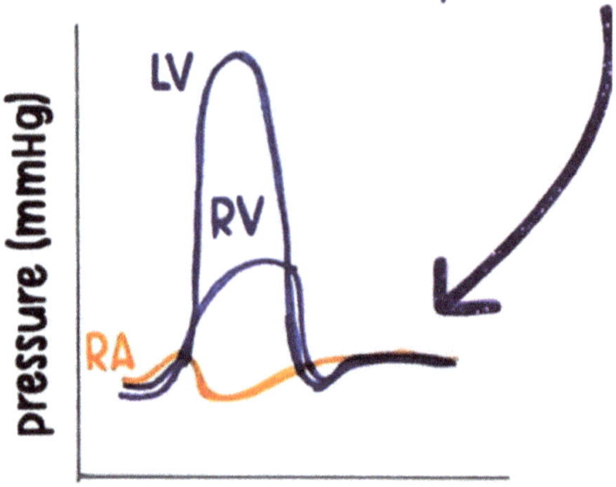

★ = Beck's Triad (JVD, muffled heart sounds, & hypotension)

PULSUS PARADOXUS

An excessive drop in the systolic blood pressure (> 10 mmHg) during inspiration that is most commonly associated c̄ **cardiac tamponade** (although it can occur c̄ other physiology).

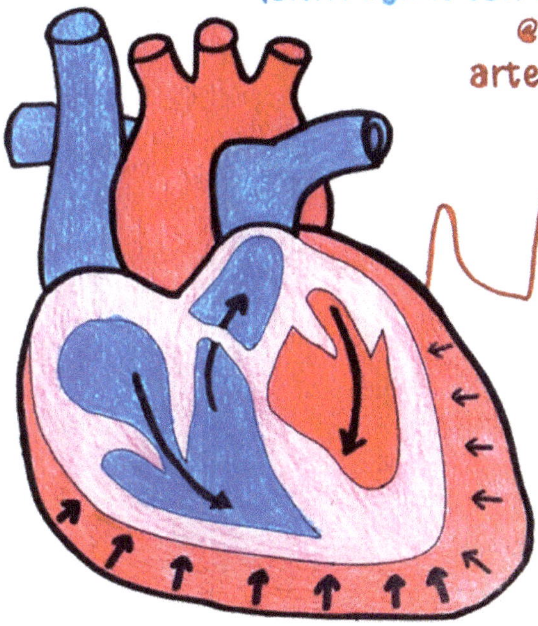

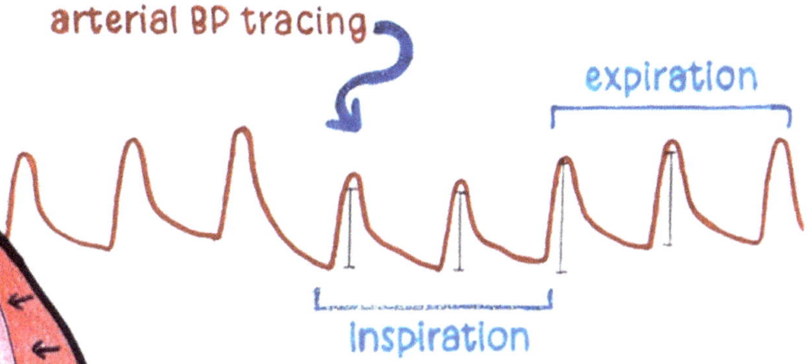

PATHOPHYSIOLOGY

UNDERSTAND THE NORMAL

Normally, arterial blood pressure fluctuates throughout the respiratory cycle: it ↓ s c̄ inspiration & ↑ s c̄ expiration. Inspiration ↓ s the intrathoracic pressure, which creates a pressure gradient that favors venous return (preload) to the right side of the heart and, at the same time, the pulmonary vasculature dilates & holds on to more blood. This generalized pooling of venous blood during inspiration causes a normal physiological ↓ in LV filling that results in an expected drop in systolic blood pressure by no more than 10 mmHg.

...BEFORE YOU UNDERSTAND THE ABNORMAL!

In the setting of cardiac tamponade, fluid accumulates in the pericardial space, ↑ intrapericardial pressure. This pressure limits the ability of the right ventricle to expand & accommodate the ↑ venous return that normally occurs during inspiration. To compensate, the interventricular septum shifts further into the left ventricle, causing compression & impaired LV filling during diastole. This leads to a greater ↓ in the LV diastolic volume (preload) & LV stroke volume (and therefore systolic blood pressure) during inspiration.

ELECTRICAL ALTERNANS

electrical alternans

Beat-to-beat alternations in the amplitude (height) of the QRS complexes that is most often associated c̄ a large pericardial effusion & impending tamponade, although it's rare.

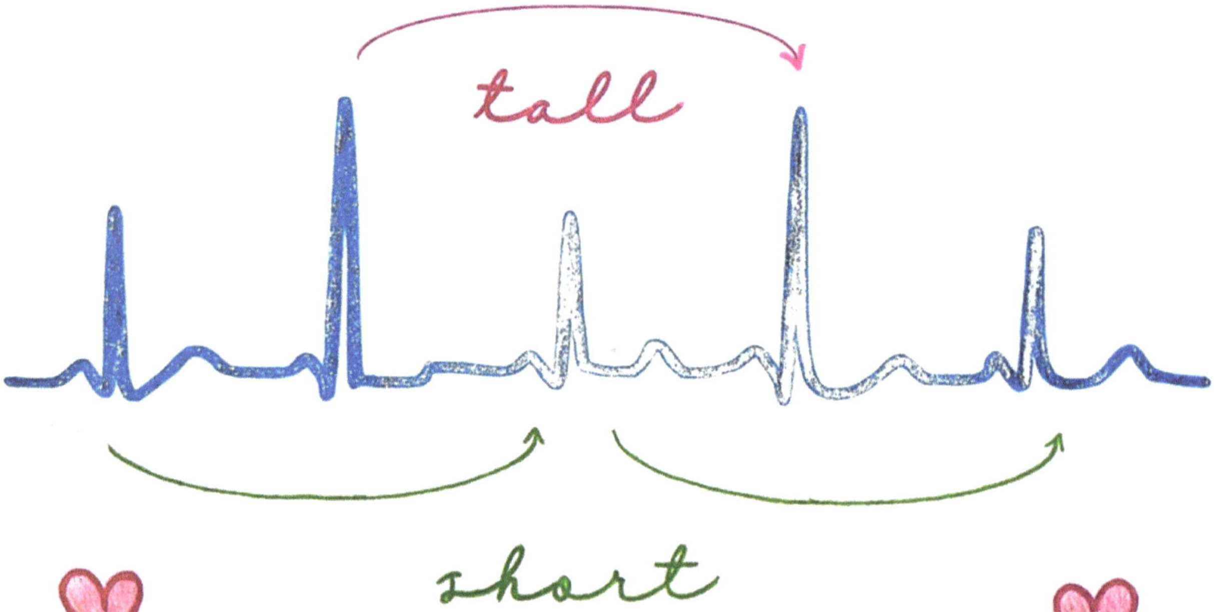

PATHOPHYSIOLOGY

Electrical alternans is thought to be caused by the back-and-forth "swinging" of the heart within the fluid-filled pericardium c̄ each contraction. During some beats, the heart is closer to the anterior chest wall (taller QRS) & at times it is farther (shorter QRS), resulting in a beat-to-beat variation in the QRS amplitude.

@icunursingnotesbycaitlyn

Kussmaul's Sign

A paradoxical ↑ in jugular venous pressure (JVP) during inspiration that often indicates impaired right ventricular filling 2/2 RV dysfunction.

PATHOPHYSIOLOGY:

Normally, inspiration causes a ↓ in intrathoracic pressure which, in turn, enhances the flow of blood from the vena cava into the right atrium (venous return/preload). This causes the JVP to ↓. The walls of the RV can normally expand freely & easily to accommodate the extra volume but, if it can't, then blood is displaced into the SVC & IVC & right atrial pressure (RAP) exceeds the inspiratory ↓ in pleural pressure, causing visible jugular venous distention (JVD) & a subsequent ↑ in JVP during inspiration.

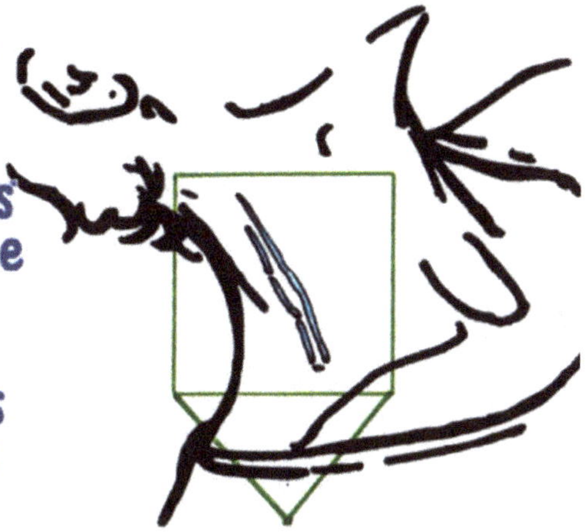

↑JVP & visible JVD during inspiration

♡ ETIOLOGY ♡

Kussmaul's sign is usually caused by ↑venous return (preload) in the setting of a constricted/non-compliant RV.

- RV infarct
- severe heart failure
- restrictive cardiomyopathy
- constrictive pericarditis
- tricuspid stenosis
- cardiac tamponade
- cor pulmonale
- massive PE

@icunursingnotesbycaitlyn

PERICARDIOCENTESIS

A procedure, done either electively or emergently, in which a needle is inserted percutaneously into the pericardial space to drain fluid as treatment for a worsening effusion or tamponade.

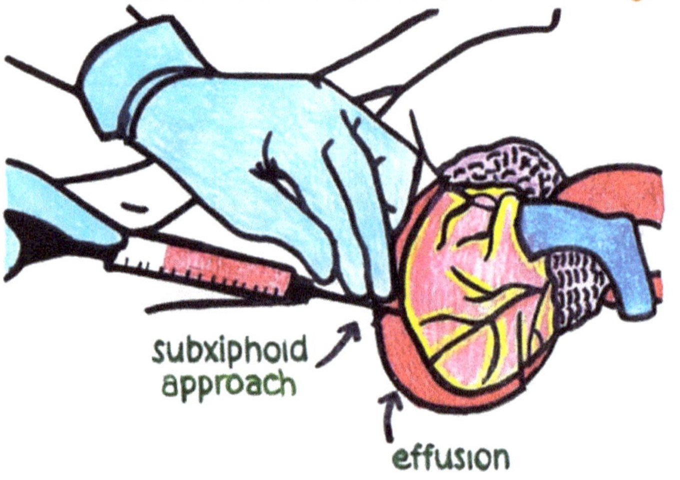

performed under echocardiographic &/or fluoroscopic guidance

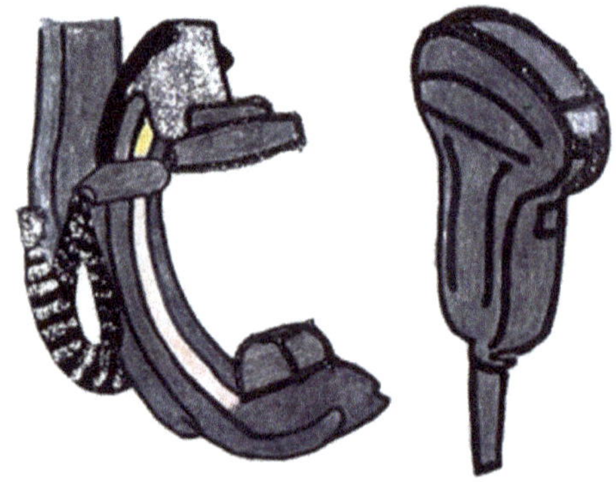

NURSING CONSIDERATIONS:

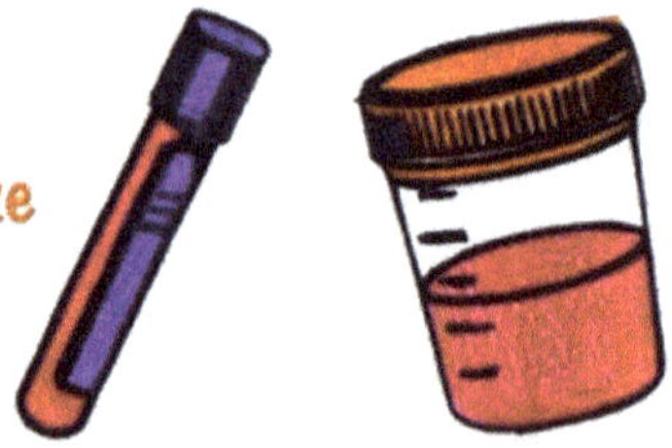

- Position the patient using a wedge to ↓ WOB & to maximize fluid removal.
- Ensure a pre-procedure type & screen has been drawn.
- Treat pain.
- During/after fluid removal, anticipate an improvement in blood pressure (↑), heart rate (↓), & cardiac output, and a ↓ in intracardiac pressures (measured via a Swan-Ganz/PA catheter), & a ↓ in pericardial pressure.
- Monitor for ECG changes (specifically PVCs &/or ST-elevation), as both suggest that the needle is in contact c̄ the epi/myocardium (inserted too far).
- Large volume fluid removal (> 1 L) can precipitate acute LV failure. A pericardial drain typically remains in place for continuous fluid removal.
- Know the complications & be prepared for each: ventricular perforation, pneumothorax, dysrhythmias, etc.
- Samples of pericardial fluid are collected to identify the etiology/cause of the pericardial effusion.

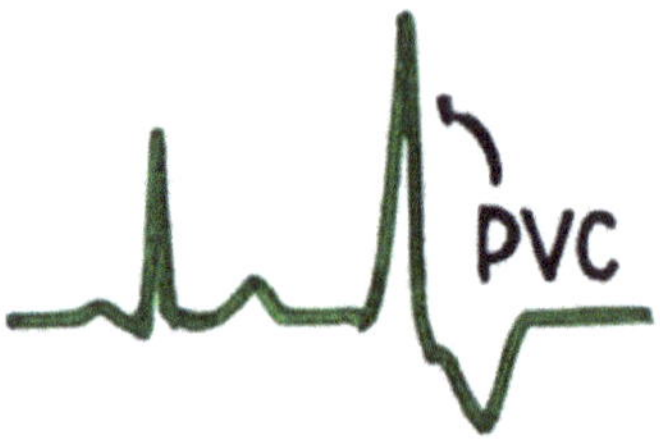

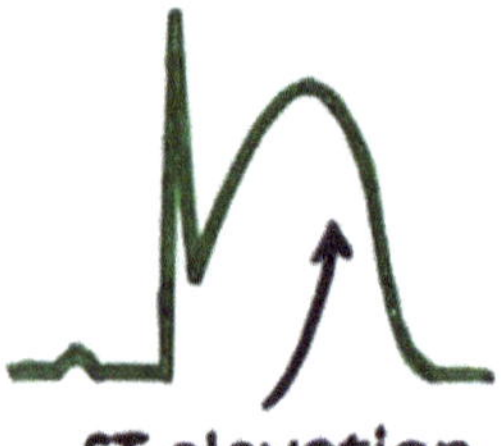

Pericardial Decompression Syndrome

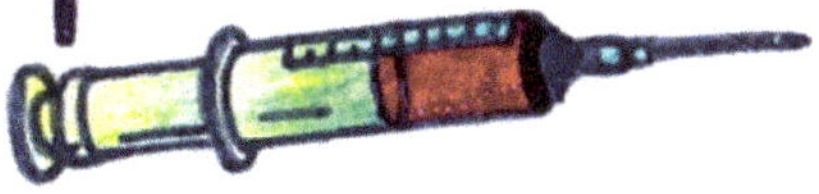

A rare but often fatal complication of a pericardiocentesis characterized by acute hemodynamic instability, pulmonary edema, & cardiogenic shock that develops immediately or up to 48 hours post-procedure.

THE PATHOPHYSIOLOGY: it's not entirely understood!

HEMODYNAMIC SHIFTS

Drainage of pericardial fluid relieves pressure on the RV, leading to a sudden ↑ in the venous return (preload). The RV expands at the expense of the LV and, the ↑ in preload, combined c̄ the residually ↑ afterload/SVR (compensatory response), causes a preload-afterload mismatch that may precipitate LV overload & subsequent failure.

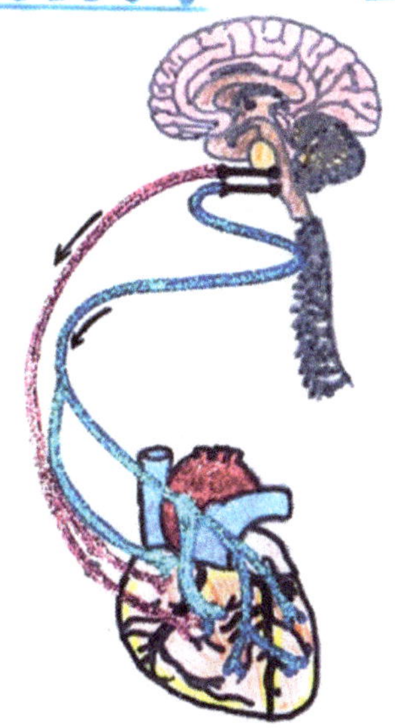

ISCHEMIC Δs

A high intrapericardial pressure ↓s coronary perfusion, which can cause global ischemia that results in transient myocardial stunning that persists after the removal of pericardial fluid, causing transient LV dysfunction.

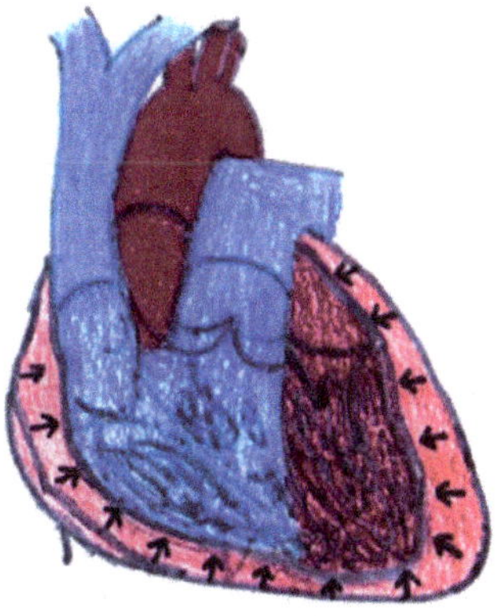

AUTONOMIC IMBALANCE

Removal of the sympathetic stimulus s/p pericardiocentesis reveals pre-existing/underlying myocardial dysfunction that was previously compensated for by high endogenous catecholamine levels (stress response).

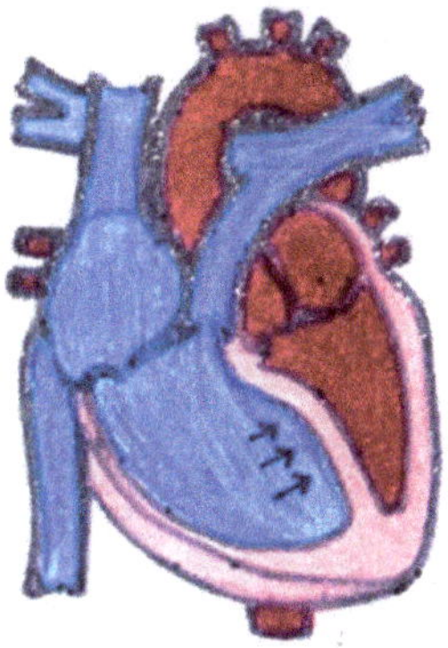

RISK FACTORS:

- malignancy-related effusion
- chronic pericardial effusion
- pulmonary hypertension
- pre-existing RV dysfunction
- rapid removal of a large volume of pericardial fluid
- females

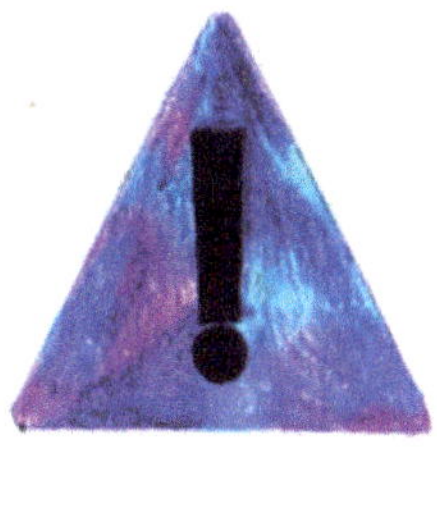

MANAGEMENT:

- mechanical circulatory support (MCS)
- vasopressor support
- + inotropic support (i.e. dobutamine)
- aggressive diuresis

Ejection Fraction

the % of blood ejected from the left ventricle (LV) c̄ each contraction: it's used to measure contractility (the effectiveness of the ♥ as a pump)

$$EF = \frac{\text{stroke volume (SV)}}{\text{end-diastolic volume (EDV)}}$$

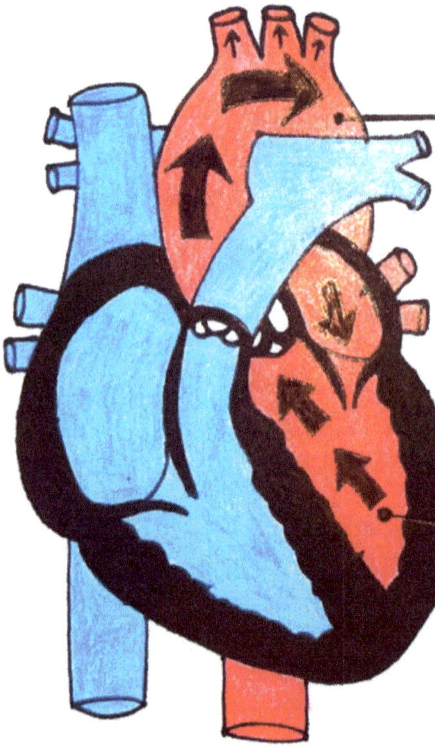

SV — the volume (mL) of blood ejected c̄ each beat; SV = EDV − ESV

÷

EDV — volume (mL) of blood in the LV at end-diastole (ventricular filling)

★ A.K.A. preload!

EF can be measured via an echocardiogram, cardiac cath, cardiac MRI or CT & via a cardiac nuclear medicine scan.

@icunursingnotesbycaitlyn

Classification

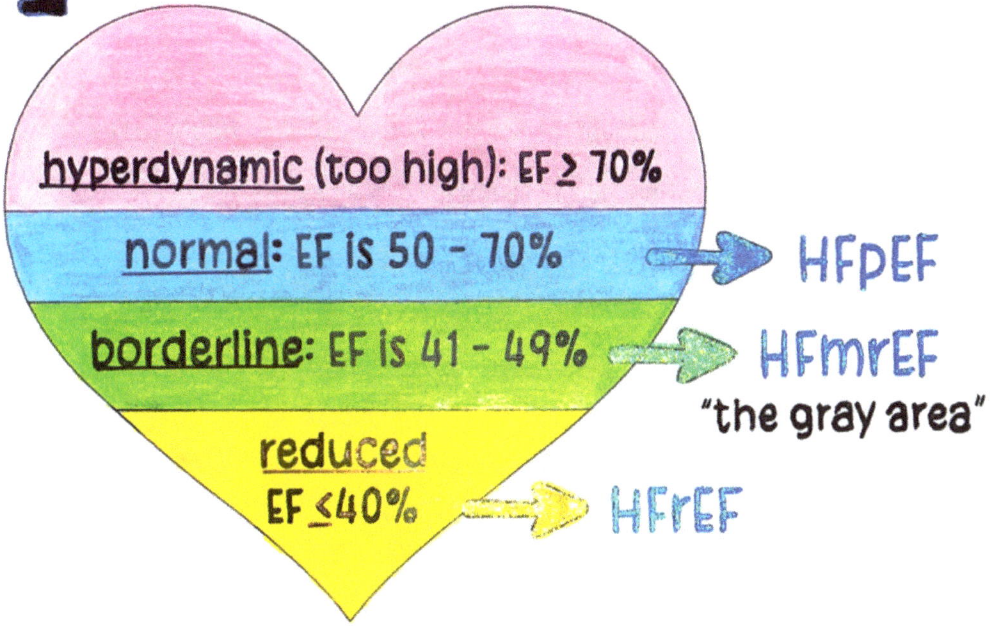

- HFpEF: heart failure c̄ preserved EF
- HFmrEF: heart failure c̄ moderately-reduced EF
- HFrEF: heart failure c̄ reduced EF

* Be on the lookout for upcoming cheat sheets that will go into more detail on each of these! *

A patient can have heart failure and still have a normal EF (HFpEF)! With HFpEF, the problem is diastolic dysfunction. With HFrEF, the problem is systolic dysfunction.

@icunursingnotesbycaitlyn

A patient c̄ a low EF (especially c̄ a PMH of a MI/CAD) may benefit from an ICD because of the ↑ risk for sudden cardiac death (SCD/SCA).

Frank Starling Law

Ventricular contraction is altered by changes in venous return. The greater the stretch of the cardiac muscle (within limits), the greater the resulting contraction.

PATHOPHYSIOLOGY

Heart muscle fibers stretch in response to the increased end-diastolic volume (preload) before contracting. Stretching of the muscle fibers allows the heart to eject the additional volume c̄ ↑ force, thereby ↑ stroke volume (SV). The greater the preload (EDV), the stronger the force of ventricular contraction & the greater the SV, resulting in an increased cardiac output.

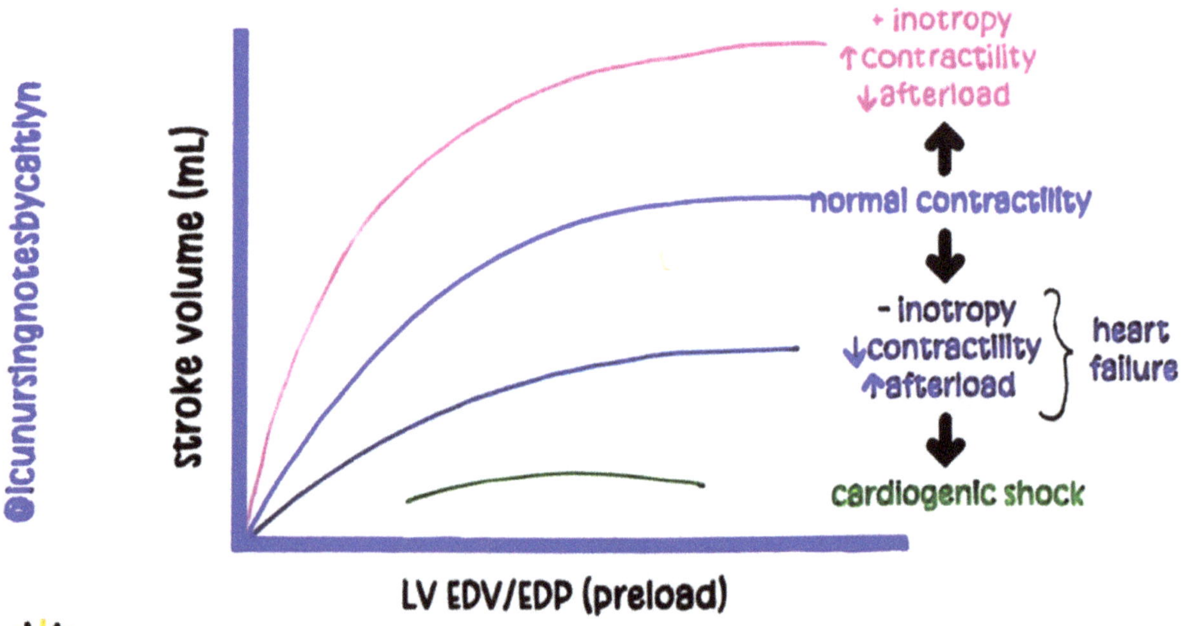

A water balloon is a great visual analogy for the Frank-Starling Law. The more water inside a water balloon, the more the balloon has to stretch. The water inside will create a greater force of ejection (like the heart) when you pop it!

HEART FAILURE

HFrEF

systolic dysfunction

EF < 40%

"pump failure" - a problem c̄ contractility!

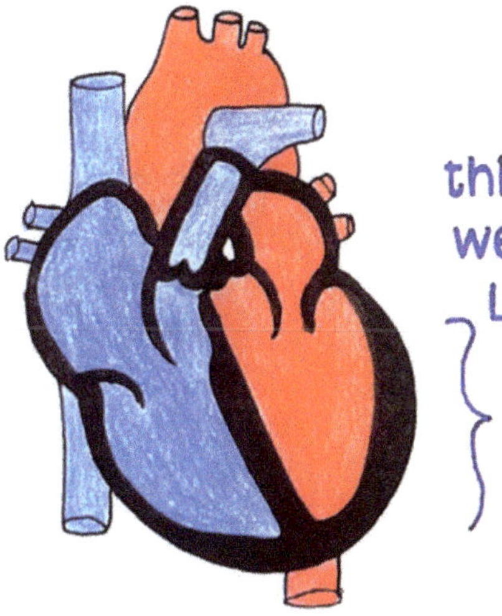

thin & weak LV

HFpEF

diastolic dysfunction

EF > 50%

"filling failure" - a problem c̄ ventricular filling!

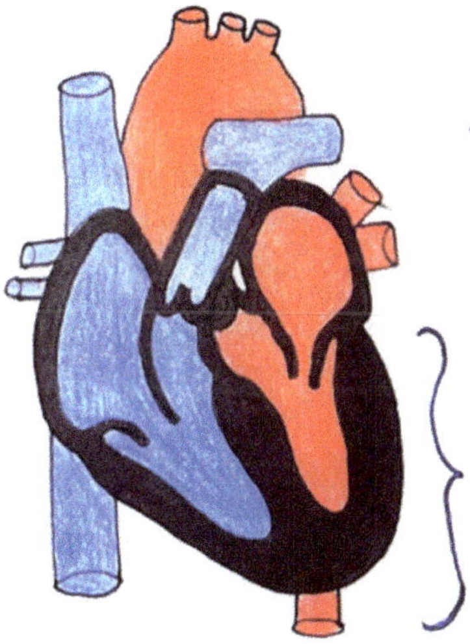

thick & stiff LV

CAUSES

HFrEF:

- *CAD/MI
- *chronic conditions (HTN, DM, etc)
- *valvular ❤ disease
- *cardiomyopathies
- *arrhythmias
- *CHD

HFpEF:

- *myocarditis
- *medications (methamphetamines, antineoplastics, etc)
- *infiltrative diseases (amyloidosis/sarcoidosis)

↑ vs. ↓ Output Heart Failure

High-Output

high demand c̄ a high output (CO > 8 L/min) & a low SVR

Low-Output

normal demand c̄ a low output & a high SVR

- HFrEF
- HFpEF

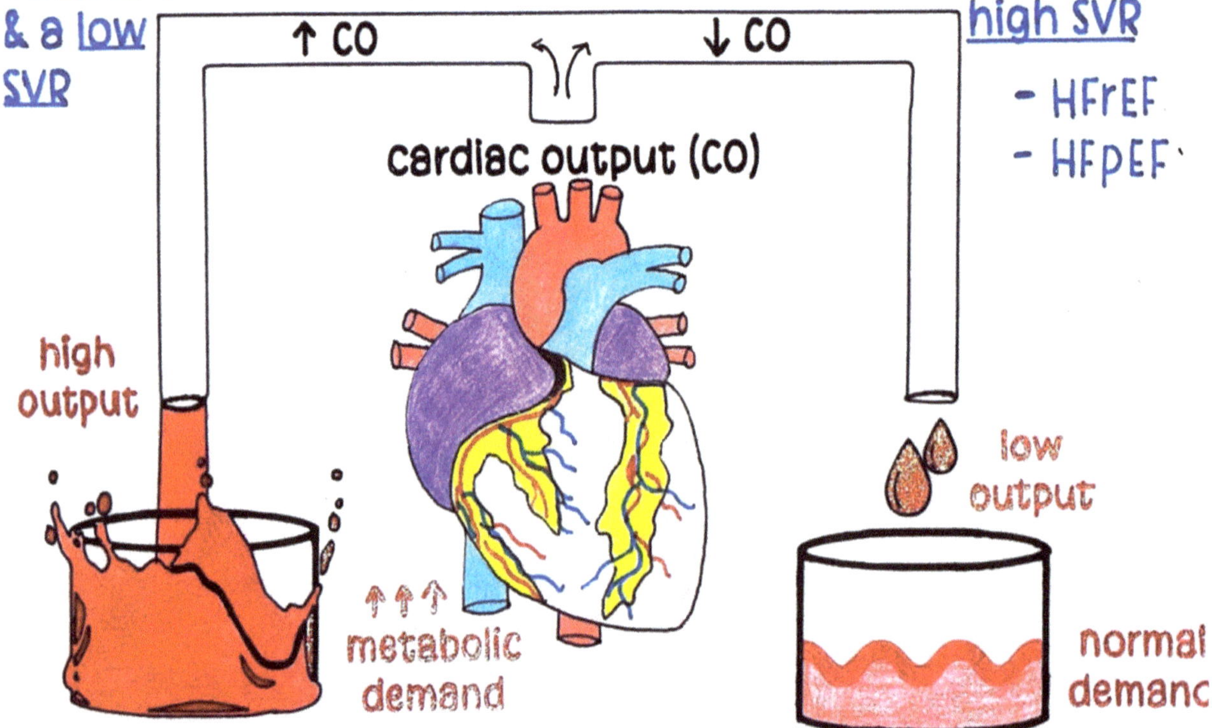

Causes:

- severe anemia
- thyrotoxicosis
- sepsis*
- AV fistula c̄ shunting
- beriberi
- Paget's disease
- pregnancy
- multiple myeloma

Causes:

- CAD
- HTN
- cardiomyopathies
- valvular disease
- idiopathic

@icunursingnotesbycaitlyn

Acute Decompensated Heart Failure

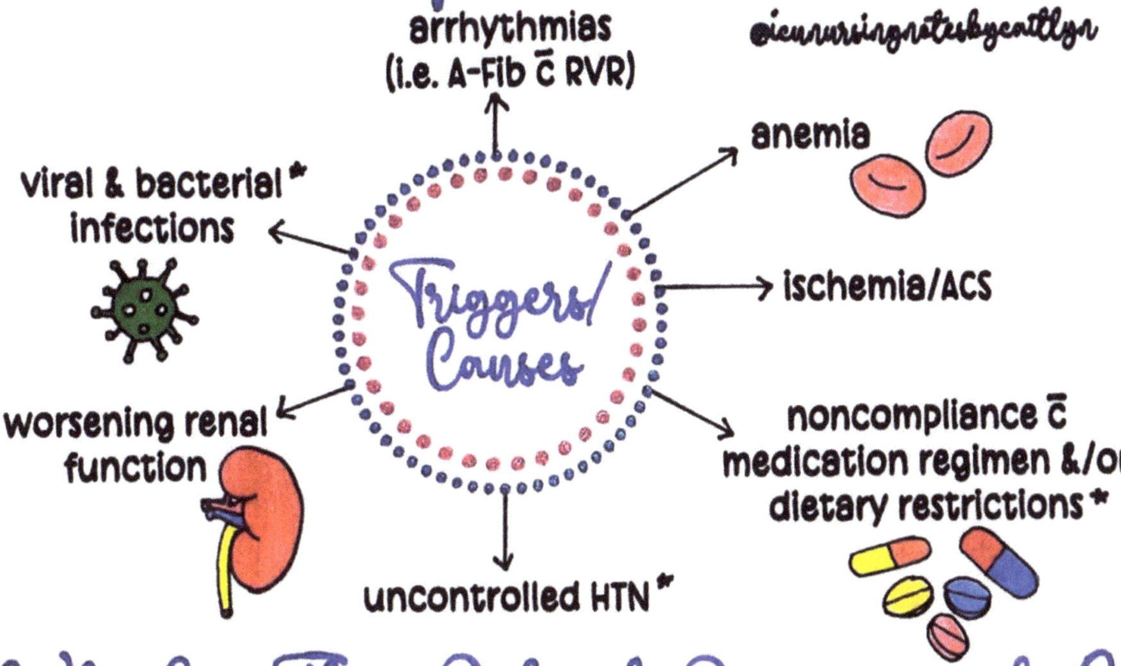

Why Can These Patients Decompensate So Quickly?

Treatment of ADHF focuses on interrupting this downward spiral!

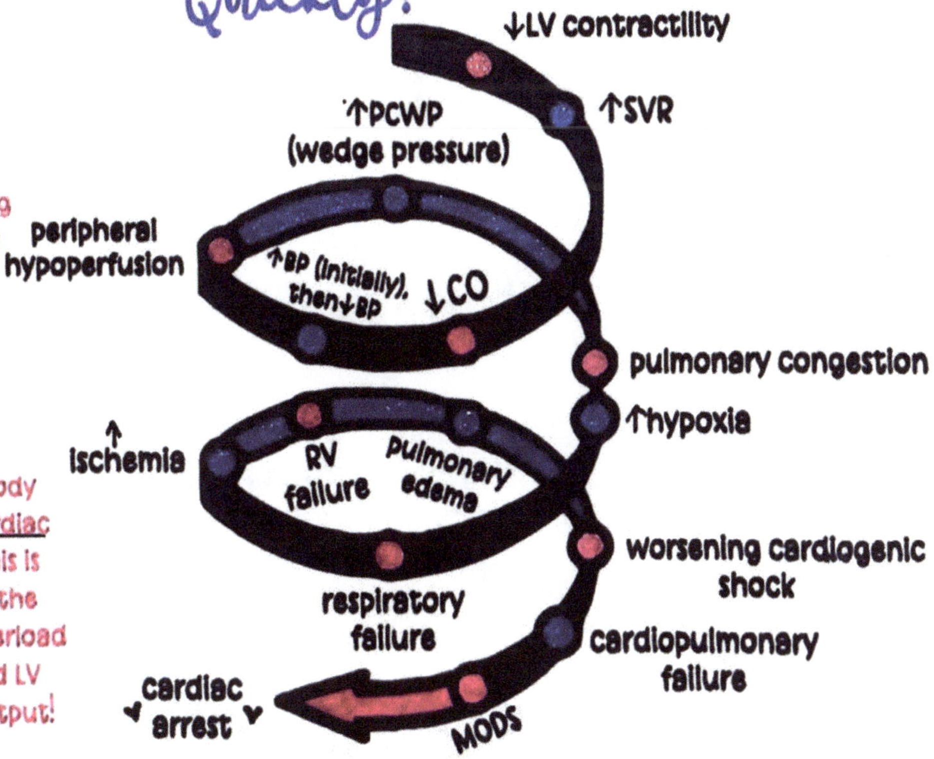

Remember that the body compensates for a ↓cardiac output by ↑SVR, but this is counterproductive in the setting of ADHF. ↑the afterload for an already impaired LV will further ↓cardiac output!

Acute Decompensated Heart Failure

@icunursingnotesbycaitlyn

well-perfused s̄ congestion

"compensated"

"warm & dry"

- PO medication management

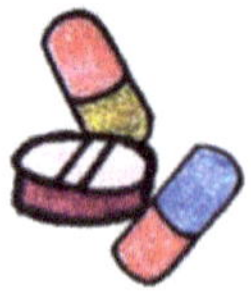

well-perfused c̄ congestion

"pulmonary edema"

"warm & wet"

- NIPPV (i.e. BIPAP)
- IV vasodilator
  - NTG
  - Natrecor
- IV diuretics
  - Lasix
  - Bumex
  - Diuril

hypoperfusion s̄ congestion

"hypovolemic"/ "overdiuresed"

"cold & dry"

- fluid challenge &/or
- + inotrope
  - dobutamine
  - milrinone

hypoperfusion & congestion

"cardiogenic shock"

"cold & wet"

- mechanical ventilation
- + inotrope
- vasopressors
- IV diuretics/CRRT
- MCS (IABP, Impella, ECMO, LVAD)

Remember that ♥ failure & renal dysfunction often coexist! ADHF ↑s a patient's risk for worsening renal function & diuretic resistance (the fancy term for this is "cardiorenal syndrome")!

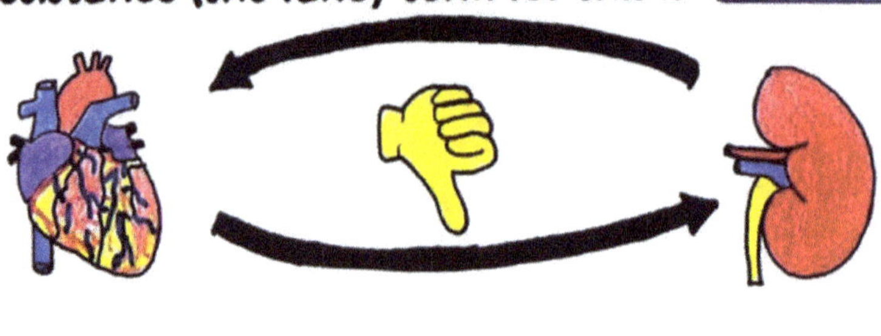

Nursing Care

- Strict hourly I&O (don't forget to include IV gtts in the hourly intake!), daily weights, & frequent assessment of volume status.
- Know your patient's IV diuresis goal (typically, net negative 1 to 2 L in 24 hrs).
- Monitor labs (CBC, Cr/BUN, ABG/VBG, BNP/NT-proBNP, LFTs, electrolytes, etc).
- Try to identify & treat the cause of the CHF exacerbation.
- Focused cardiac & pulmonary assessments!
- Invasive hemodynamic monitoring (i.e. art line &/or Swan-Ganz catheter) is helpful, but don't forget that your assessment is just as important ("treat the patient, not the monitor").
- If your patient has a PA line/Swan, monitor & trend hemodynamics. Is the patient responding well to treatment?
- Avoid calcium channel & beta-blockers in decompensated HF.
- Anticipate holding a patient's ACE-I/ARB c̄ worsening renal function.
- Care & maintenance of mechanical circulatory support devices (i.e. IABP, Impella, etc) & CRRT for severe cases of ADHF/cardiogenic shock - see my previous cheat sheets for more info on these!
- Foley & central line care & maintenance, oral care for intubated patient DVT/PUD prophylaxis, PI prevention, etc.
- Consider if your patient & his/her family would benefit from palliative care (remind your patient that this is different from hospice!!).
- Goals of care conversations

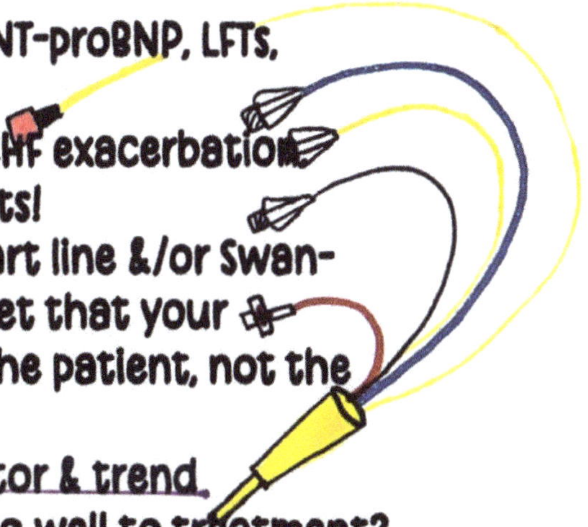

@icunursingnotesbycaitlyn

While an IV nitrate (i.e. NTG) may be used for preload & afterload reduction, you wouldn't want to give this to a patient who is preload-dependent (i.e. aortic stenosis/AS, HOCM, inferior MI c̄ RV involvement, etc)!

Hypertrophic Obstructive Cardiomyopathy (HOCM)

A genetic condition in which asymmetrical septal hypertrophy & systolic anterior motion (SAM) of the mitral valve obstruct the left ventricular outflow tract (LVOT), impeding blood flow to the body.

PATHOPHYSIOLOGY

Thickening (hypertrophy) of the interventricular septum (IVS) causes narrowing of the left ventricular outflow tract (LVOT). Systolic anterior motion (SAM) of the mitral valve occurs when the mitral valve leaflets move toward the septum during systole, resulting in a dynamic LVOT obstruction & mitral regurgitation. Diastolic dysfunction occurs 2/2 a stiff & non-compliant LV, leading to ↑ LV filling & pulmonary venous pressures!

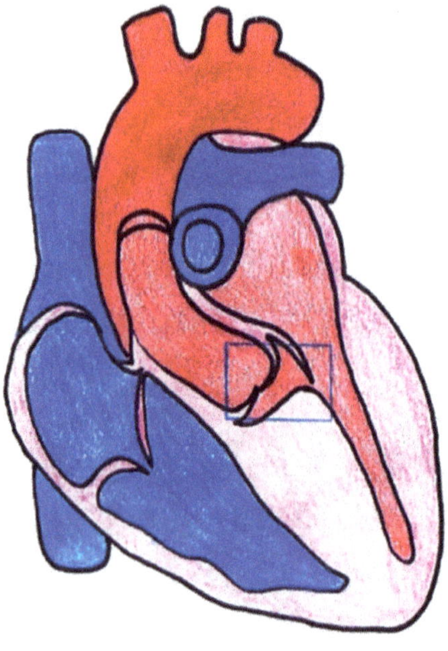

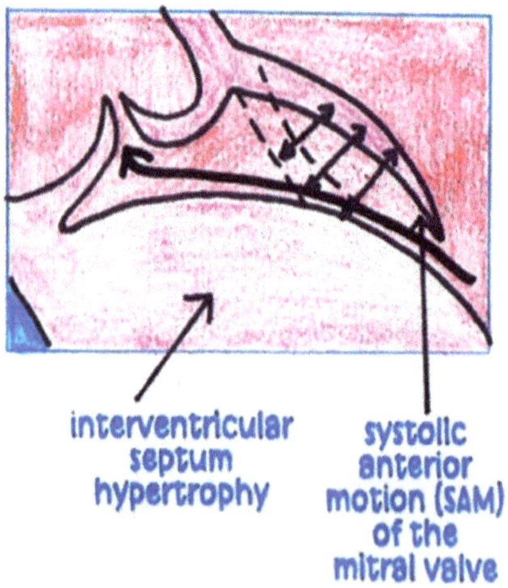

@icunursingnotesbycaitlyn

Hypertrophic Obstructive Cardiomyopathy

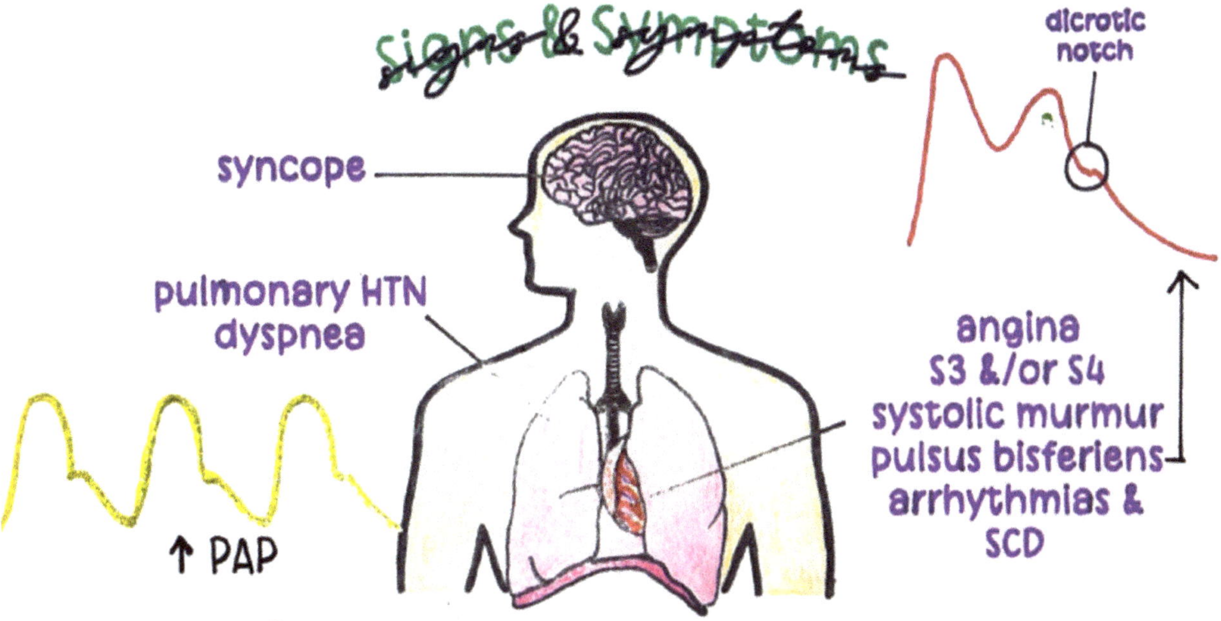

The DOs & DON'Ts of HOCM Management

- beta blockers
- verapamil & diltiazem (CCBs)
- disopyramide (Norpace)
  - ↳ adjunct to BB & CCBs
- IV fluids + phenylephrine/Neo
  - ↳ (cardiogenic shock c̄ HOCM)
- ICD for SCD prevention
- dual-chamber pacing
- septal myectomy
- alcohol septal ablation
- heart transplant

- + inotropes
- cardiac glycosides (Digoxin)
- ACE inhibitors & ARBs
- nifedipine (Procardia)
- vasodilators & nitrates
- high-dose diuretics
- mechanical circulatory support devices

@icunursingnotesbycaitlyn

Brockenbrough Braunwald Morrow Sign

@icunursingnotesbycaitlyn

A ↓ in pulse pressure after a PVC due to ↑ outflow obstruction produced by ↑ contractility of the post-PVC beat in patients c̄ hypertrophic obstructive cardiomyopathy (HOCM).

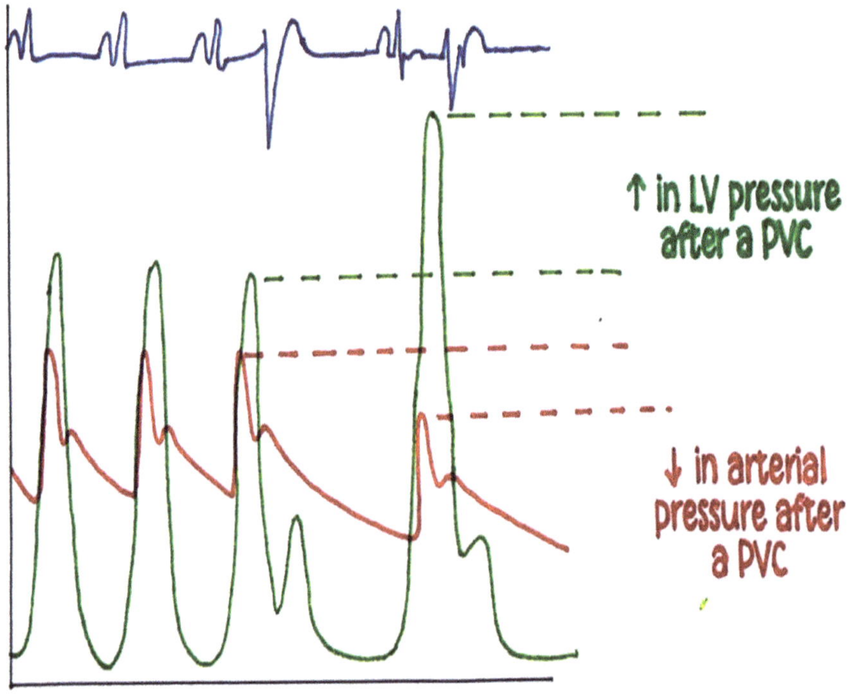

Physiology!

Normally, a premature ventricular contraction (PVC) results in a compensatory pause, ↑ventricular filling & ↑contractility. In patients c̄ HOCM, the post-PVC beat worsens the LVOT obstruction 2/2 ↑ contractility. This ↑ s the LV systolic pressure & the systolic gradient, but it ↓ s aortic systolic pressure, narrowing the pulse pressure.

Systolic Anterior Motion of the Mitral Valve

@xcunursingnotesbycaitlyn

Displacement of the anterior mitral valve leaflet towards the left ventricular outflow tract (LVOT) & interventricular septum during systole, resulting in a transient LVOT obstruction & mitral regurgitation (MR)

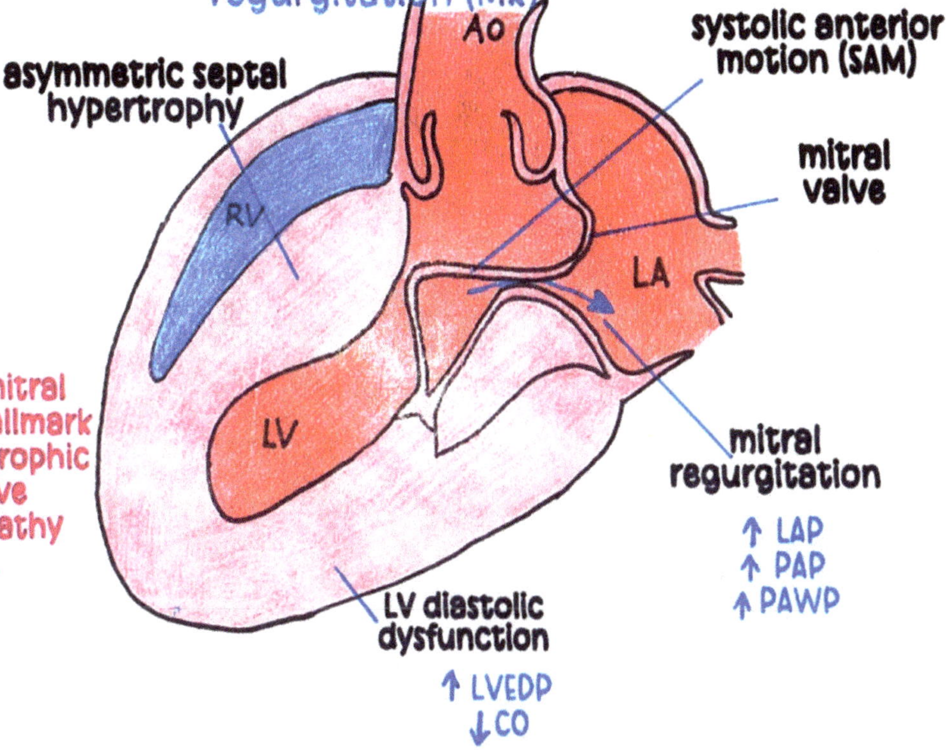

SAM of the mitral valve is the hallmark sign of hypertrophic obstructive cardiomyopathy (HOCM).

HEMODYNAMIC GOALS IN SAM

↑ preload	↓ contractility
↑ afterload	maintain NSR

CORONARY ARTERY DISSECTION

coronary artery dissection

A split or tear in the tunica intima layer of one of the coronary arteries; depending on the severity of the dissection, it can also involve the artery's medial layer.

The tear creates a false lumen between the vessel walls, leading to the formation of a hematoma. The ↑ pressure of the false lumen by an enlarging hematoma causes compression of the true coronary lumen, resulting in ↓ coronary blood flow. Depending on severity, a coronary dissection can lead to abrupt vessel closure, MI, side branch closure, & cardiac tamponade.

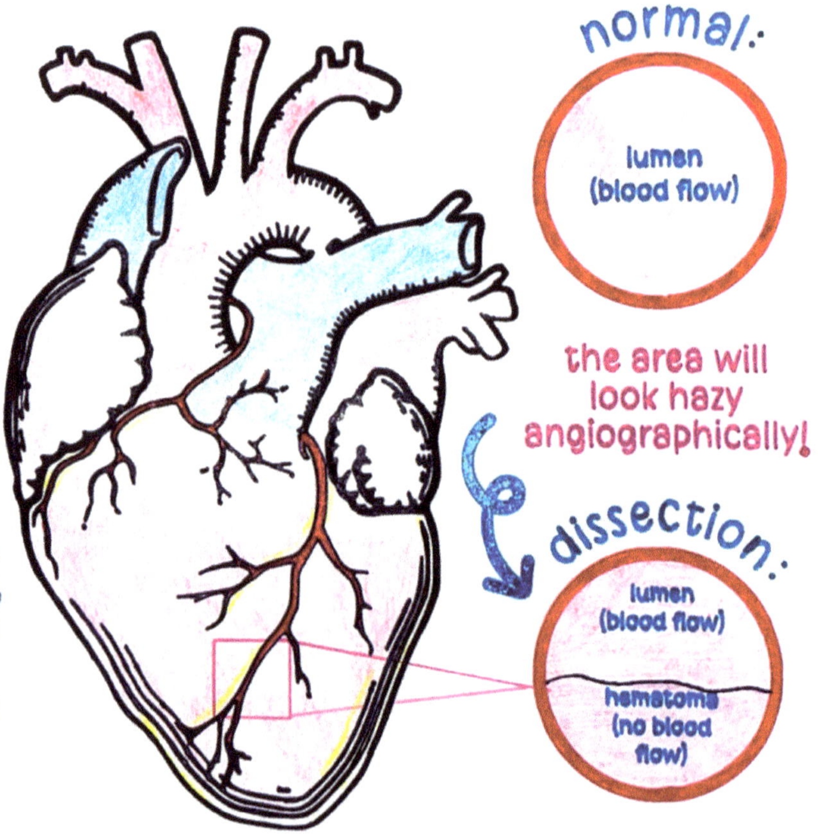

CAUSES:

- spontaneous (SCAD)
- contrast injection c̄ dampened pressure
- oversized balloon/stent & ↑ inflation pressures
- catheter, wire, ballon, & stent manipulation

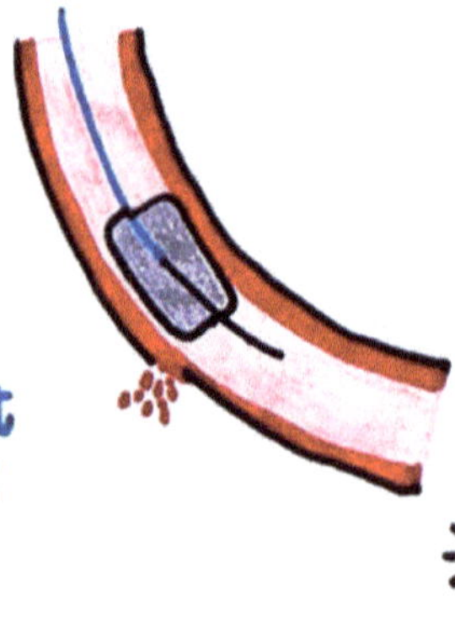

TREATMENT:

- additional stenting (PCI)
- emergent CABG (if an extensive dissection is not treatable c̄ stents)

It's critical to achieve adequate BP control in these patients!

Spontaneous Coronary Artery Dissection (SCAD)

The leading cause of acute coronary syndrome (ACS) in women ≤50 years-old who have no apparent risk factors for coronary artery disease (CAD).

@icunursingnotesbycaitlyn

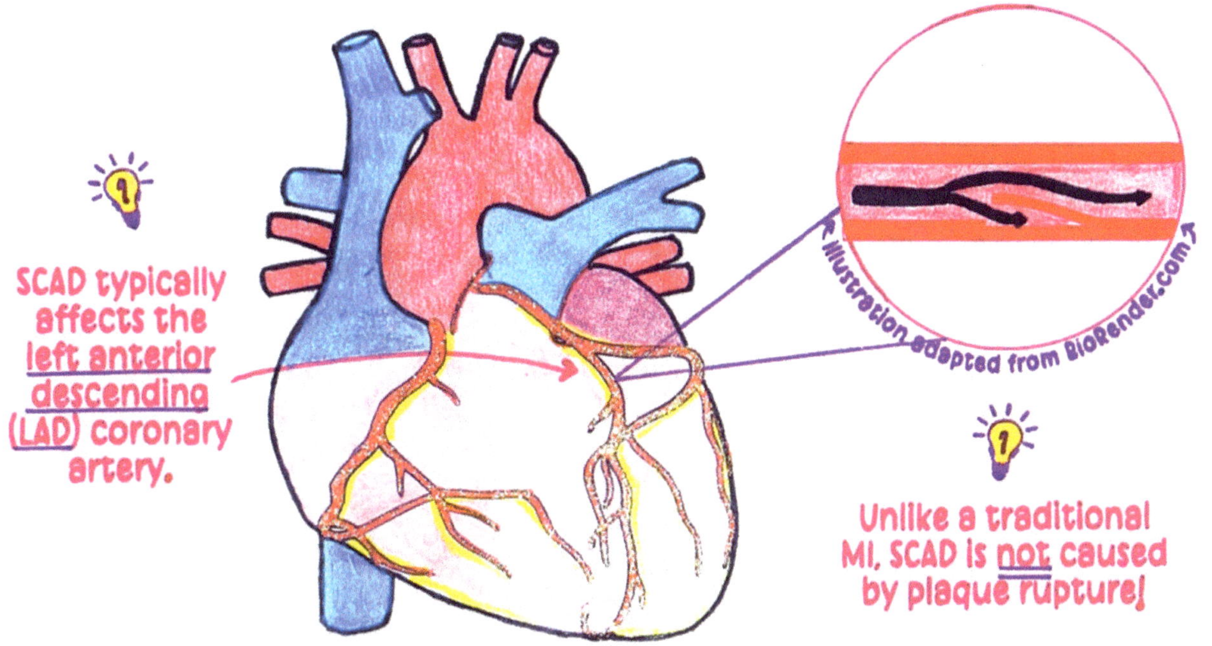

Pathophysiology:

When a coronary artery spontaneously dissects, its inner layers split apart. Blood continues to flow, but it travels in between these layers, creating a "false lumen." This new "pathway" (false lumen) compresses the true arterial lumen, reducing or completely obstructing blood flow to the heart muscle. This leads to myocardial ischemia (partial obstruction) or infarction (complete obstruction)!

Risk Factors:

- pregnancy
- emotional stress
- anorexia nervosa
- connective tissue disorders
- fibromuscular dysplasia
- autoimmune disorders
- hypertension

Treatment:

- conservative management (ASA, beta blocker, & BP control)
- PCI is typically only done in the setting of hemodynamic instability, left main dissection, ongoing ischemia, &/or sustained ventricular arrhythmias

LEFT MAIN DISEASE

The highest-risk subset of ischemic heart disease that occurs when there is ≥ 50% stenosis (narrowing) of the left main coronary artery (LMCA).

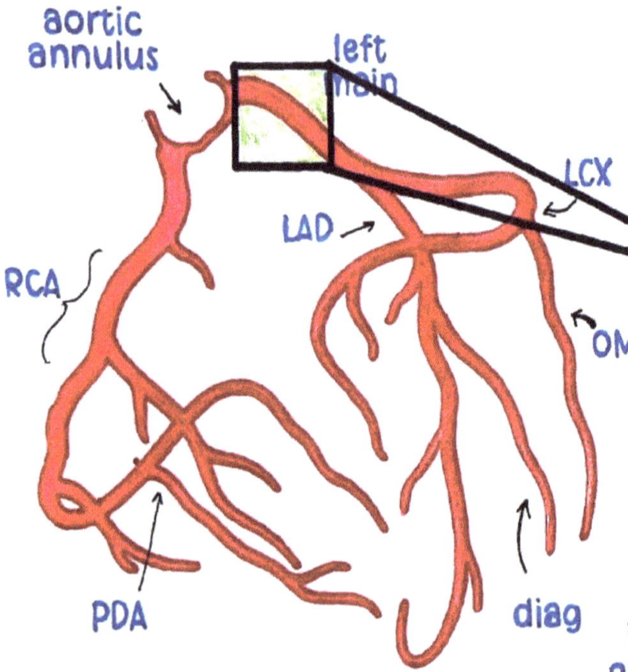

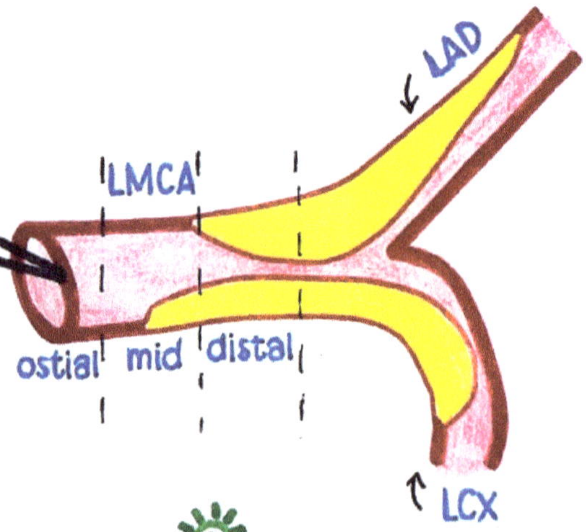

The LMCA usually bifurcates into the LAD & the LCX, but in ≈ 20 of patients, the LM trifurcates into the LAD, LCX, & the ramus intermedius.

Depending on coronary dominance, the LMCA supplies blood to ≈ 75-100% of the heart muscle; this is why LM disease is associated c̄ ↑ morbidity & mortality!

MANAGEMENT:

REVASCULARIZATION!

- coronary artery bypass grafting
- high-risk PCI (non-surgical candidates)

\+

- medication management (beta blockers, statins, DAPT, & ACE-I/ARBS)

Coronary In Stent Restenosis (ISR)

Re-narrowing of a previously stented coronary artery segment due to an abnormal healing response to angioplasty-induced arterial wall injury (neointimal hyperplasia).

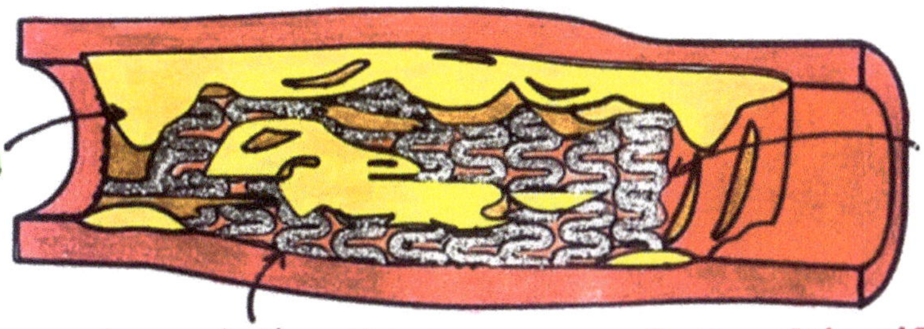

Pathophysiology

ISR is caused by neointimal hyperplasia – a phenomenon in which scar tissue overgrows within the stent, & causes re-narrowing of the arterial lumen. Various inflammatory mediators & growth factors stimulate uncontrolled vascular smooth muscle cell proliferation & extracellular matrix production within the inner layer of the artery, leading to in-stent luminal narrowing 3-6 months s/p PCI.

Treatment

- aggressive GDMT
- repeat PCI
- drug-coated balloon (DCB)
- cutting/scoring balloons
- laser atherectomy
- vascular brachytherapy

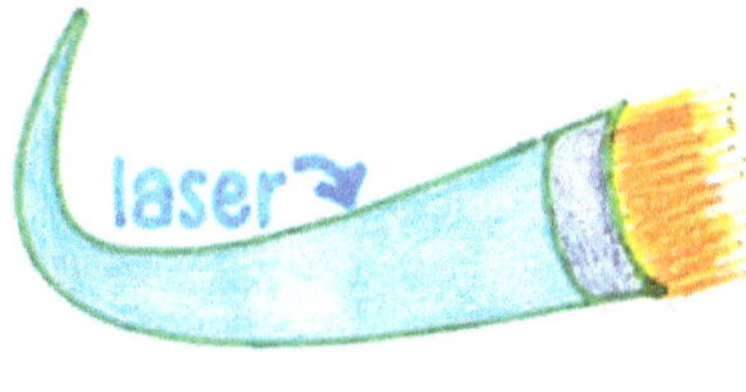

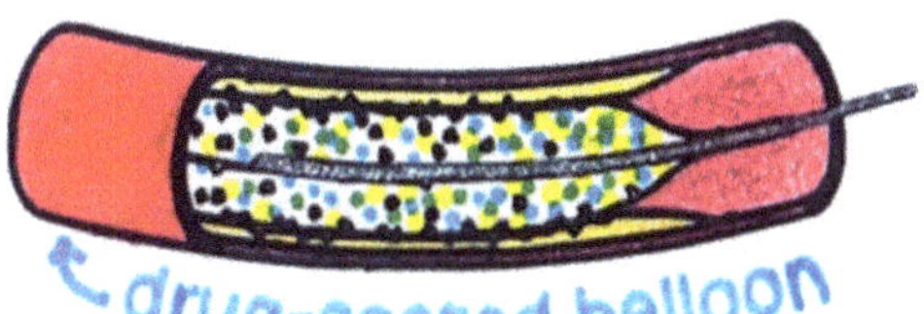

Images from Mind the Graph.

Risk Factors

- bifurcation lesion
- complex lesion
- ostial lesion
- stent underexpansion
- longer stent length
- non-compliance c̄ DAPT
- Plavix non-responder
- small vessel lumen
- DM, CKD & HTN
- previous CABG
- older & female

@icunursingnotesbycaitlyn

AGENT™ DRUG-COATED BALLOON

The first FDA-approved drug-coated coronary balloon in the US for the treatment of coronary in-stent restenosis (ISR).

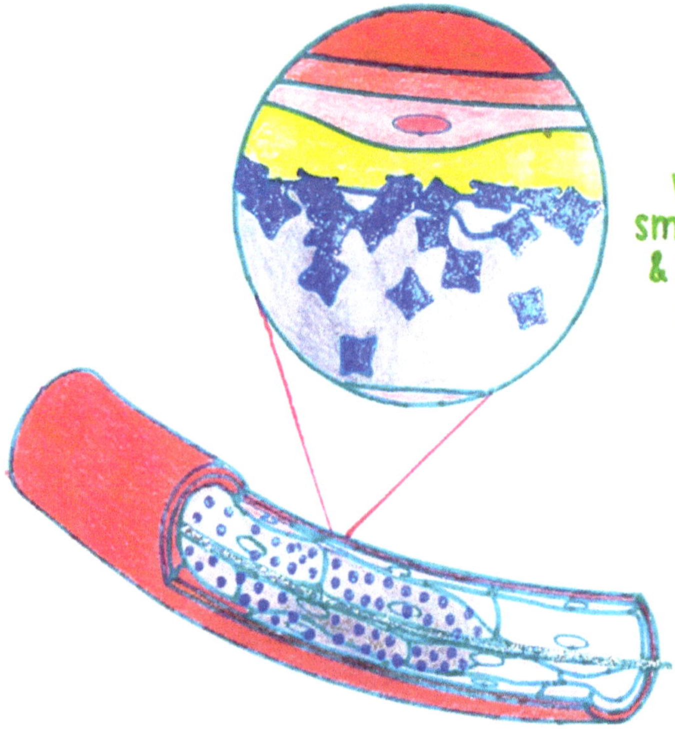

The balloon is coated c̄ low-dose paclitaxel (an antiproliferative agent), which inhibits the excessive smooth muscle cell proliferation & migration (neointimal hyperplasia) that contributes to coronary ISR.

DCBs serve as an alternative to traditional treatments for ISR like additional layers of stenting, brachytherapy, & laser!

Once the balloon is inflated, paclitaxel is released & is transferred to the arterial wall. To ensure adequate drug delivery, lesion preparation (i.e. calcium modification c̄ IVL, cutting/scoring ballons, etc) is key to ensure adequate drug delivery!

Shockwave (intravascular lithotripsy)

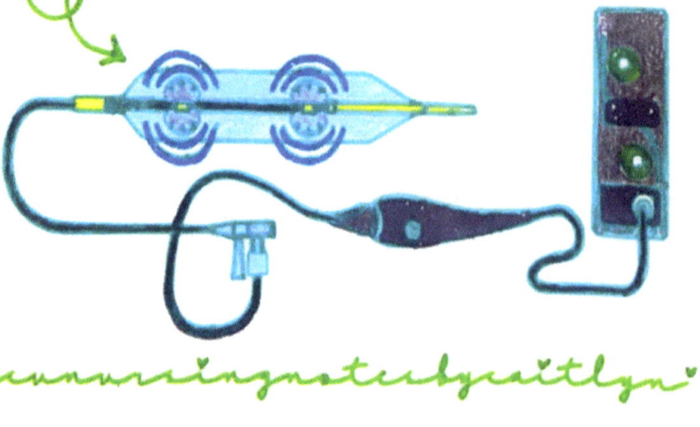

SHOCKWAVE

(coronary intravascular lithotripsy)

A new technique used as an alternative to an atherectomy to treat severely calcified coronary lesions requiring stenting.

How Does It Work?

Intravascular lithotripsy (IVL) of a coronary artery is performed through a cardiac catheterization. It involves threading a catheter over a guidewire via the radial or femoral artery to the location of the calcified coronary lesion. Once the catheter's balloon is positioned across the lesion, it generates a series of pulsatile sonic pressure waves ("shockwaves") that help crack & break up the calcified plaque. Once the calcium is successfully cracked, the artery can be expanded at low pressure & a stent can then be placed to improve blood flow to the ♥ muscle (myocardium).

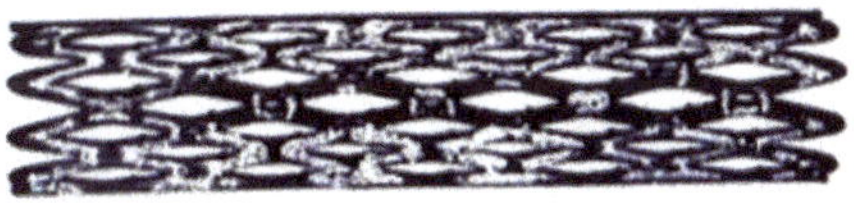

drug-eluting stent

Pay attention to the aortic (Ao) pressure waveform & ECG tracing.

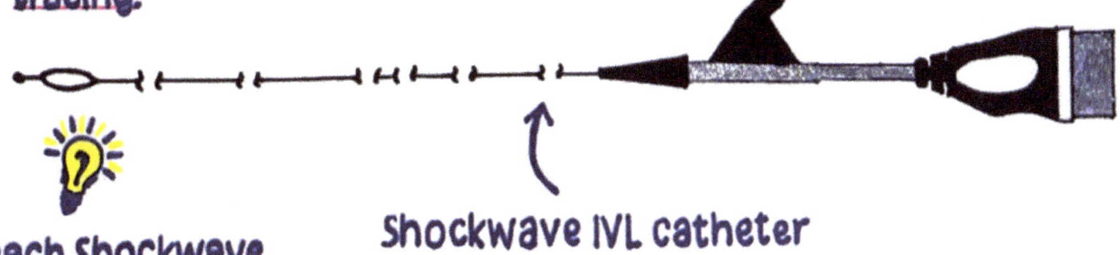

Shockwave IVL catheter

With each Shockwave cycle, you may see electrical signals that mimic pacing spikes on the ECG tracing! This is expected!

@icunursingnotesbycaitlyn

Coronary Microvascular Dysfunction

Structural & functional alterations in the coronary microcirculation that lead to impaired coronary blood flow, myocardial ischemia, & angina, despite patent epicardial coronary arteries (American College of Cardiology, 2022).

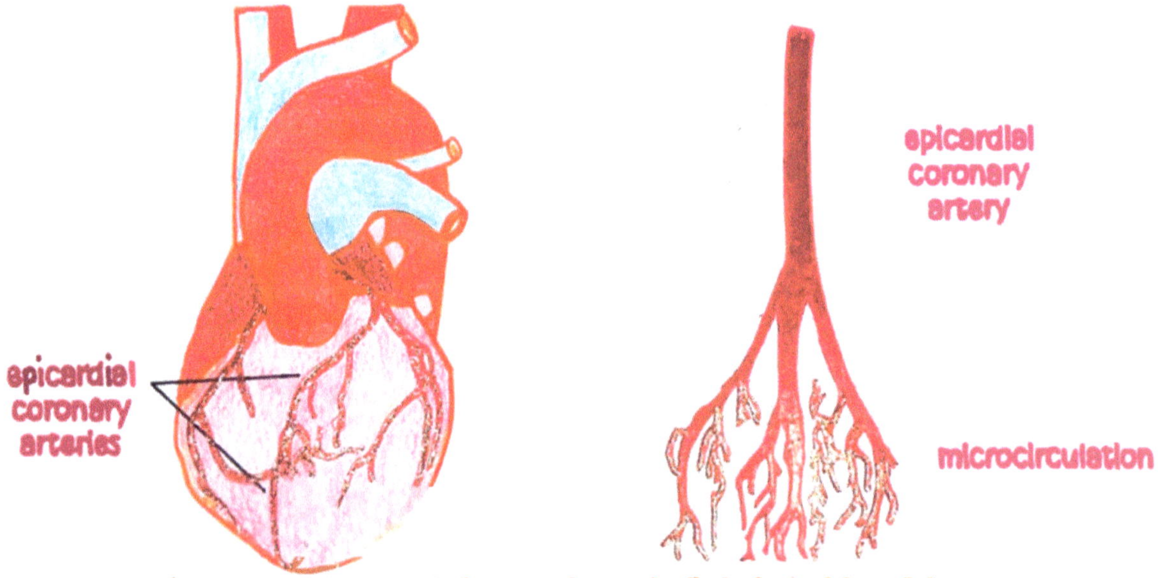

Illustration adapted from: Lynch, P.J. & Jaffe, C.C. Drawing coronary arteries & circulation of the heart. Creative Commons

The Pathophysiology

The coronary microcirculation can develop a number of structural & functional changes, particularly in patients c̄ pre-existing cardiovascular risk factors, that limit the ability of the microvasculature to adapt to changes in myocardial oxygen demand, leading to regional ischemia. The pathophysiology is complex, but endothelial dysfunction, ↑ sympathetic tone, insulin resistance, vascular remodeling, inflammation, & estrogen deficiency in women are believed to play a role in coronary microvascular dysfunction.

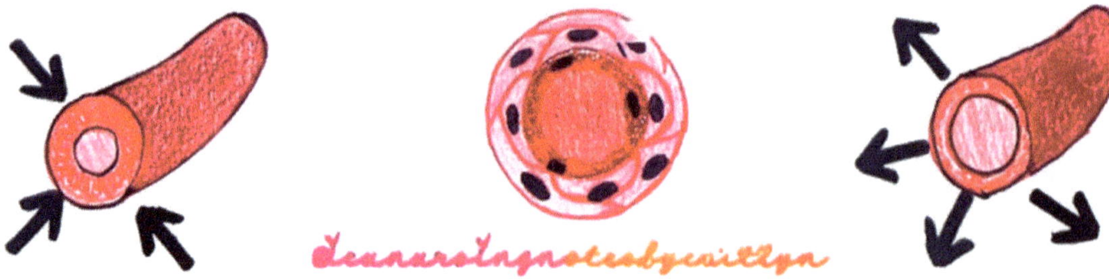

@icunursingnotesbycaitlyn

CORONARY MICROVASCULAR DISEASE:

PART II

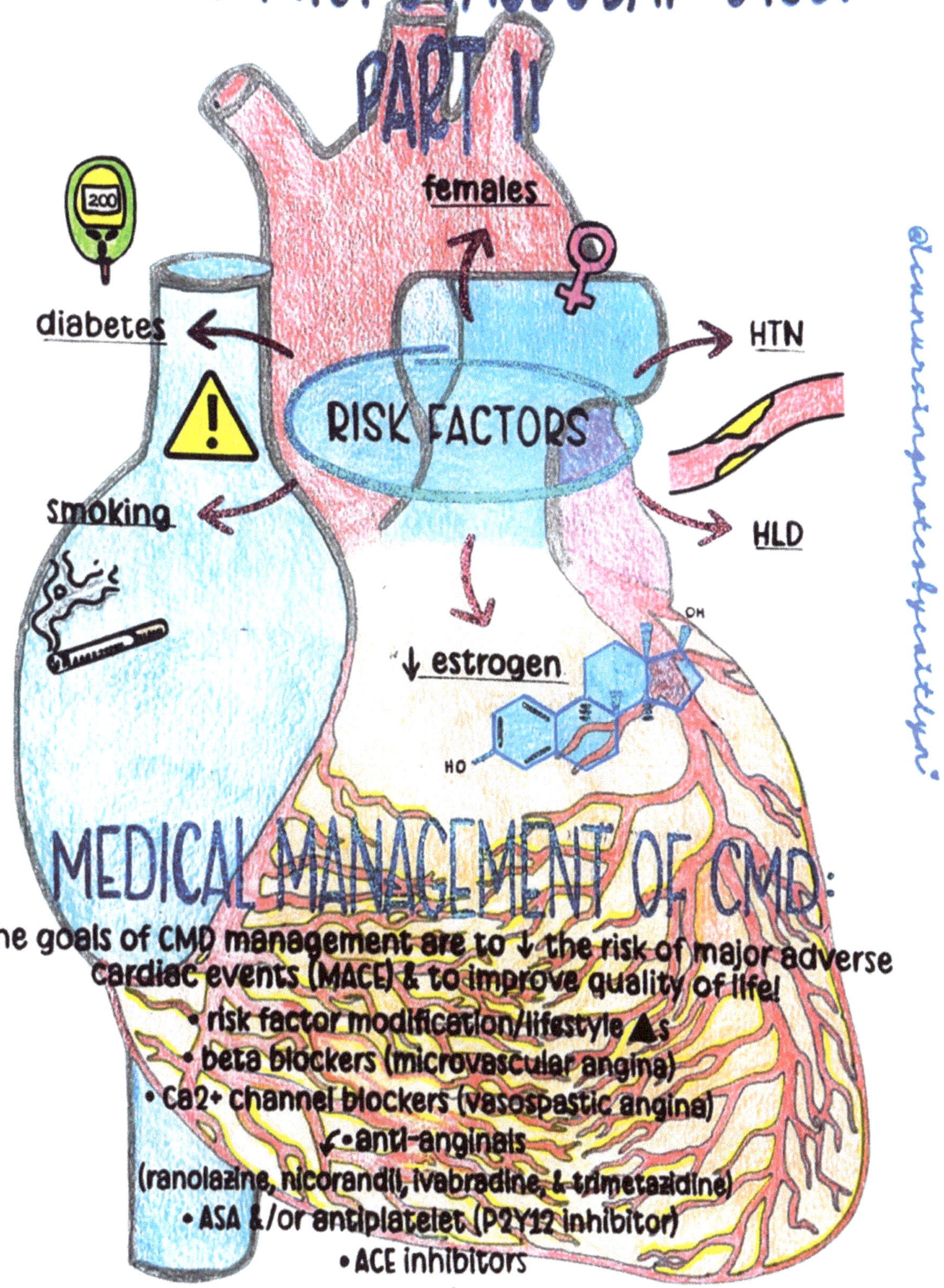

MEDICAL MANAGEMENT OF CMD:

the goals of CMD management are to ↓ the risk of major adverse cardiac events (MACE) & to improve quality of life!

- risk factor modification/lifestyle ▲s
- beta blockers (microvascular angina)
- Ca2+ channel blockers (vasospastic angina)
- anti-anginals (ranolazine, nicorandil, ivabradine, & trimetazidine)
- ASA &/or antiplatelet (P2Y12 inhibitor)
- ACE inhibitors
- statins

MINOCA

(MYOCARDIAL INFARCTION C̄ NON-OBSTRUCTIVE CORONARY ARTERIES)

An umbrella term used to classify patients who present c̄ clinical evidence of a MI (ischemic ECG changes, + troponin, new RWMA, etc), but who are found to have angiographically normal/near-normal coronary arteries.

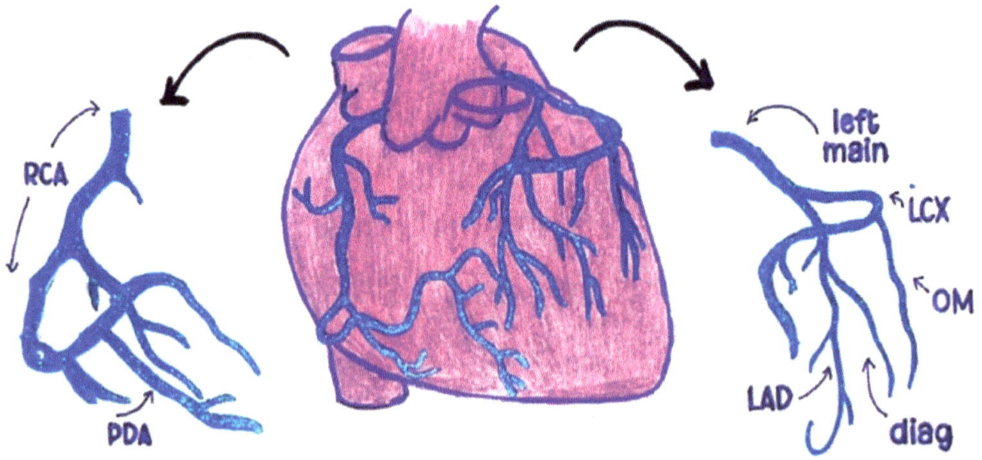

Etiology & Pathophysiology

Typical MIs are caused by a culprit lesion - an overt blockage that obstructs blood flow & oxygen delivery to the myocardium 2/2 thrombus formation inside an epicardial coronary artery. Although the pathophysiology of MINOCA isn't entirely understood, myocardial ischemia, in the absence of a coronary blockage, is attributable to epicardial & microvascular mechanisms.

Epicardial Causes

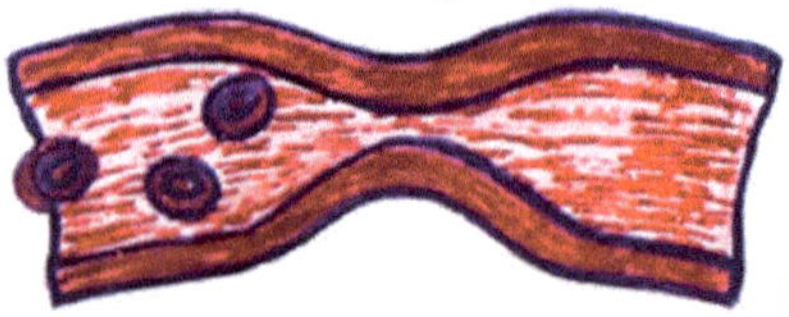

- plaque erosion/rupture
- spontaneous coronary artery dissection (SCAD)
- coronary artery spasm
- coronary thromboembolism
- myocardial bridging

Microvascular Causes

- coronary microvascular dysfunction (CMD)
- Takotsubo/stress-induced cardiomyopathy
- viral myocarditis

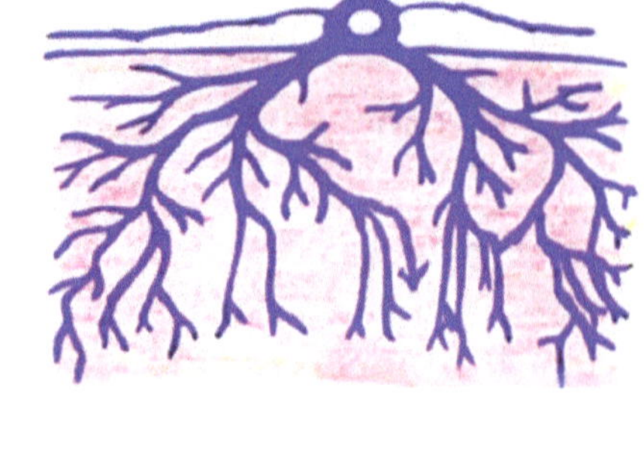

@cunursingnotesbycaitlyn

NO-REFLOW PHENOMENON

A PCI-related complication in which there is an acute↓in myocardial blood flow despite the re-opening of the culprit epicardial coronary artery 2/2 microvascular obstruction.

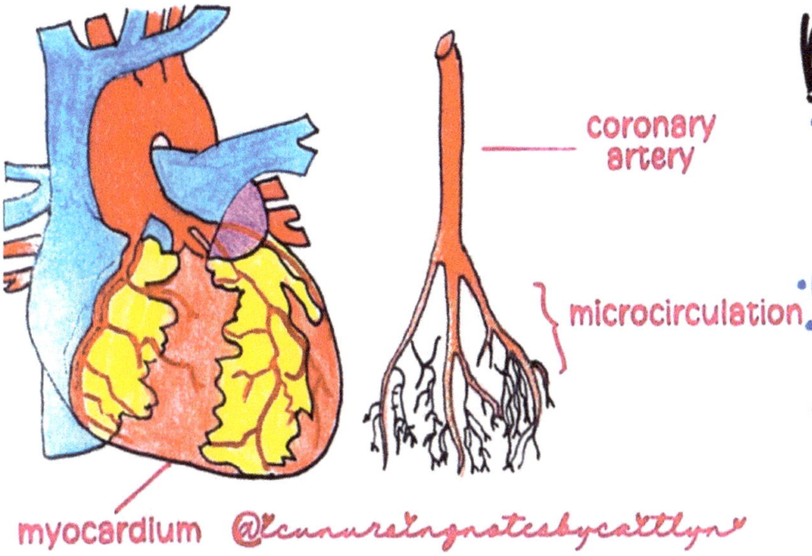

RISK FACTORS

- saphenous vein graft (SVG) PCI
- acute myocardial infarction (MI)
- rotational atherectomy
- high thrombus burden
- plaque composition
- delayed presentation
- longer lesions

PATHOPHYSIOLOGY

No-reflow is suspected to result from a combination of endothelial damage, platelet & fibrin embolization, vasospasm, & tissue edema that overwhelms the coronary microcirculation. Reperfusion-related injury is also thought to contribute to no-reflow via infiltration of the coronary microvasculature c̄ neutrophils & platelets.

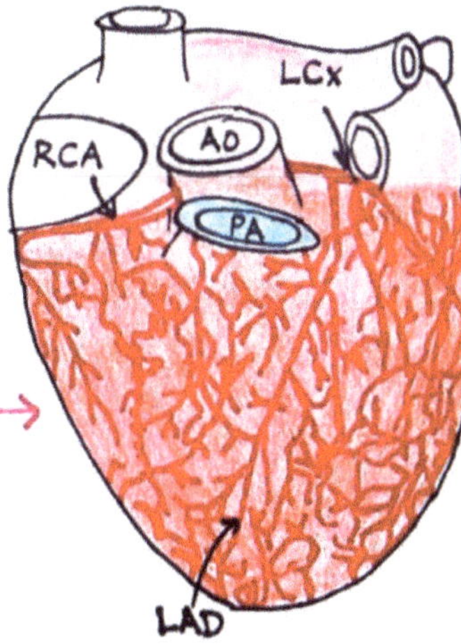

TREATMENT OF NO-REFLOW

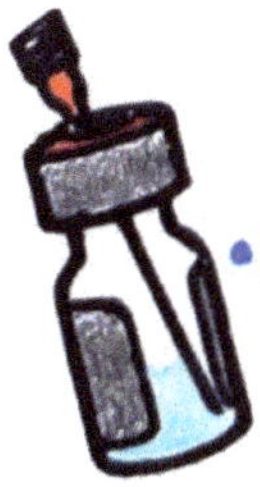

- Intracoronary (IC) administration of nitroprusside, epinephrine, adenosine, nicardipine, verapamil, or diltiazem.
- Consider the use of IV glycoprotein IIb/IIIa receptor inhibitors: eptifibatide (Integrilin) & tirofiban (Aggrastat).
- Additional hemodynamic support may be needed.
- Maintain an activated clotting time (ACT) > 250 seconds.

Takotsubo Cardiomyopathy

Broken Heart Syndrome

ETIOLOGY

- significant stressor
  - physical or emotional
- post-menopausal women
- * typically no underlying cardiac disease

"Takotsubo" is a Japanese term for "octopus trap" used by Japanese fishermen. Stress cardiomyopathy/ "broken heart syndrome" is also known as "Takotsubo cardiomyopathy because the left ventricle changes shape during systole (a 'ballooned' apex c̄ a narrow base) that resembles the Japanese octopus trap.

PATHOPHYS

"Takotsubo Cardiomyopathy" is characterized by acute left ventricular (LV) systolic dysfunction that is triggered by severe emotional stress (hence why it's also called stress-induced cardiomyopathy / broken-heart syndrome). It often occurs in patients with no underlying cardiac disease. Severe emotional stress ⟶ excessive release of catecholamines in the body ⟶ microvascular dysfunction & myocardial stunning that creates the classic "ballooning" appearance of the left ventricle.

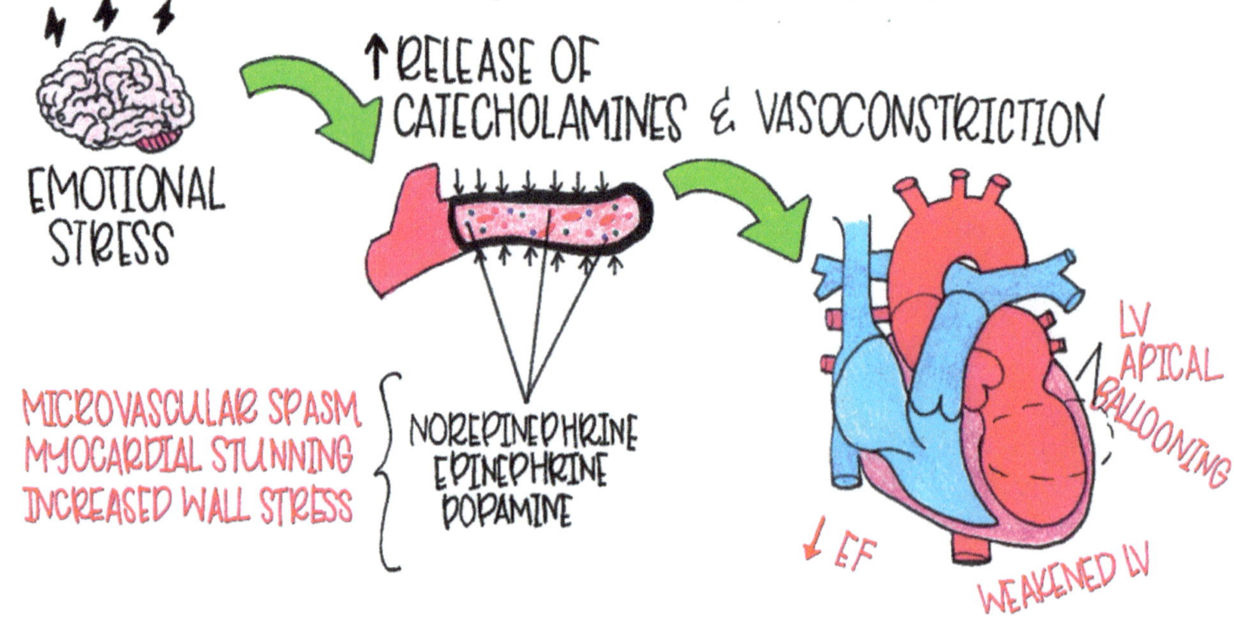

S/S

S/S of Takotsubo cardiomyopathy mimic acute coronary syndrome (ACS).

- substernal chest pain
- dyspnea
- N/V
- ST-segment elevation
- elevated troponin levels

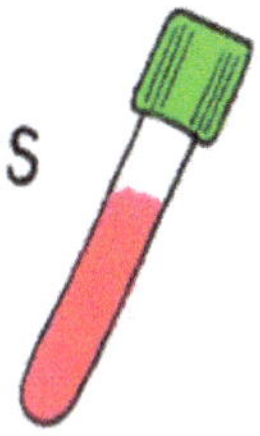

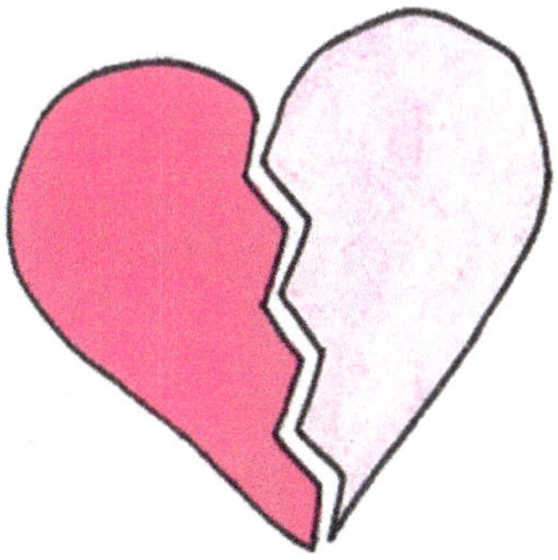

DX

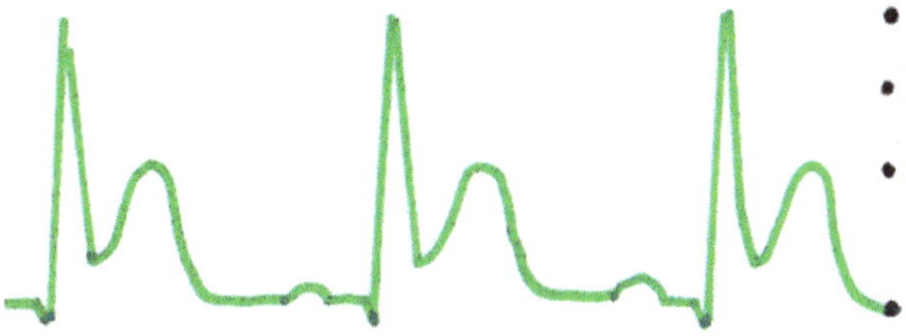

- coronary angiogram } clean coronaries
- left heart cath } clean coronaries
- echocardiogram (apical ballooning & systolic dysfunction)
- ECG (ST-elevations/T-wave inversion)
- R/O phenochromocytoma or myocarditis

TREATMENT

- Typical HFrEF medications may be used (only until cardiac function has recovered).
  - diuretics
  - ACE-I
  - BB
- Stress management therapy

Takotsubo cardiomyopathy is generally a transient & reversible syndrome with a good prognosis that resolves with supportive therapy.

Atrial Fibrillation

RISK FACTORS:

- post-CABG
- valvular heart disease
- MI/CAD
- diabetes
- HTN
- rheumatic heart disease

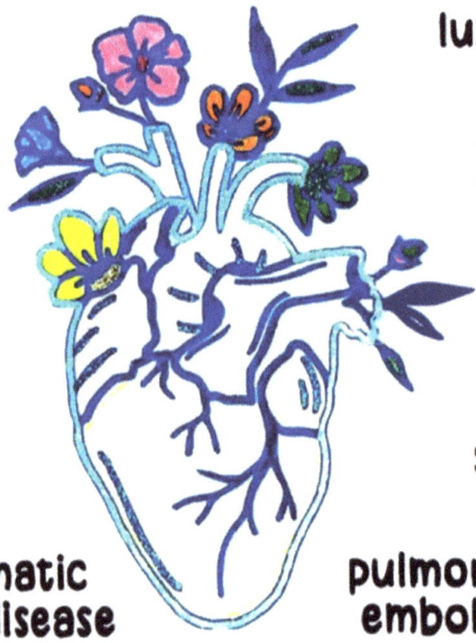

- lung disease
- obstructive sleep apnea
- ETOH abuse
- sepsis
- pulmonary embolism

ECG CHARACTERISTICS:

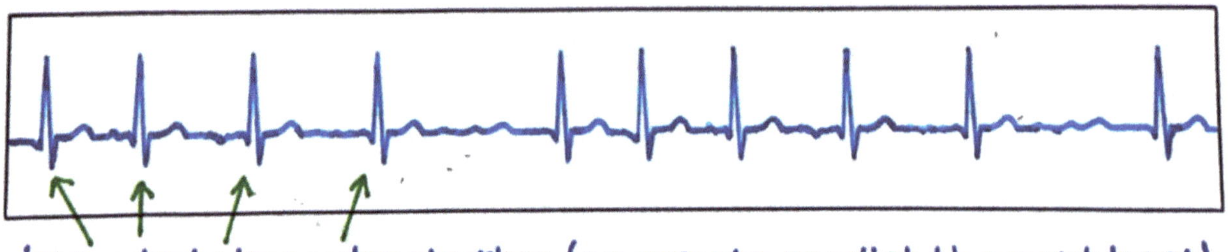

- irregularly irregular rhythm (no way to predict the next beat)
- no discernible P waves
- variable heart rate

@icunursingnotesbycaitlyn

Atrial Kick

the amount of blood pumped into the ventricles by contraction of the atria, which accounts for ≈ 20% of total cardiac output (& up to 40% in patients c̄ LV dysfunction)

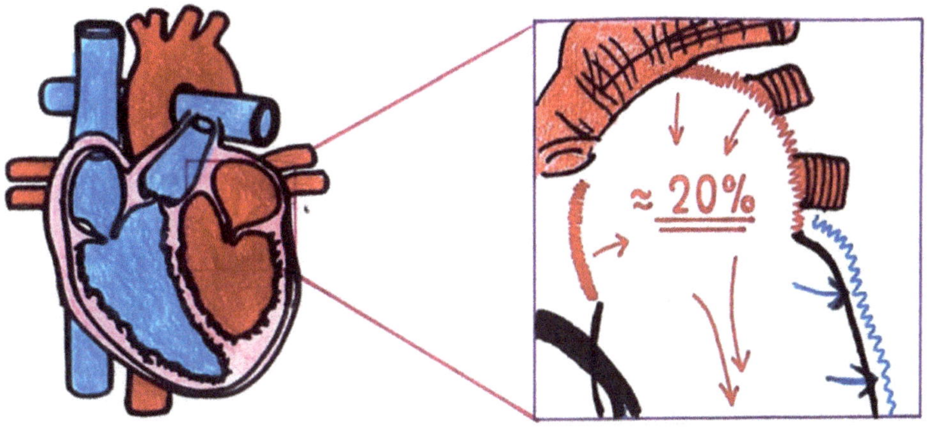

Loss of Atrial Kick = ↓ Cardiac Output

high ventricular rate

↑HR = ↓diastolic filling time = ↓ cardiac output

A-Fib/flutter & complete ♥ block

lack of coordinated atrial contraction = ↓LV end-diastolic volume (preload) = ↓stroke volume = ↓cardiac output

In the setting of left ventricular hypertrophy (LVH), aortic stenosis, mitral stenosis, & diastolic dysfunction, atrial kick is essential to maintain stroke volume & cardiac output because a ↑ LVEDP is needed to maintain the same volume of cardiac output. Loss of atrial kick in these patients can result in acute hemodynamic decompensation (this is why maintenance of normal sinus rhythm is so critical)!

Drawing inspired by the work of Tyler Scanlon, RN (@thevisualnurse)

THE LEFT ATRIAL APPENDAGE

An extension of the left atrium that functions as a decompression chamber during ventricular systole (contraction), releases atrial natriuretic peptide (ANP) in response to ↑cardiac filling pressures to promote diuresis, & is the most frequent site of clot formation in patients c̄ non-valvular atrial fibrillation.

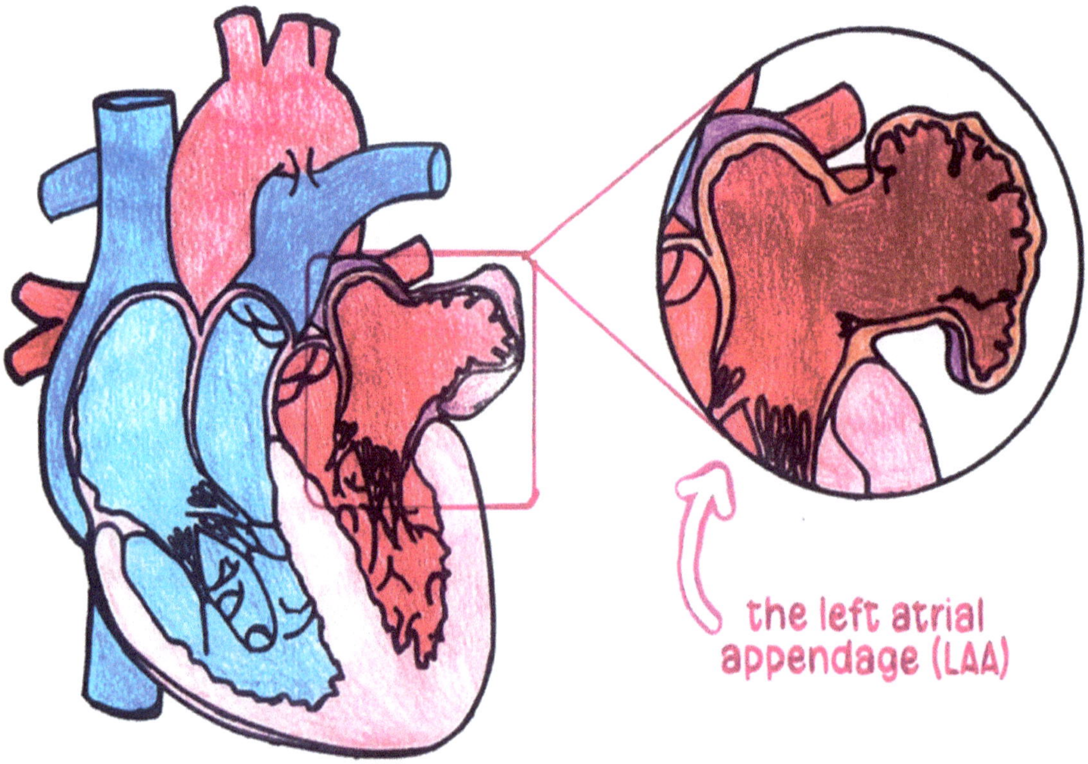

In patients c̄ non-valvular A-Fib, more than 90% of stroke-causing blood clots originate in the LAA (Journal of the American College of Cardiology, 2022).

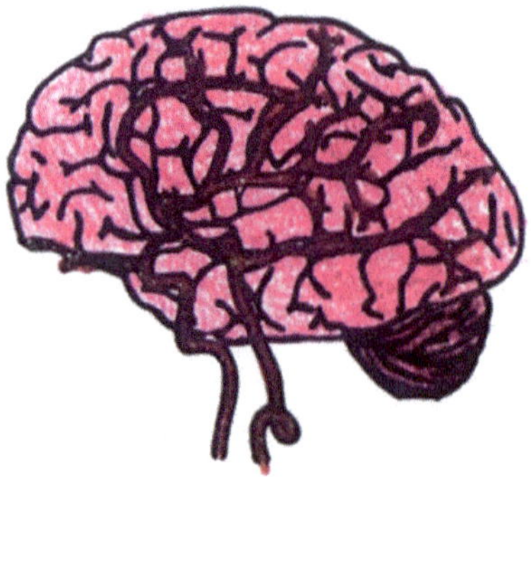

LEFT ATRIAL APPENDAGE

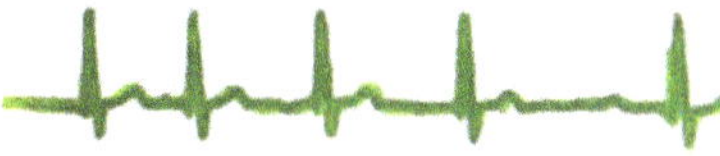

OCCLUSION

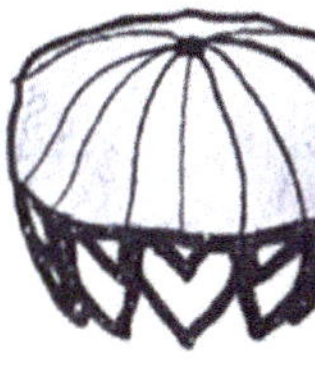

(WATCHMAN™)

A percutaneous, catheter-based procedure for stroke risk reduction in patients c̄ A-Fib who cannot tolerate long-term anticoagulation (i.e. recurrent GI bleeds, prior ICH, high fall risk, non-compliance, etc).

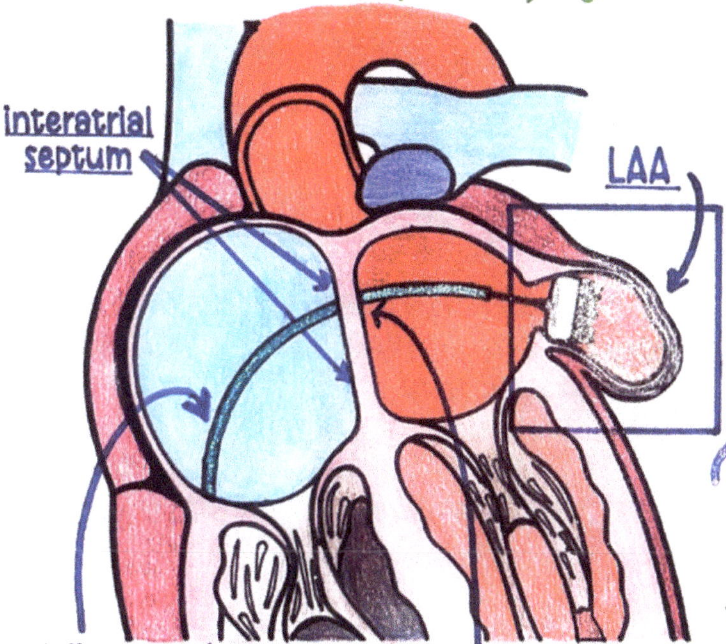

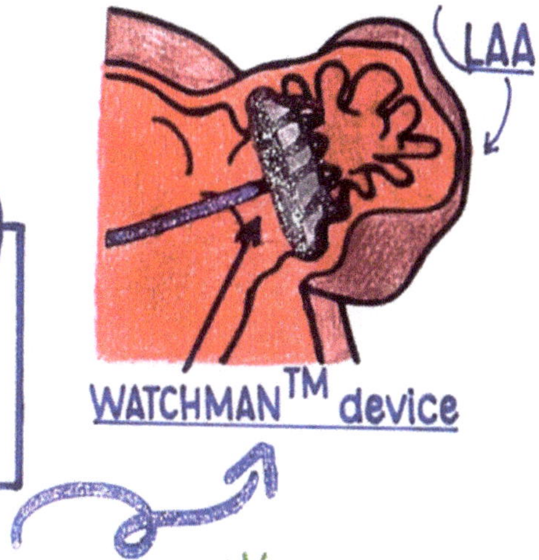

Because the wall of the LAA is thin, it can be easily perforated during device delivery, leading to a **pericardial effusion** - the most common procedural complication!

UNDERSTANDING HOW IT WORKS

The Watchman device acts as a "plug" by closing off the left atrial appendage (LAA) to **prevent clots from entering systemic circulation, thereby ↓ cardioembolic stroke risk.** Inserted percutaneously via the **femoral vein,** the device is delivered under fluoroscopic & echocardiographic guidance (typically TEE, but sometimes ICE) to the LAA via a transseptal puncture into the left atrium. After it's implanted, it takes **≈ 45 days** for endothelial tissue to grow over the device & make a complete seal (confirmed by TEE), so **anticoagulation + ASA is typically continued for up to 45 days post-procedure.** Dual-antiplatelet therapy (DAPT) c̄ ASA & clopidogrel (Plavix) is recommended x 6 months after the device is implanted. A daily ASA is continued indefinitely.

PATENT FORAMEN OVALE (PFO)

A congenital ♥ defect that occurs when the foramen ovale, a small, flap-like opening between the left & right atrium that exists in utero, fails to close at birth.

PATHOPHYS:

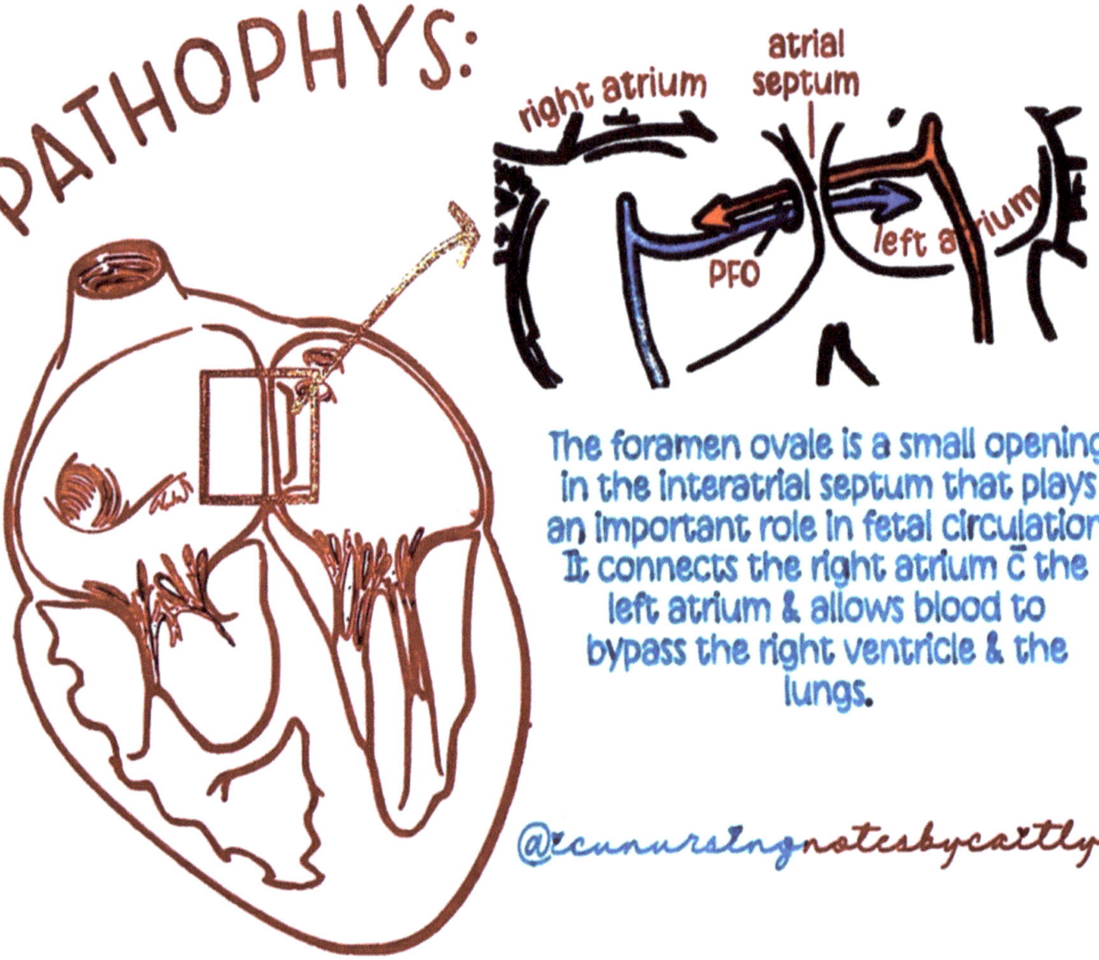

The foramen ovale is a small opening in the interatrial septum that plays an important role in fetal circulation. It connects the right atrium c̄ the left atrium & allows blood to bypass the right ventricle & the lungs.

@icunursingnotesbycaitlyn

At birth, the abrupt ↓ in pulmonary vascular resistance or PVR (due to lung expansion) & the ↑ in systemic vascular resistance or SVR (due to cord clamping) causes the left atrial pressure (LAP) to exceed right atrial pressure (RAP); these pressure Δs usually result in closure of the foramen ovale during infancy. In 25-30% of the adult population (1 in 4 people), the foramen ovale fails to close after birth (Jones & Kucia, 2022); the medical term for this is a "patent foramen ovale" or PFO!

Drawing inspired by the work of Tyler Scanlon, RN (@thevisualnurse)

ETIOLOGY

The causes of a PFO are primarily idiopathic, although research studies support that patency of the foramen ovale may be related to other ♥ defects, genetics, & conditions that ↑ right atrial pressure (Ferri, 2022).

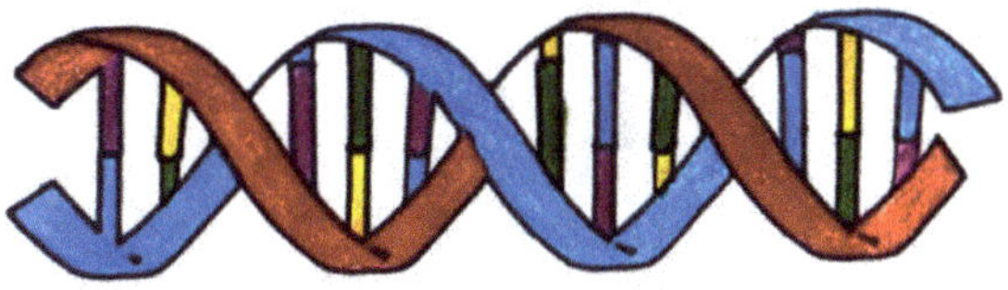

S/S

- generally asymptomatic
- cryptogenic stroke
- migraine H/A

(Mojadidi et al., 2020)

If a PFO is present, it creates a "doorway" for a clot to cross from the right side of the ♥ to the left, enabling the clot to pass through the aorta & up to the brain, causing a stroke (Morrison, 2021).

A transesophageal echocardiogram (TEE) c̄ bubble study is the gold standard for identifying & diagnosing a PFO (Ferri, 2022).

@icunursingnotesbycaitlyn

TREATMENT

for asymptomatic patients c̄ a PFO as an incidental finding → no treatment is necessary

for patients c̄ cryptogenic stroke or TIA & a PFO → percutaneous transcatheter closure

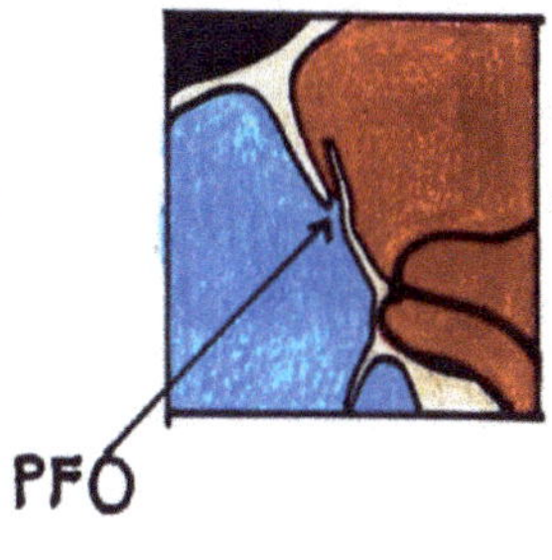

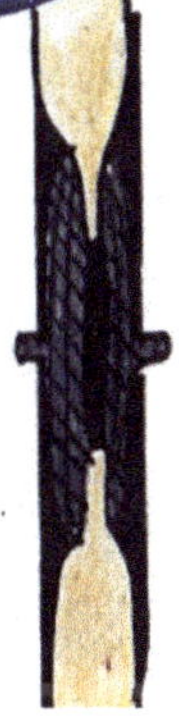

Bubble Study

@icunursingnotesbycaitlyn

Injecting agitated saline (microbubbles) into a peripheral IV to assess for intracardiac shunt(s), such as a PFO or ASD, &/or pulmonary arteriovenous malformations (PAVMs) during an echocardiogram (specifically, a TEE).

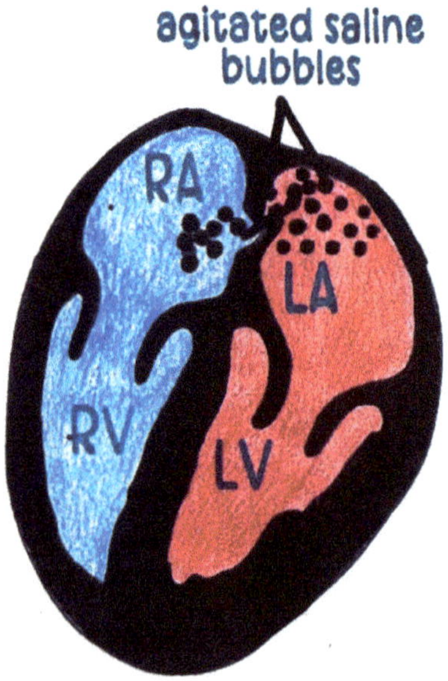

PHYSIOLOGY:

After agitating the saline c̄ 2 syringes & a stopcock, it's injected into a peripheral vein. "Microbubbles" enter the right side of the heart. In the absence of a right-to-left shunt (normal), most bubbles are filtered out by the lungs and, therefore, don't enter the left heart chambers. If the patient has an intracardiac or an intrapulmonary shunt, then the bubbles will appear in the left atrium/ventricle.

Intracardiac or Intrapulmonary?

intracardiac shunt (PFO or ASD)

early appearance of saline bubbles in the left heart chambers (within 3 beats of injection)

intrapulmonary shunt

delayed appearance of saline bubbles in the left heart chambers (5 to 7 beats after injection).

Critical care 101: It's important to identify & close an ASD or PFO prior to left ventricular assist device (LVAD) placement. Even a small PFO can result in significant lef left-to-right shunting & severe hypoxemia in these patients!! (Bacich et al., 2020).

Shunt Run

A technique that is used during a right heart (Swan-Ganz) catheterization to detect & localize a left-to-right intracardiac shunt.

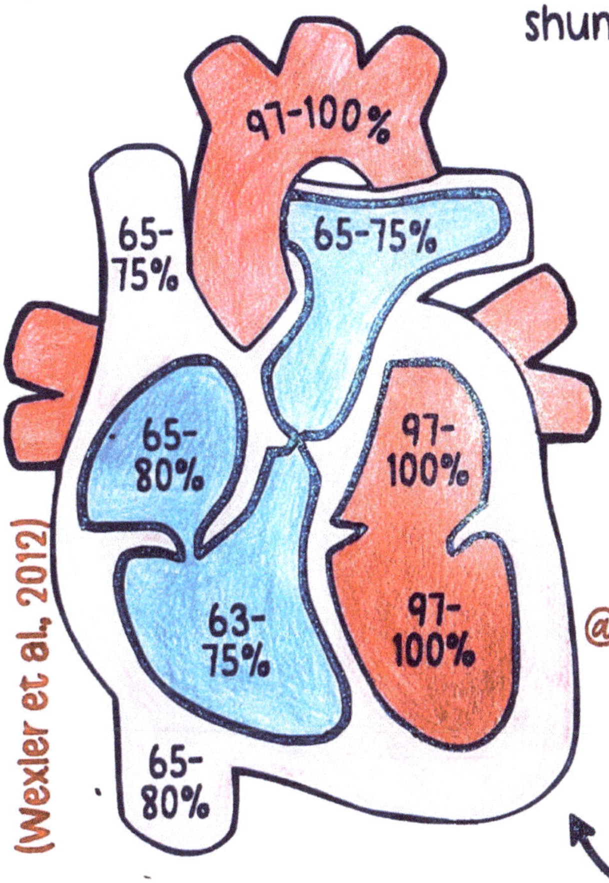

HOW?

The oxygen saturation of blood is measured by obtaining blood samples from all right-sided locations, including the pulmonary artery (PA), right ventricle (RV), low/mid/high right atrium (RA), & the inferior vena cava (IVC) and superior vena cava (SVC)!

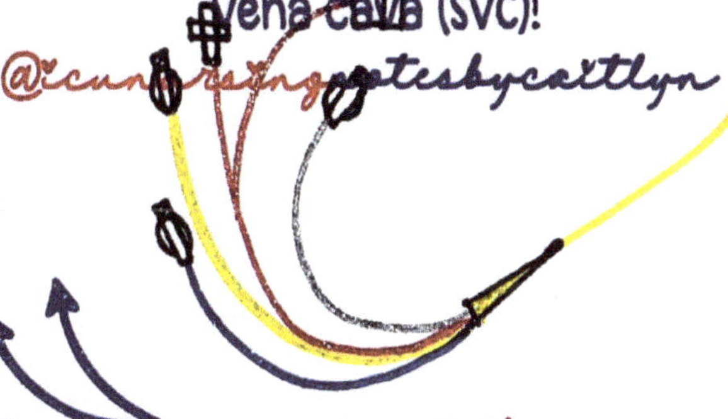

average normal intracardiac oxygen saturations

PHYSIOLOGY

Blood oxygen saturations in the chambers of the right side of the normal heart are similar. In the presence of a left-to-right shunt, there is a "step up," or ↑, in the oxygen saturation because oxygenated blood (left side of the heart) mixes c̄ venous blood (right side of the heart), increasing the oxygen saturation.

A significant "step-up" (increase) in oxygen saturation levels is characteristic of intracardiac shunts (Layon et al., 2017).

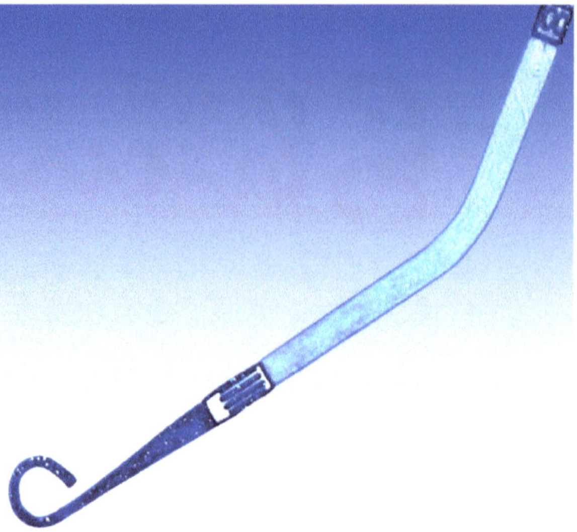

CRITICAL CARE DEVICES

critical care devices

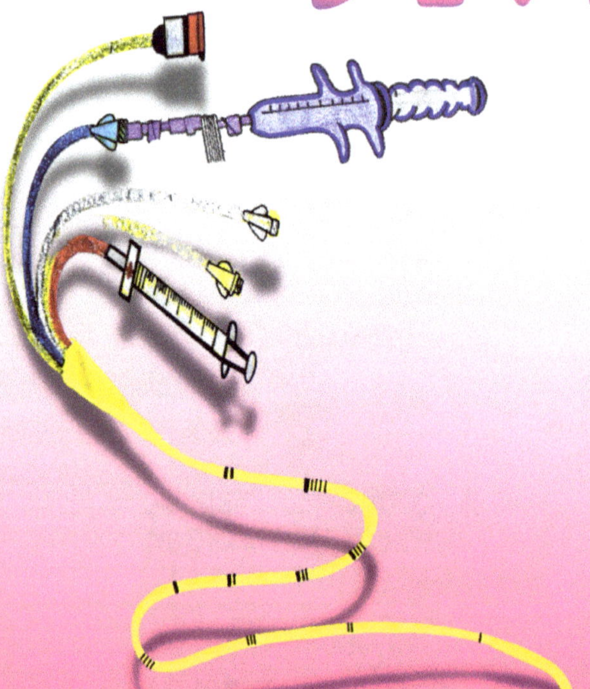

TARGETED TEMPERATURE MANAGEMENT

(therapeutic hypothermia)

A standard, evidence-based treatment used to preserve neurologic function in resuscitated cardiac arrest patients who remain unconscious after ROSC.

TTM is the deliberate cooling of a patient to 33-36°C (varies by hospital) x 24 hours to improve neurological outcomes p̄ a cardiac arrest c̄ ROSC. Hypothermia ↓ cerebral metabolism & ↓ cerebral oxygen consumpiton (the brain needs less O2 to function).

Immediately s/p ROSC, this ↓ in O2 demand (induced by hypothermia) improves brain oxygenation. Other benefits of TTM include stabilization of cell membranes & the blood-brain barrier (BBB), ↓ free radical production during reperfusion, & a ↓ in cerebral edema!

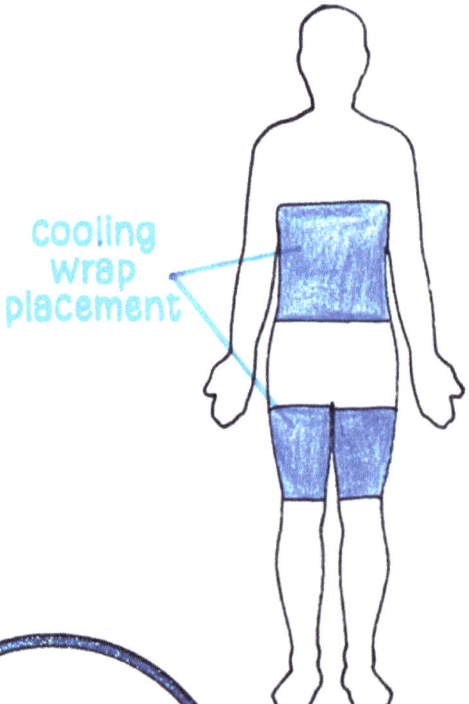

The 3 Phases:

within 4 hours of ROSC!

COOLING
core body temperature is reduced quickly to target temperature (32-36°C)

MAINTENANCE
the patient is maintained at target temperature x 24 hours

REWARMING
the patient is slowly rewarmed (0.2-0.5°C/hr) until normothermic (37°C)

@icunursingnotesbycaitlyn

TTM Devices

SURFACE-COOLING DEVICES

circulate cold or warm water through wraps/pads applied to the patient's skin

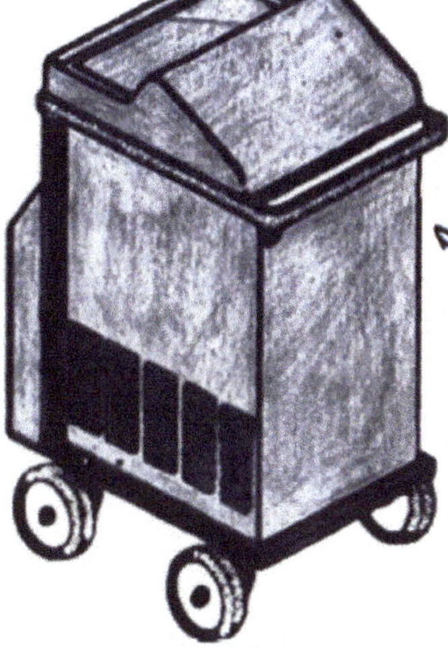

Arctic Sun
Gaymar
Blanketrol
Medi-Therm

INTRAVASCULAR COOLING CATHETERS

central venous catheters that regulate core body temperature !

Thermoguard XP
InnerCool RTx

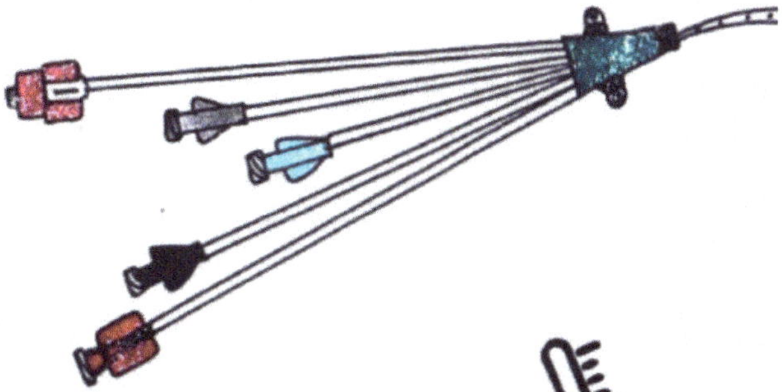

Temperature Monitoring

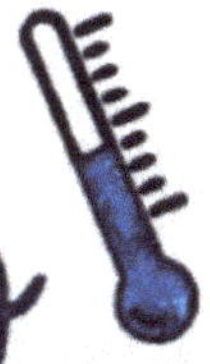

A consistent temperature site must be monitored during TTM. Use 2 of the following to monitor the patient's core temperature:

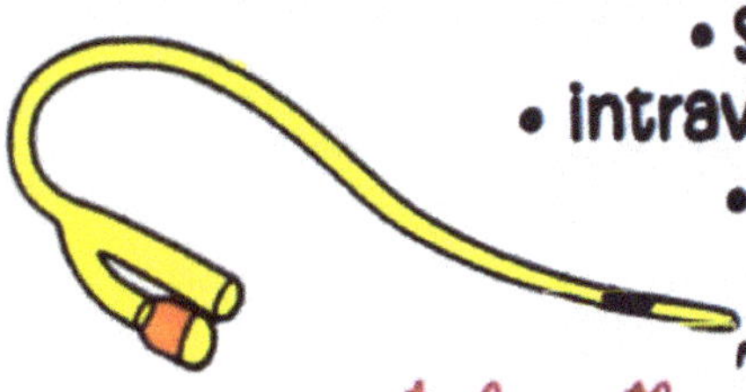

- Swan-Ganz Catheter
- intravascular cooling catheter
- esophageal probe
- Foley catheter
- rectal probe

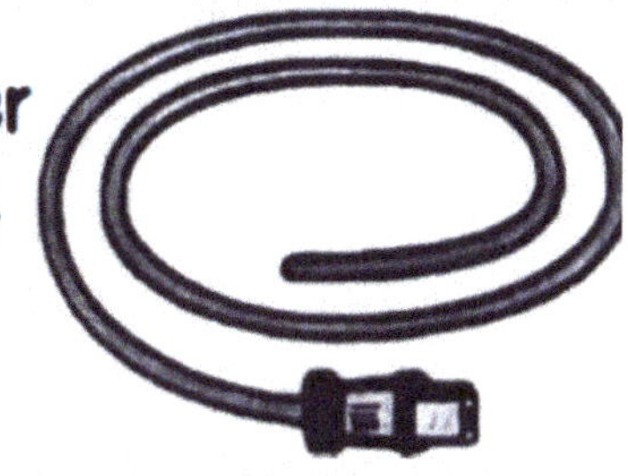

@icunursingnotesbycaitlyn

Nursing Care

@icunursingnotesbycaitlyn

TTM is typically a 1:1 nursing assignment!

- Initiate TTM & achieve target temperature (33-36°C) within 4 hours of ROSC (ideally); maintain goal x 24 hrs. After 24 hours at goal, slowly rewarm the patient to a target of 37°C.
- Obtain initial labs & track/trend (CBC, BMP, ABG/VBG, trop, lactate, PT/aPTT/INR, D-dimer, CPK, fibrinogen, LFTs, lipase, UA, etc).
- Have a good baseline nursing assessment p̄ initiating TTM & frequently monitor ongoing neurologic status!
- Continuously monitor core body temperature at 2 different sites.
- Monitor for ECG changes: bradycardia is common during TTM.
- Assess the patient's electrolytes, glucose (TTM causes insulin resistance & hyperglycemia), arterial blood gas & coags.
- Do not pause sedation to do your neuro assessment (as you normally would for a typical intubated patient).
- Strict I&O: hypothermia induces diuresis, so anticipate the need to administer IVF & replete lytes during the cooling phase.
- Monitor for electrolyte depletion when cooling but ↑K+ when rewarming. Be cautious c̄ K+ repletion p̄ rewarming (hyperkalemia risk).
- Assess for shivering using the Bedside Shivering Assessment Scale (BSAS). An ideal BSAS is 0-1.
- If BSAS >1, put a Bair Hugger on the patient, socks on the hands & feet, & follow your hospital's shivering protocol: common medications used include Tylenol, buspirone, Demerol, IV mag, & clonidine.
- Use Train of Four monitoring if administering IV paralytics for refractory shivering (last resort).
- Monitor for hypotension, especially when rewarming (vasodilation).
- Rewarm slowly (0.5 C/hr) to ↓ the risk of hemodynamic instability
- Standard care for any intubated patient (DVT/PUD prophylaxis, PI prevention, oral care, central line care and maintenance, & VAP/CLABSI/CAUTI prevention). TTM also causes immunosuppression & linfection risk.
- Keep the HOB at 30 to ↓ ICP & ↓ aspiration risk.
- Assess for TTM-related complications: ECG changes (bradycardia, prolonged QTc), fluid & electrolyte imbalances, seizures (continuous EEG monitoring should be in place), coagulopathy & shivering.
- Don't forget to involve the patient's familyi n the plan of care: this is scary for them!

TTM is uncomfortable! Ensure that your patient is adequately sedated (sedative + analgesic). Remember that sedatives (i.e. propofol) are NOT analgesics!!

Anatomy of an Intra-Aortic Balloon Pump!

Remember that the IABP inflates when the heart relaxes (diastole) & pushes blood flow back toward the coronary arteries. It deflates just a the heart contracts (systole) & ↓ afterload!

An IABP is inserted by an interventional cardiologist in the cath lab under fluoroscopy

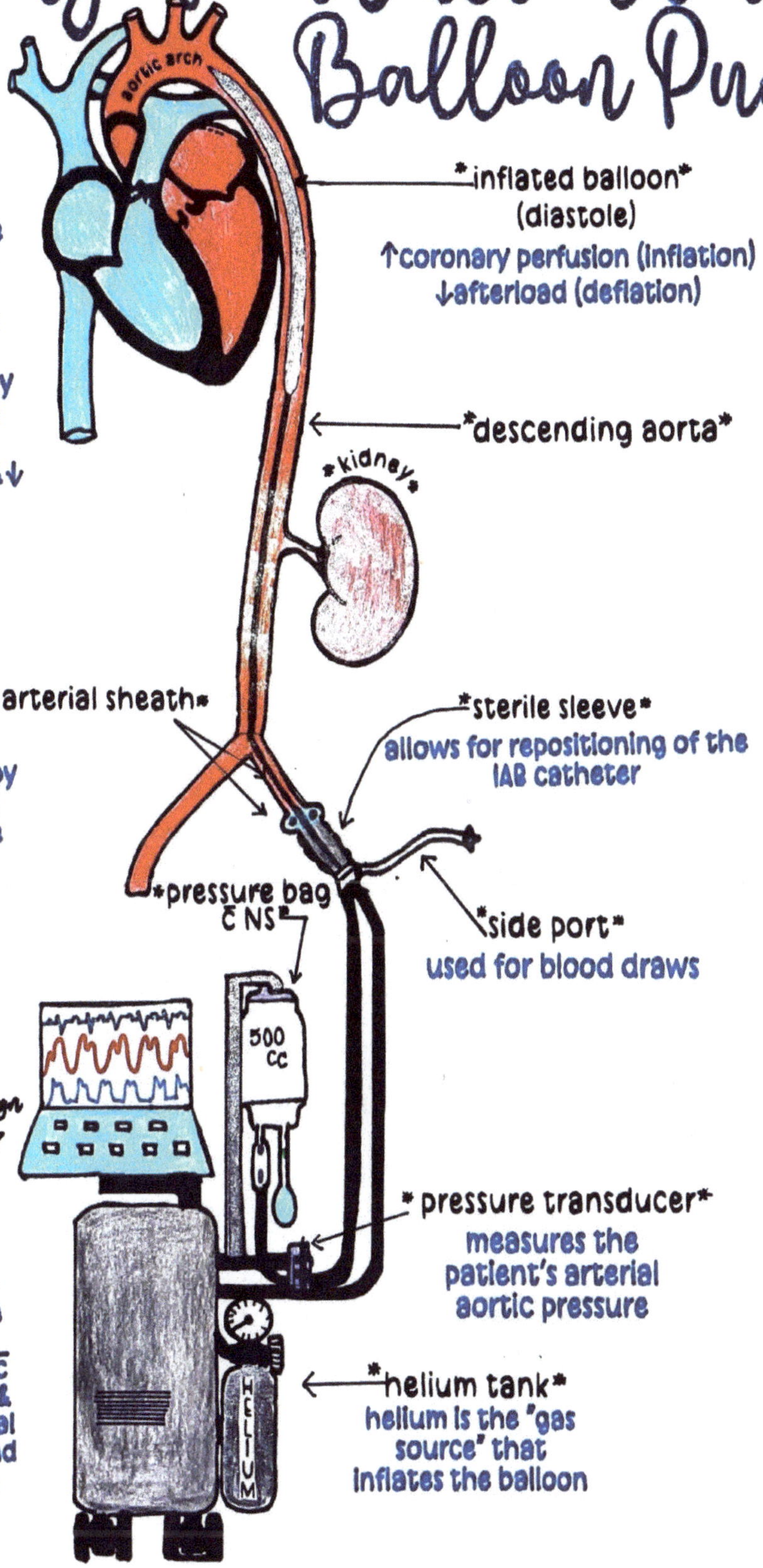

* the console *
regulates balloon inflation and deflation in sync c̄ the cardiac cycle & displays the arterial waveforms, ECG, and balloon inflation waveform.

INTRA-AORTIC BALLOON PUMP:
THE MONITOR SCREEN

ECG TRACING

This is generated from the IABP leads that are on the patient. We can trigger the IABP by syncing it c̄ the patient's cardiac cycle. The ECG triggers balloon inflation at the middle of the T-wave (diastole) & triggers deflation at the peak of the R wave (systole).

BALLOON PRESSURE WAVEFORM

This waveform tells you whether the balloon is inflating & deflating properly. It represents helium movement between the console & the intra-aortic balloon catheter. Compare this waveform c̄ the arterial pressure waveform to assess the effect of balloon inflation on the augmented arterial pressure.

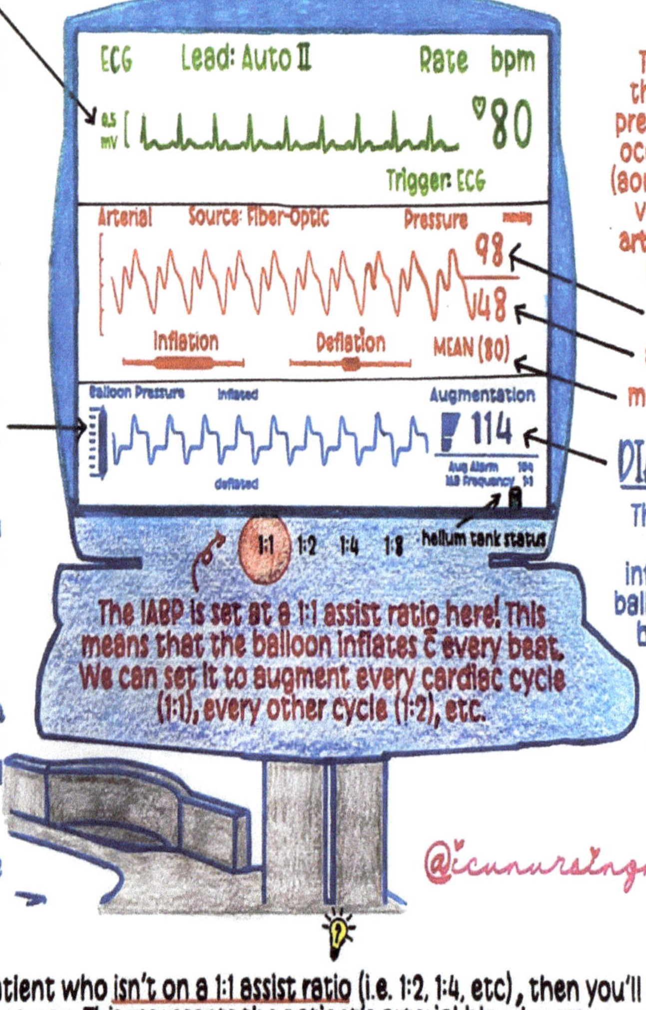

CENTRAL AORTIC ARTERIAL PRESSURE

This waveform represents the patient's central aortic pressure (Ao). Balloon inflation occurs at the dicrotic notch (aortic valve closure & onset of ventricular diastole) if the arterial waveform (instead of ECG) is used as a trigger.

- aortic systolic pressure
- aortic diastolic pressure
- mean arterial pressure (MAP)

DIASTOLIC AUGMENTATION

This represents the patient's diastolic blood pressure c̄ inflation of the intra-aortic balloon catheter. It should be higher than the patient's systolic blood pressure.

This is a number, not a waveform!

@icunursingnotesbycaitlyn

If you're caring for a patient who isn't on a 1:1 assist ratio (i.e. 1:2, 1:4, etc), then you'll see an "unassisted pressure" reading on the monitor screen. This represents the patient's arterial blood pressure on beats that are NOT assisted by inflation of the intra-aortic balloon catheter!

Intra-aortic Balloon Pump: Timing Errors

The Normal IABP Waveform (1:2):

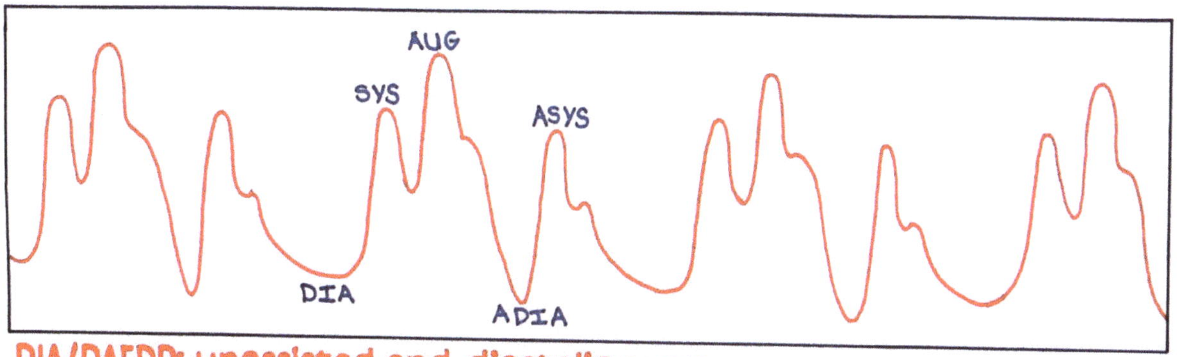

DIA/PAEDP: unassisted end-diastolic pressure
SYS/PSP: unassisted peak systolic pressure
AUG/PDP: diastolic augmentation
ADIA/BAEDP: assisted end-diastolic pressure
ASYS/APSP: assisted peak systolic pressure (systole after IAB deflation)
DN: dicrotic notch

Remember the goal of IABP inflation & deflation; The goal of inflation is to rapidly ↑ aortic pressure (optimizes diastolic augmentation) & ↑ coronary artery perfusion. The goal of deflation is to ↓ afterload, ↓ MVO2, & ↑ cardiac output!

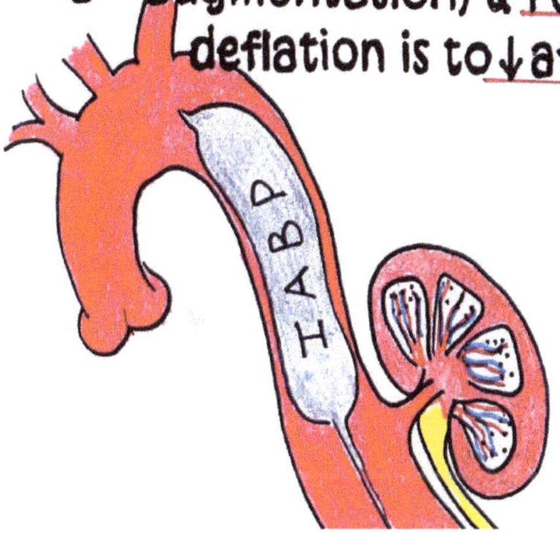

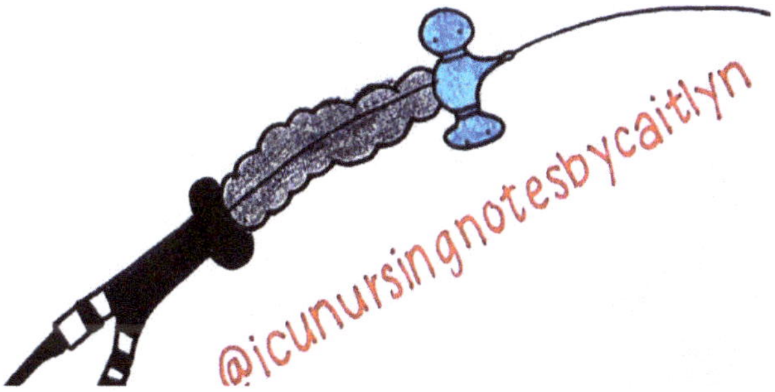

Timing Errors

early inflation	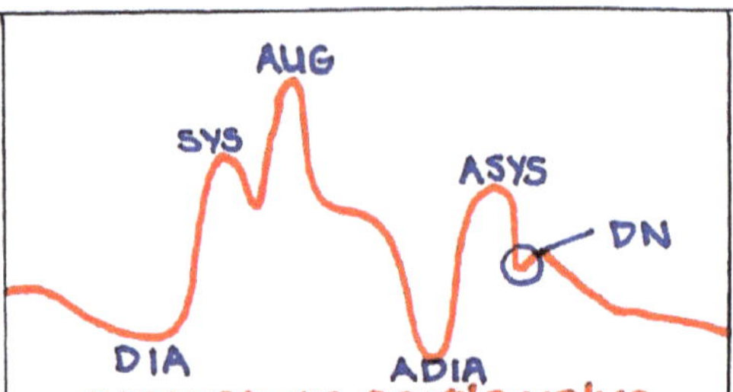 premature aortic valve closure	↑afterload ↓diastolic perfusion ↓cardiac output/SV ↑LVEDP
early deflation	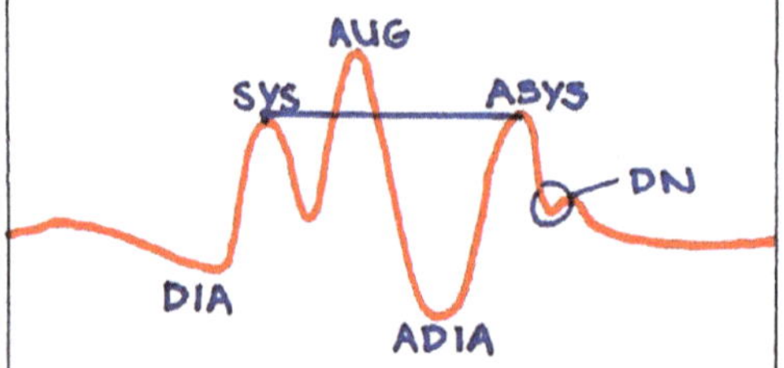 ASYS = SYS: U shaped	No afterload reduction
late inflation	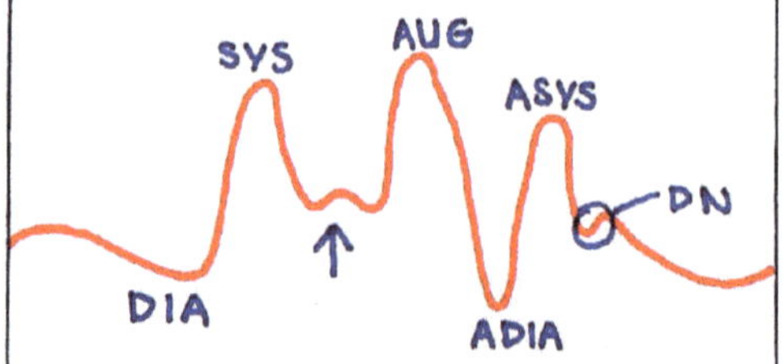 dicrotic notch is visible between SYS/AUG	↓diastolic augmentation = ↓coronary artery perfusion
late deflation	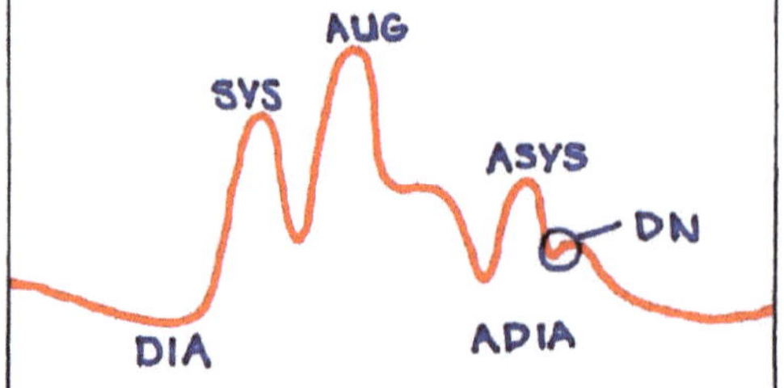 ADIA > DIA: W shaped	↑afterload ↑myocardial O2 demand (MvO2)

Nursing Considerations

-Always assess the timing of the IABP at a 1:2 ratio; if the patient is at 1:1, then turn the pump to 1:2, print the strip, & turn the pump back to 1:1.

-Assess the timing of the IABP c̄ the arterial waveform.

-Hourly check of arterial tracing & ECG, triggers, timing frequency & ratio.

-Regular check of pressure bag, IABP lines, & helium tank.

-Reassess timing c̄ any significant patient changes (i.e. change in rhythm, hemodynamics, etc).

-If balloon augmentation is less than the patient's systolic pressure, then consider that the patient may be hypovolemic or tachycardic, the balloon may be positioned too low, or the balloon volume is set too low.

-Consider setting the timing & the frequency of the IABP to optimize hemodynamic status (i.e. if the patient is tachycardic, the IABP may need to be set to a 1:2 frequency).

Remember that timing is always assessed at a 1:2 ratio so that you can compare the assisted & unassisted arterial waveforms.

The balloon must be timed accurately to give the full benefit of augmentation to the patient; incorrect timing will cause the heart to work harder.

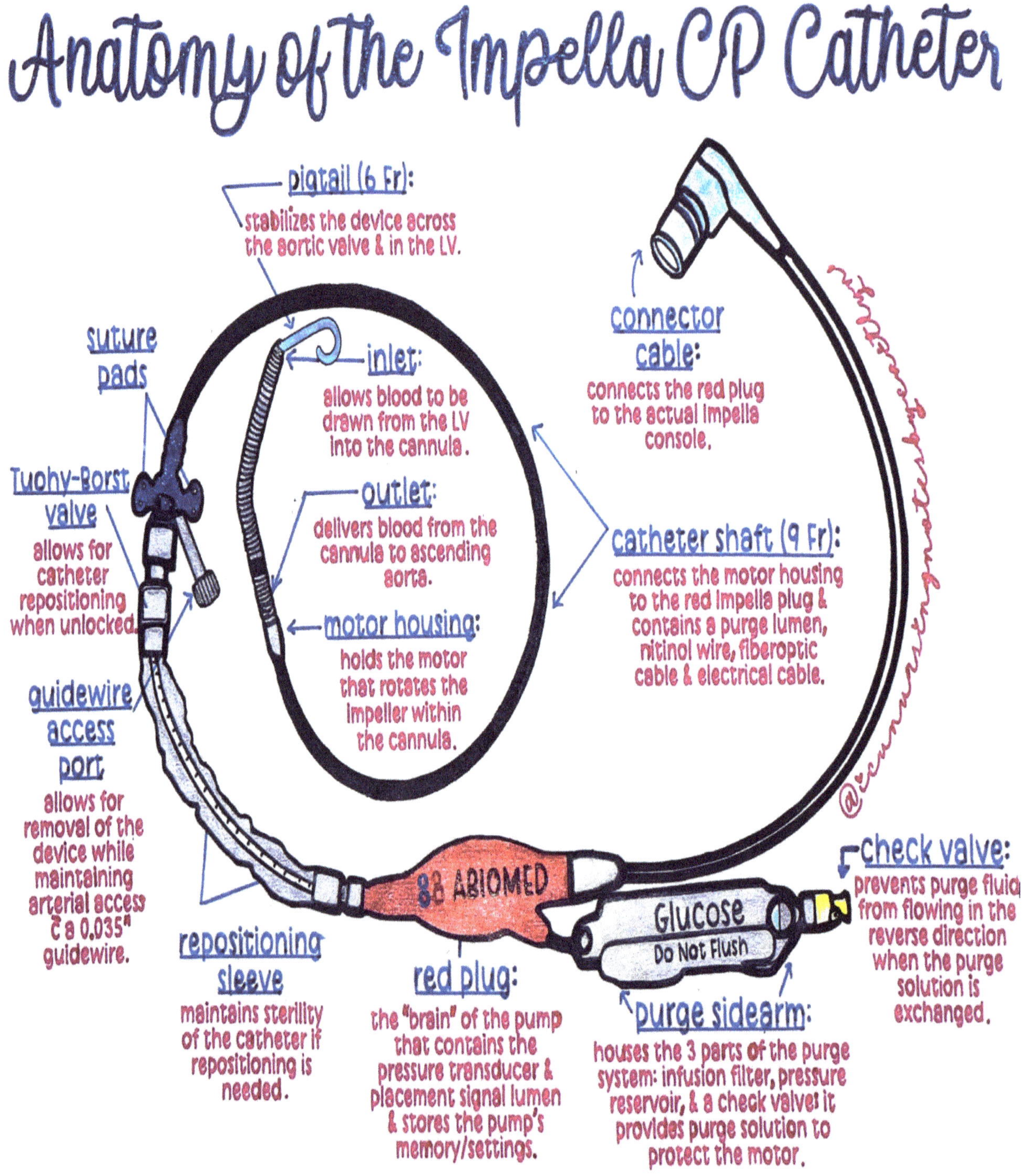

Drawing inspired by David Convissar, MD (@countbackwardsfrom10)

UNDERSTANDING THE VARIOUS TYPES OF IMPELLA CATHETERS

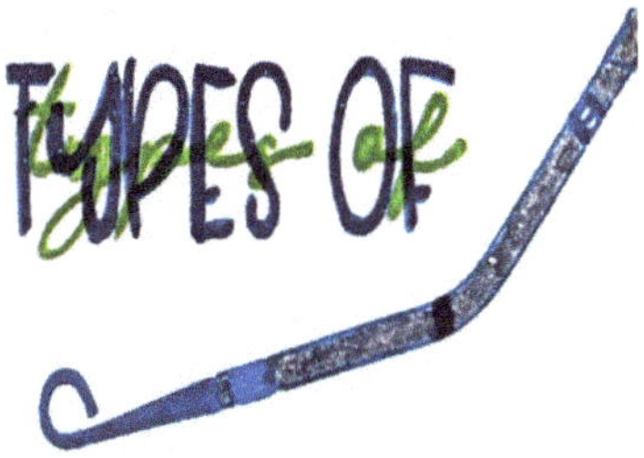

percutaneous insertion			surgical insertion		
Impella 2.5	**Impella CP**	**Impella RP**	**Impella 5.0**	**Impella LD**	**Impella 5.5**

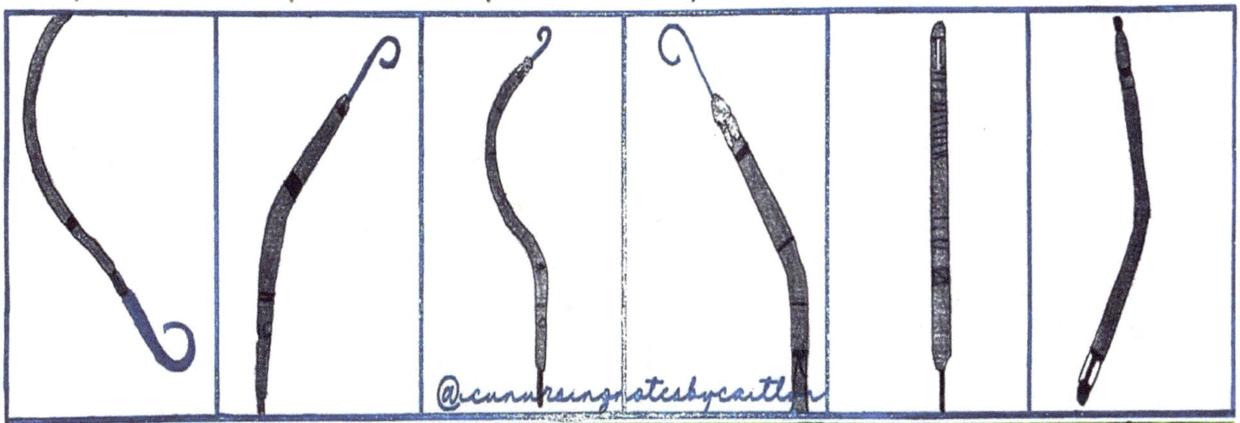

Impella 2.5	Impella CP	Impella RP	Impella 5.0	Impella LD	Impella 5.5
• LV → aorta • percutaneous insertion via the femoral artery • flow rate up to 2.5 L/min • short-term use 9 Fr catheter, 12 Fr pump motor	• LV → aorta • percutaneous insertion via the femoral artery • flow rate up to 4.3 L/min • short-term use • SmartAssist • 9 Fr catheter, 14 Fr pump motor	• RA → PA • percutaneous insertion via the femoral vein • flow rate > 4 L/min • supports the right ventricle • can be used c̄ a left-sided Impella device for biventricular HF	• LV → aorta • surgical insertion via an axillary or femoral artery cutdown • flow rate up to 5.0 L/min • 9 Fr catheter, 21 Fr pump motor	• LV → aorta • surgically placed directly through the aorta • requires cardiac surgery • flow rate up to 5.0 L/min • 9 Fr catheter, 21 Fr pump motor • no pigtail	LV → aorta • surgical insertion via an axillary cutdown • flow rate up to 6.2 L/min • 9 Fr catheter, 19 Fr pump motor • no pigtail • SmartAssist

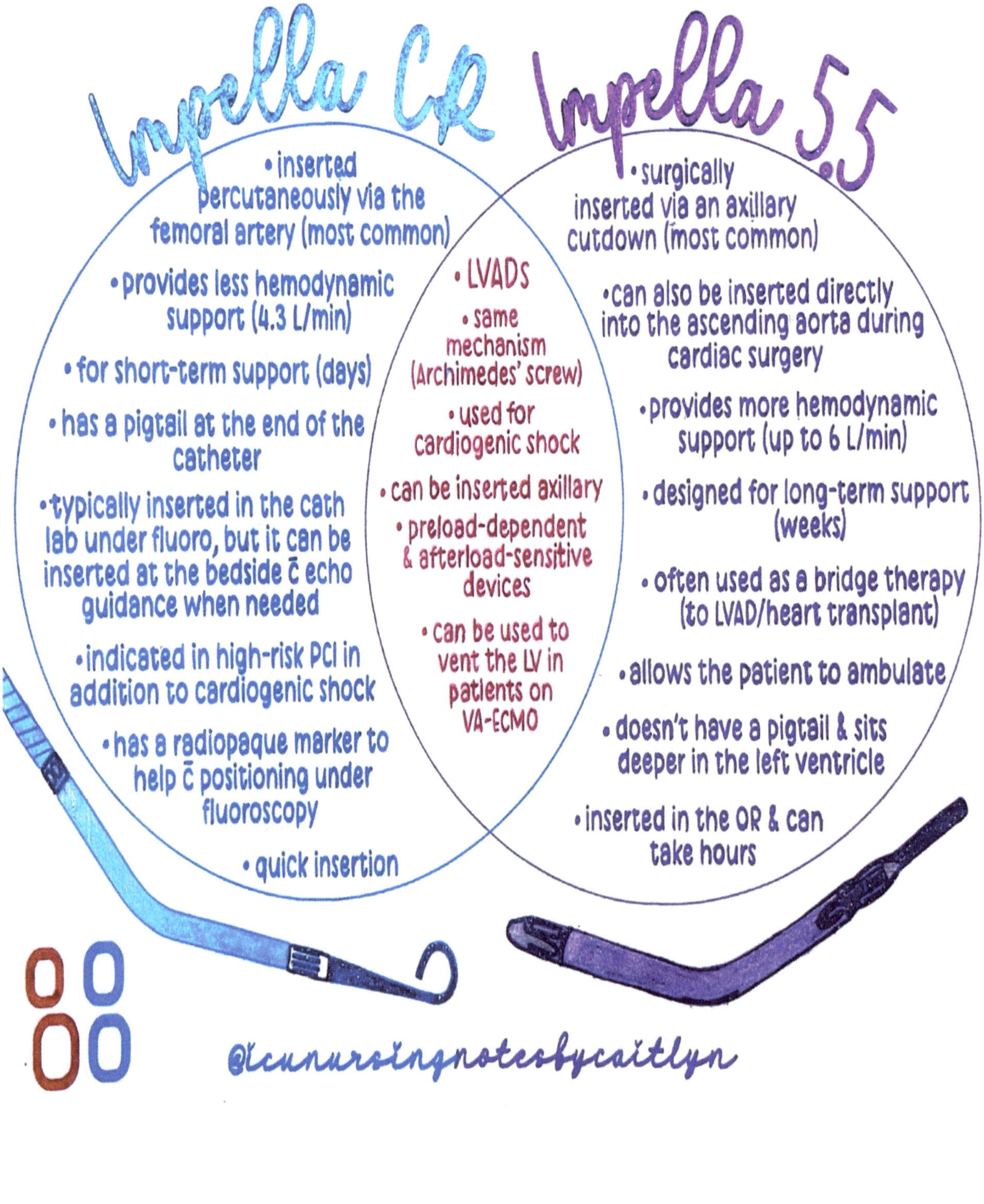
Impella CP
Impella 5.5
• inserted percutaneously via the femoral artery (most common)
• provides less hemodynamic support (4.3 L/min)
• for short-term support (days)
• has a pigtail at the end of the catheter
• typically inserted in the cath lab under fluoro, but it can be inserted at the bedside c̄ echo guidance when needed
• indicated in high-risk PCI in addition to cardiogenic shock
• has a radiopaque marker to help c̄ positioning under fluoroscopy
• quick insertion
• LVADs
• same mechanism (Archimedes' screw)
• used for cardiogenic shock
• can be inserted axillary
• preload-dependent & afterload-sensitive devices
• can be used to vent the LV in patients on VA-ECMO
• surgically inserted via an axillary cutdown (most common)
• can also be inserted directly into the ascending aorta during cardiac surgery
• provides more hemodynamic support (up to 6 L/min)
• designed for long-term support (weeks)
• often used as a bridge therapy (to LVAD/heart transplant)
• allows the patient to ambulate
• doesn't have a pigtail & sits deeper in the left ventricle
• inserted in the OR & can take hours
@icunursingnotesbycaitlyn

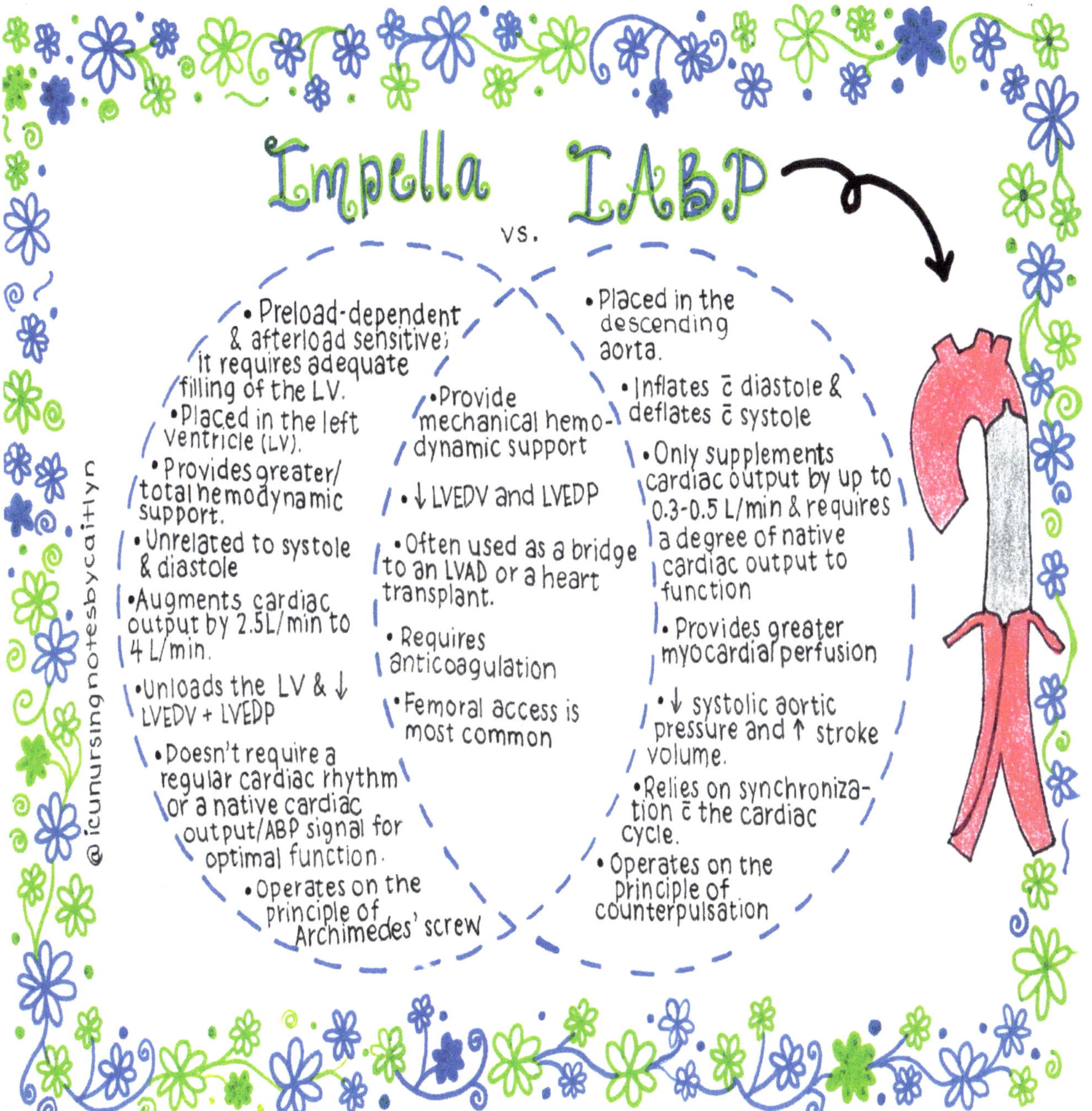
Impella vs. IABP
• Preload-dependent & afterload sensitive; it requires adequate filling of the LV.
• Placed in the left ventricle (LV).
• Provides greater/total hemodynamic support.
• Unrelated to systole & diastole
• Augments cardiac output by 2.5L/min to 4 L/min.
• Unloads the LV & ↓ LVEDV + LVEDP
• Doesn't require a regular cardiac rhythm or a native cardiac output/ABP signal for optimal function.
• Operates on the principle of Archimedes' screw
• Provide mechanical hemodynamic support
• ↓ LVEDV and LVEDP
• Often used as a bridge to an LVAD or a heart transplant.
• Requires anticoagulation
• Femoral access is most common
• Placed in the descending aorta.
• Inflates c̄ diastole & deflates c̄ systole
• Only supplements cardiac output by up to 0.3-0.5 L/min & requires a degree of native cardiac output to function
• Provides greater myocardial perfusion
• ↓ systolic aortic pressure and ↑ stroke volume.
• Relies on synchronization c̄ the cardiac cycle.
• Operates on the principle of counterpulsation
@icunursingnotesbycaitlyn

Impella Waveforms

Placement Signal:

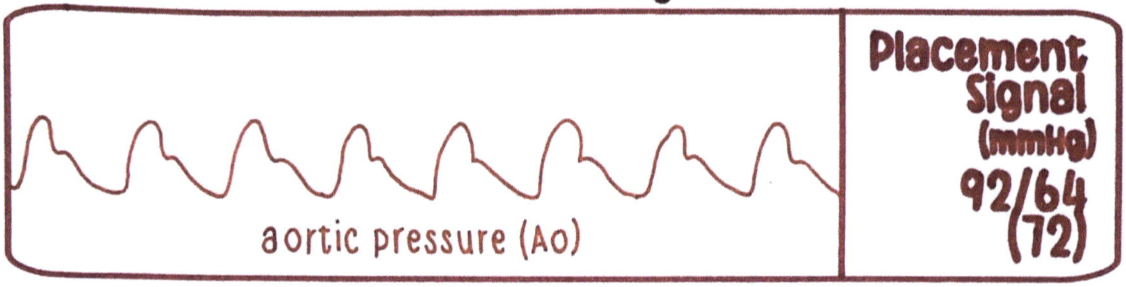

- Used to monitor whether the Impella catheter is correctly positioned across the aortic valve.
- Should see a pulsatile aortic pressure waveform (Ao)!
- If you see a ventricular waveform (rather than aortic), then the catheter needs to be repositioned under fluoro/echo guidance.
- Watch the diastolic number - if it becomes excessively low, reeassess the patient's volume status (likely dry) & ? the possibility of RV failure. If fluids don't help, then consider an echo to see how well the RV is pumping (↓the P-level to P2 when repositioning).

Motor Current:

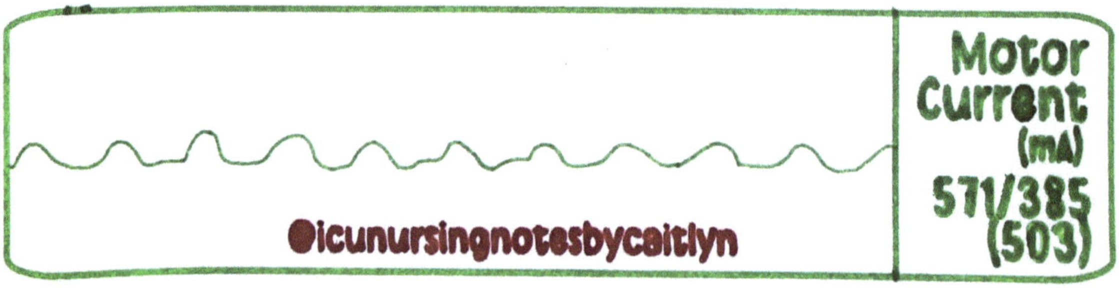

- Should be pulsatile!
- Measures how much energy is being used by the Impella (varies c̄ P-level & the LV-Ao pressure gradient).
- Provides information about catheter position relative to the aortic valve
- If the waveform is dampened or flat, then the catheter is not in the right place (it's either too far in the LV or in & up the aorta).
- If the patient is hypovolemic, there will be a↓in the motor current & the waveform will be dampened (in addition to suction alarms)!

NURSING CARE OF AN IMPELLA

a review of the Impella catheter

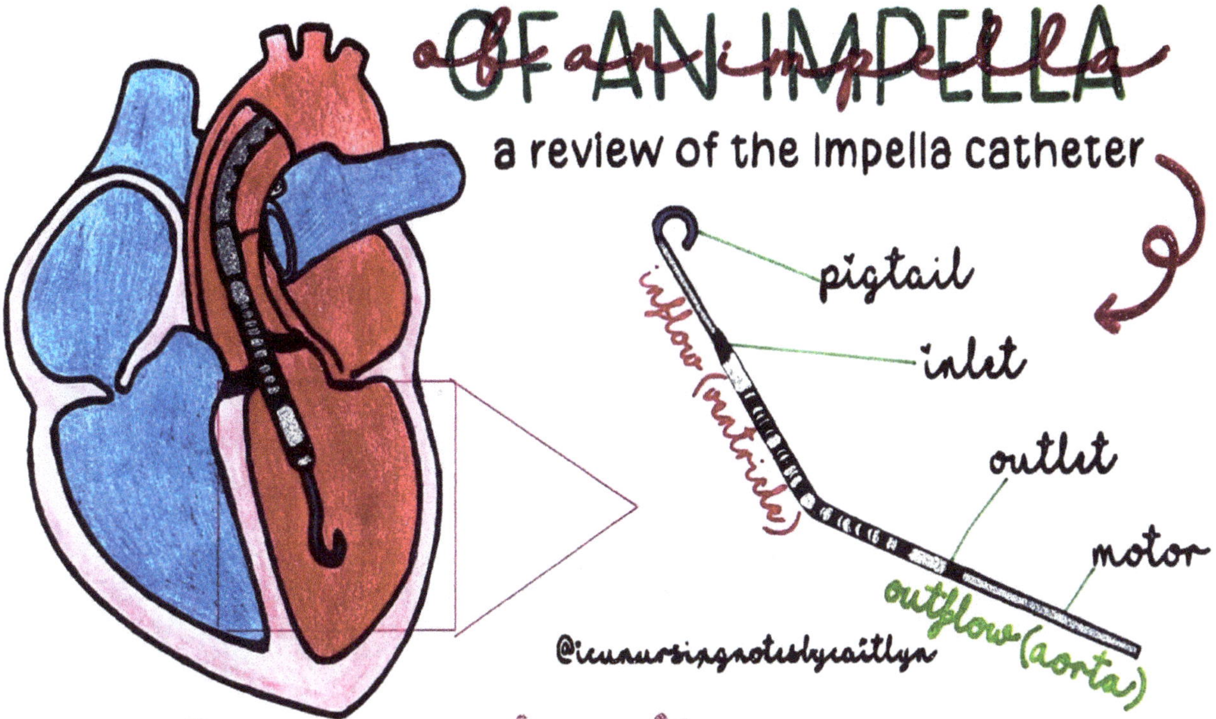

General Nursing Care

- Assess for perfusion, DP/PT pulses, & CRT distal to the access site hourly.
- Make sure that alarm limits are on & set appropriately!
- Understand the waveforms!!
- Monitor for ↑s in motor current: it can indicate impending pump failure!
- Sterile* dressing Δs, per hospital policy.
- Ensure that your patient is laying flat; don't raise the HOB. Log-roll & apply a knee immobilizer!
- Assess access site for bleeding, a hematoma, &/or S/S of infection.
- Monitor the patient's volume status, assess hemodynamics, & waveforms.
- Change the purge cassette q 4 days.
- Position assessment- you should see an aortic placement signal & a pulsatile motor current! (waveform).
- Assess & document the catheter's position (in cm) from the hub.
- Update the cardiac output on the Impella c̄ Swan thermos q 8 hrs.
- Monitor for hemolysis (↓ HgB, hemolyzed labs, hematuria) – run the Impella at the lowest P-level that the patient can tolerate.
- Work to ↓ the patient's SVR – ↑SVR can ↓ pump flow.
- During a code, ↓ P-level to P2.

Troubleshooting the Impella 101!

IMPELLA ALARM	WHAT TO LOOK FOR?	WHAT TO DO?
suction	lower than expected Impella flow rates, ↓ BP, ↓ motor current, & possible hemolysis.	1) ↓ the P-level 2) Check Impella position 3) Assess the patient's volume status (remember that an Impella is preload-dependent!).
position	ventricular (not aortic) placement signal &/or a flat (not pulsatile) motor current	1) ↓ the P-level to P-2. 2) Repositioned under echo guidance (done by a provider). 3) Return to previous P-level once position is confirmed
high/low purge pressure	leaks/kinks in the purge tubing & ↓ in the motor current.	1) Tighten any loose connections. 2) △ the concentration of the purge fluid (may be too ↑ or ↓). 3) Replace the purge cassette.

@icunursingnotesbycaitlyn

CARDIAC POWER OUTPUT (CPO)

A measure of cardiac pumping ability that accounts for both the pressure- & flow-generating abilities of the heart, and it's the most reliable hemodynamic predictor of mortality outcome in patients c̄ cardiogenic shock (Fincke, et al., 2004).

$$\text{CARDIAC POWER OUTPUT (watts)} = \frac{\text{MAP} \times \text{CO}}{451}$$

@icunursingnotesbycaitlyn

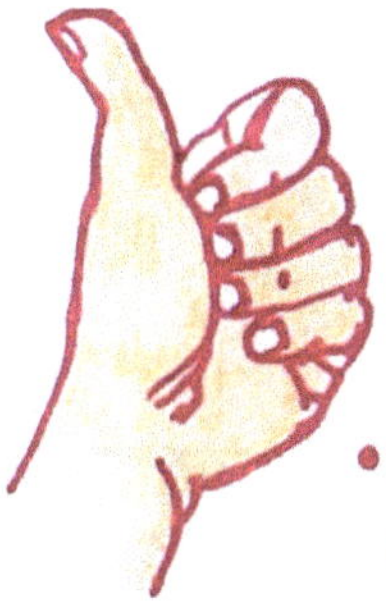

CPO > 0.6

- goal for patients c̄ cardiogenic shock
- greater chance of myocardial recovery
- required for weaning from hemodynamic support

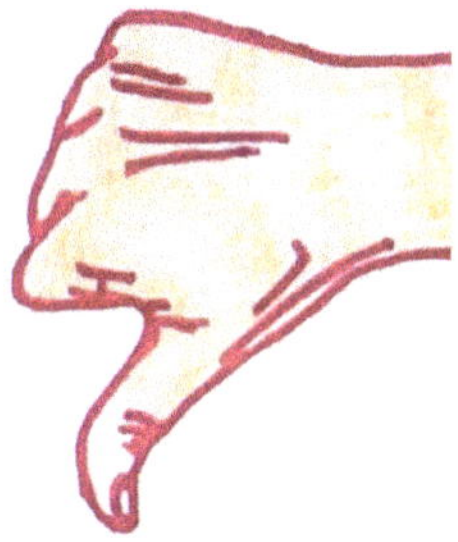

CPO ≤ 0.6

- ↑ risk of in-hospital mortality
- initiation of mechanical circulatory support (MCS) or escalation of support
- right-sided support (RVAD) if PAPi score ≤ 0.9.
- left-sided support if PAPi score is > 0.9.

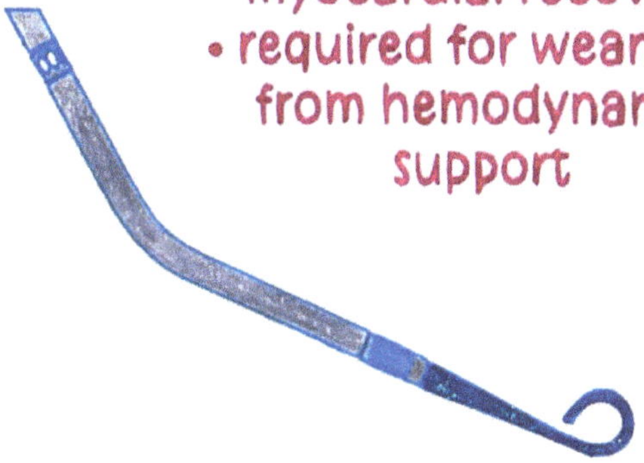

PAPi is an abbreviation for pulmonary artery pulsatility index, which tells us how the right ventricle is doing.

THE IMPELLA RP®

A percutaneous right ventricular support device (RVAD) that provides temporary RV support in patients c̄ severe RV failure s/p LVAD insertion, acute MI, heart transplant, or cardiac surgery.

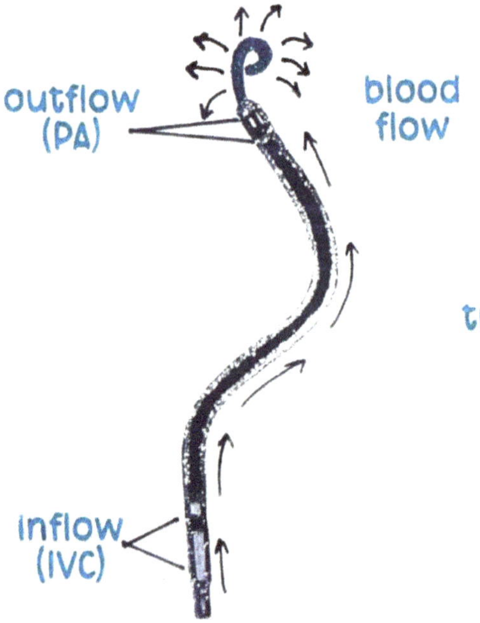

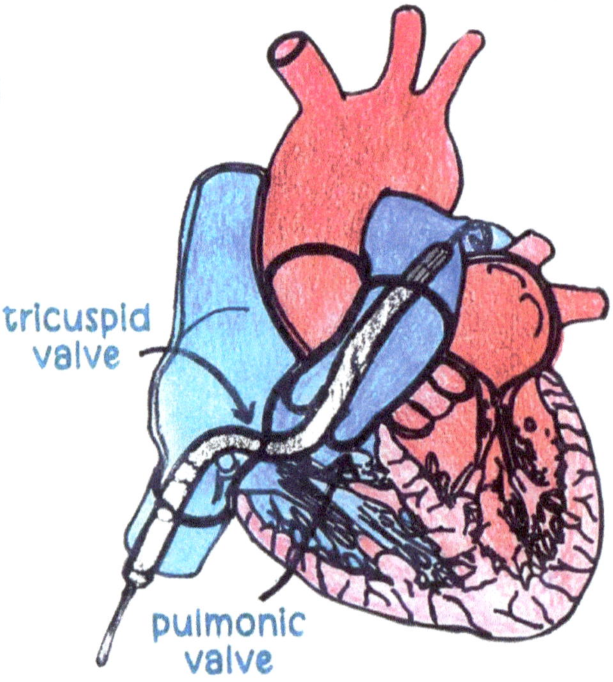

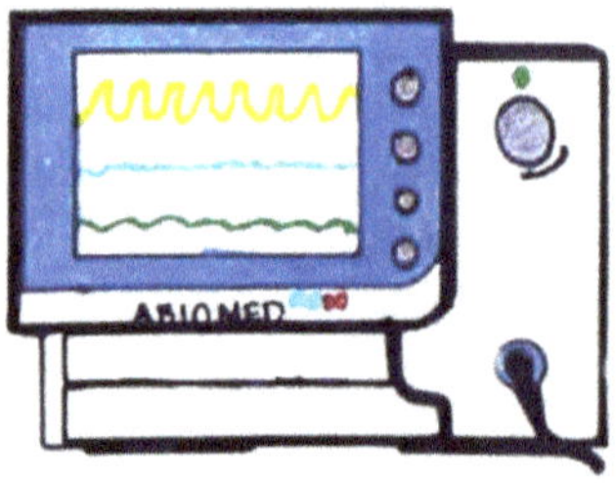

HOW IT WORKS

The Impella RP mechanically unloads the RV & generates forward flow by pumping blood from the inferior vena cava (IVC) to the pulmonary artery (PA), thereby ↓ central venous/right atrial pressures (CVP/RAP), which ↓s RV wall tension & ↓ RV workload, & ↑s overall blood flow to the left side of the heart. This, in turn, ↑s blood flow to the PA, ↑s LV preload, ↑s cardiac output/index (dependent on adequate LV function), & ↑s cardiac power output (CPO). An Impella RP can be used in tandem c̄ the Impella CP or 5.5 for biventricular support (BiPella)!

ECMO

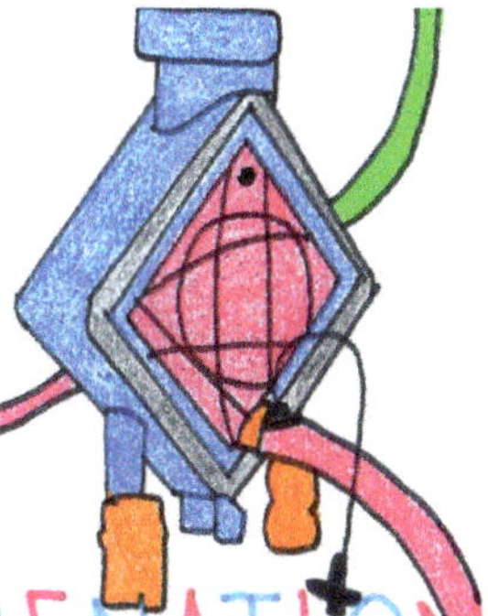

EXTRACORPOREAL MEMBRANE OXYGENATION

INDICATIONS

VV-ECMO
- ARDS
- acute respiratory failure
- bridge to a lung transplant
- trauma (pulmonary contusion)

VA-ECMO
- refractory cardiogenic shock
- inability to wean from CPB
- bridge to a heart transplant/VAD
- complicated MI
- massive PE
- cardiac arrest
- chronic cardiomyopathy
- acute myocarditis

ECMO CIRCUIT

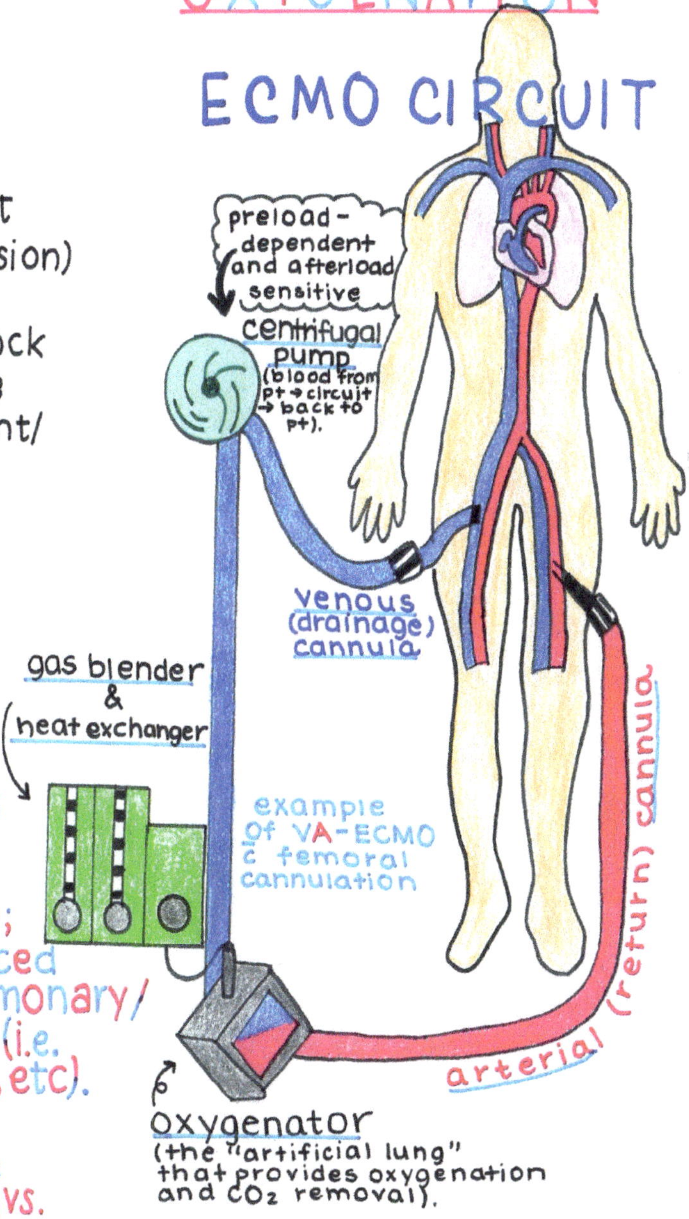

Remember: ECMO is a supportive therapy & not a treatment modality; it's a bridge to advanced therapies to support pulmonary/cardiopulmonary function (i.e. heart/lung transplant, VAD, etc).

See page 2 to learn more about veno-venous (VV) vs. veno-arterial (VA)-ECMO!

HOW IT WORKS

Think of ECMO as a modified cardiopulmonary bypass machine. ECMO provides oxygenated & ventilated blood to the body and functions as either the lungs (VV-ECMO) or both the lungs & the heart (VA-ECMO).

The ECMO circuit consists of a blood pump, a membrane oxygenator, conduit tubing cannulas, & a heat exchanger. Blood is pulled from the venous circulation through an inflow (drainage) cannula & is pumped through an oxygenator before returning to the body through an outflow (return) cannula. The gas blender delivers an air/oxygen mixture to the oxygenator, & the oxygenator removes CO_2 from the blood and oxygenates it. The term "sweep" refers to the oxygen flowing through the oxygenator, & it can be modified to either ↑ or ↓ CO_2 clearance. Positioning of the outflow cannula into arterial circulation creates a veno-arterial (VA) circuit, whereas venous return creates a veno-venous (VV) circuit. VV-ECMO & VA-ECMO have different indications (see page 1).

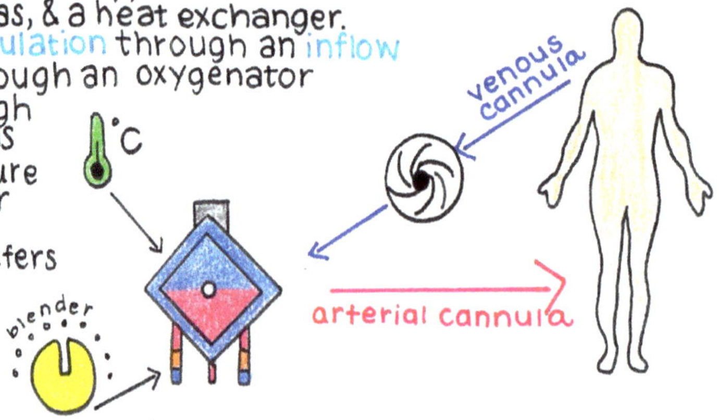

VA-ECMO VS. VV-ECMO

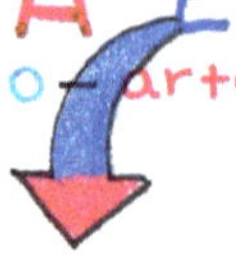

VA-ECMO (veno-arterial)

- Provides complete respiratory & cardiac support without assistance from the native heart.
- ↓ myocardial workload & oxygen consumption.
- Requires both arterial & venous cannulation.
- ↓ RV preload, ↓ RV afterload, ↓ LV preload, ↑ LV afterload
- Lower perfusion rates are needed
- Higher PaO_2 is achieved.
- Ø risk of recirculation
- Risk for North-South (Harlequin) Syndrome with peripheral VA-ECMO.

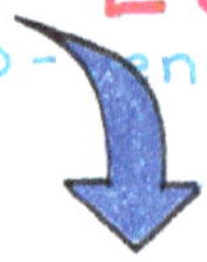

VV-ECMO (veno-venous)

- Provides respiratory support only & relies on native cardiac function.
- Requires only venous cannulation.
- 1 or 2 vessel cannulation.
- Maintains pulmonary blood flow.
- Higher perfusion rates are needed.
- Lower PaO_2 is achieved.
- Risk of recirculation.

@ icunursingnotesby caitlyn

ECMO VS. CPB

ECMO

* Essentially a modified/simplified form of CPB.
* Longer-term support (days to weeks).
* Allows time for intrinsic recovery of the lungs and/or heart.
* More dependent on preload and afterload.
* Requires less anticoagulation.

CPB

* Short-term support intraoperatively (hours).
* Provides support during cardiac surgery.
* Requires more anticoagulation.
* Has a different circuit with additional reservoirs.

General Nursing Care

- Team approach is key!
- Assess for "chattering" or "chugging" of the ECMO circuit tubing; this often indicates hypovolemia. ? the patient's volume status.
- Trace all lines from the patient, ensuring that all connections are secure.
- Assess for clots & air bubbles within the circuit & oxygenator tubing.
- Ensure plasma levels for anticoagulation (i.e. Anti-Xa - depending on facility policy) are therapeutic.
- Monitor for signs of bleeding & hemolysis (CBC, LDH, free hemoglobin, haptoglobin, pink-tinged urine).
- Frequent neurovascular assessments to assess perfusion (pulses, skin color/temp, CRT, S/S of compartment syndrome).
- For patients on peripheral VA-ECMO, monitor for S/S of North-South (Harlequin) Syndrome (hallmark sign: cyanotic upper extremities & well-perfused lower extremities).
- Frequently assess VS, hemodynamics, cardiac/pulmonary status, etc.
- Pain & sedation management.
- Strict I&O & daily weights
- Maintain sterile dressings on all invasive lines/cannula sites; assess all access sites for S/S of infection.
- PI prevention, PUD prophylaxis & VAP prevention.

ECMO "chugging" or "chattering" refers to pulsations in the circuit tubing. Usually, it's caused by hypovolemia. Assess the patient's volume status. ↓ the pump's RPM & blood flow rate is a temporary solution to the problem, but the underlying problem should be corrected in the meantime.

@icunursingnotesbycaitlyn

NORTH-SOUTH (HARLEQUIN) SYNDROME

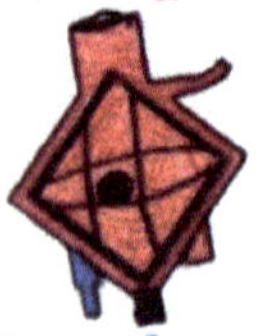

A complication of peripheral VA-ECMO in which oxygenated blood from the ECMO circuit mixes c̄ deoxygenated blood ejected from the heart, leading to significant differences in oxygen saturation between the upper & lower extremities (differential hypoxia).

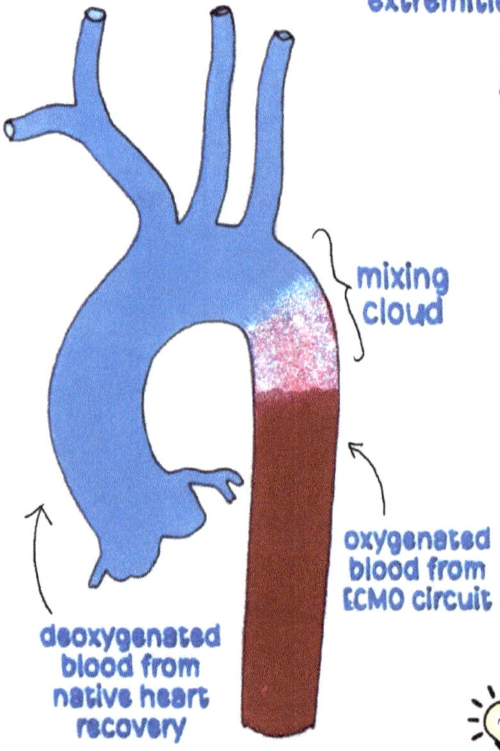

PATHOPHYSIOLOGY

North-South Syndrome is unique to femoral VA-ECMO (doesn't affect patients being treated c̄ central VA-ECMO), & it occurs when native cardiac function returns, but pulmonary function remains impaired. As left ventricular (LV) function recovers, the native cardiac output competes c̄ the ECMO circuit. The LV pumps out deoxygenated blood that mixes c̄ well-oxygenated blood (from the arterial ECMO cannula) in the descending aorta. Recovery of native cardiac function pushes the "mixing point" of the two circulations more distally along the aorta, which causes the patient's native cardiac output to take over perfusion of the cerebral & coronary circulations. Since lung function is still impaired, the heart & brain receive deoxygenated blood, resulting in the hallmark "blue head, red legs" appearance & cardiac and cerebral ischemia.

Think of it as a "tug of war" contest between native cardiac output (antegrade flow) & ECMO flow (retrograde flow).

MANAGEMENT

- ↑VA-ECMO pump flow (if able) to ↑ flow through the lungs
- Optimize ventilator settings (↑FIO2 & PEEP) - this will only help if the lungs are somewhat functional
- Wean & D/C inotropes as cardiac function improves
- Switch to central or VAV ECMO

@icunursingnotesbycaitlyn

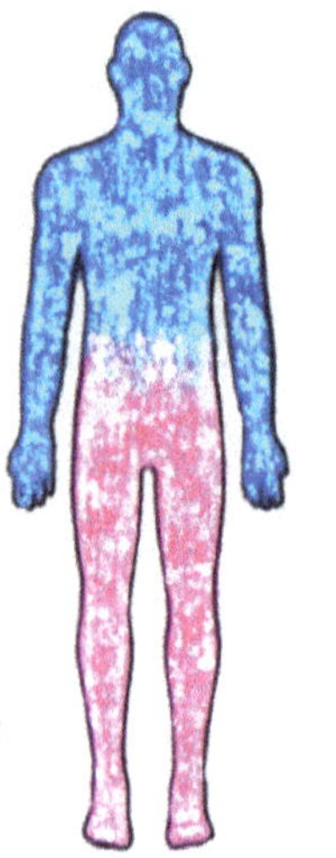

Another sign of LV recovery is a widening pulse pressure on the arterial line - remember that ECMO flow is NOT pulsatile!

EcPella

The use of an Impella device as a left ventricular (LV) venting strategy to unload the LV in patients on VA-ECMO for severe cardiogenic shock.

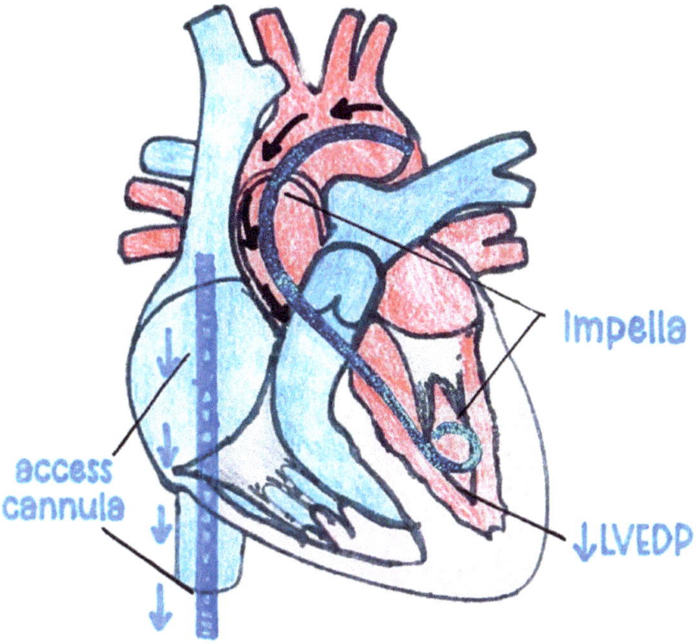

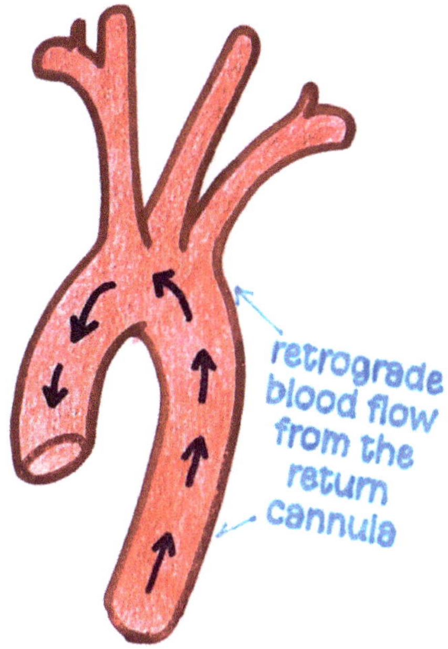

How Does it Work?

When the return cannula is placed in the femoral artery for peripheral VA-ECMO, there is a dramatic ↑ in LV afterload because blood is ejected retrograde within the aorta towards the heart!

In patients c̄ severe LV dysfunction, the LV is unable to generate enough pressure to open the aortic valve against the ↑ afterload generated by the ECMO circuit, resulting in ↓ forward flow & LV distension, which leads to more myocardial damage, acute pulmonary edema (2/2 ↑ LVEDP & ↑ LAP), & LV thrombus (due to blood stasis in the LV). Some warning signs to look for: a narrowing pulse pressure, ↑ PAP & PAWP, & ↓ LV wall motion on echo!

This is where LV venting strategies, like EcPella, are useful. The Impella helps c̄ direct LV unloading by ↓ the pressure & volume within the left ventricle (LVEDP & LVEDV). Because LV wall stress is now reduced, there is ↓ myocardial oxygen demand and, in the setting of a poorly contracting and failing heart, there is a better balance between myocardial oxygen supply & demand!

@icunursingnotesbycaitlyn

INITIATING CVVH

@icunursingnotesbycaitlyn

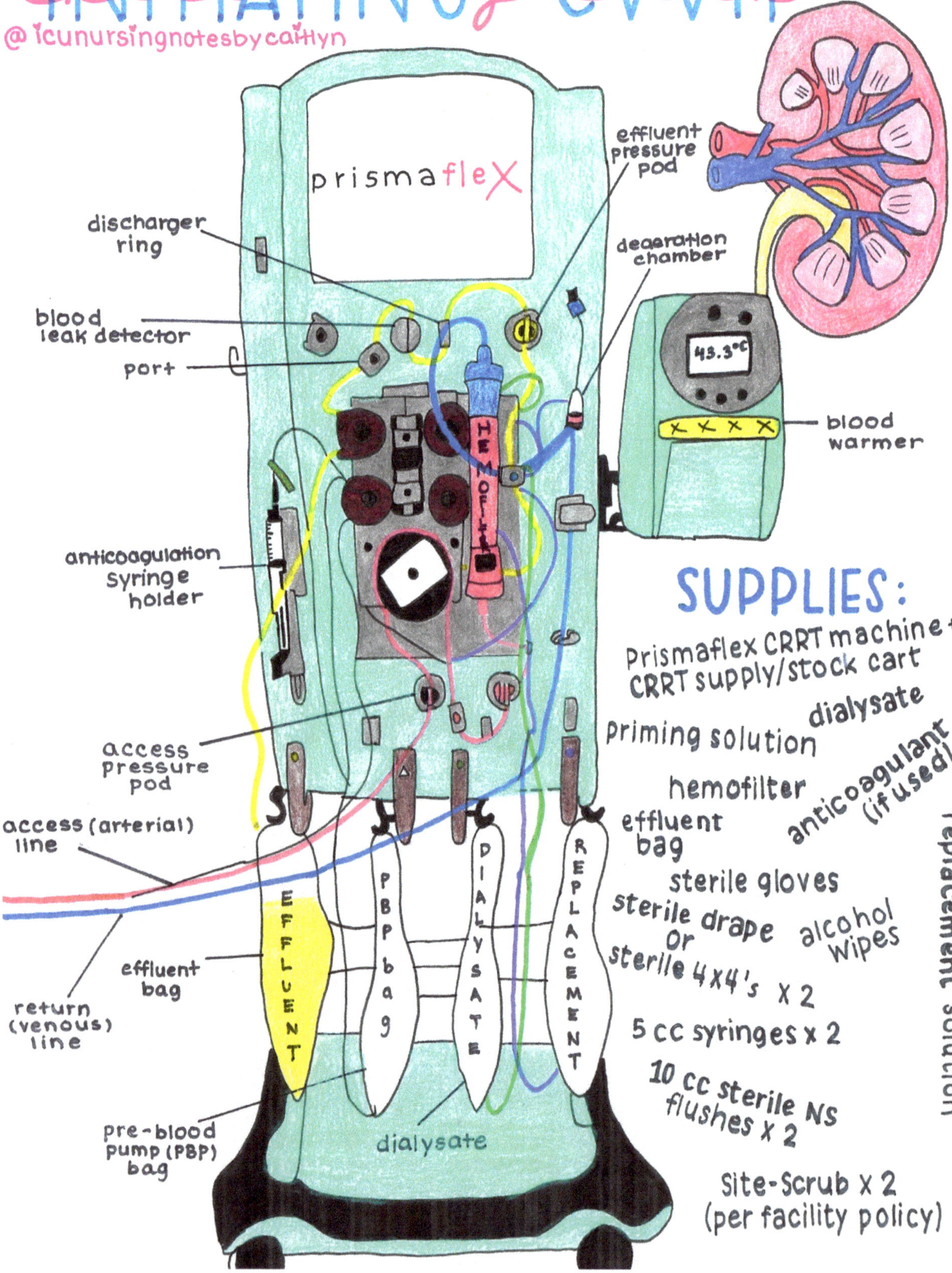

SUPPLIES:

Prismaflex CRRT machine + CRRT supply/stock cart

dialysate

priming solution

hemofilter

anticoagulant (if used)

effluent bag

replacement solution

sterile gloves

sterile drape or sterile 4x4's x 2

alcohol wipes

5 cc syringes x 2

10 cc sterile NS flushes x 2

Site-Scrub x 2 (per facility policy)

INITIATING CVVH: THE STEPS!

PRISMAFLEX MACHINE SET UP OVERVIEW

- Enter treatment settings (blood flow rate, PBP rate, dialysate rate, replacement fluid rate, dialysate rate, replacement fluid rate, patient fluid removal rate, etc) & verify c̄ another RN.
- Load the filter set, attach all pressure pods, route lines (see below for color coordination) & prime the circuit by following the prompts on the screen.
  - → PBP (white), dialysate (green), replacement solution (purple), & effluent (yellow)
- Inspect the circuit for air and manually prime, if needed.
- Adjust the deaeration chamber, ensuring that the fluid is level with the frosted line.
- Prepare to access the dialysis catheter.

ACCESSING THE CATHETER (UDALL/TRIALYSIS)

1. Gather supplies (see pg. 1 of cheat sheet)
2. Establish a sterile field & place a sterile barrier (drape or 4x4 sterile gauze) under the ports on the dialysis catheter.
3. Drop supplies onto the sterile field (syringes, flushes, etc).
4. Put on sterile gloves.
5. Ensuring that the line is clamped, remove the dead-end cap on the arterial (red) port/lumen.
6. Perform a 30 second friction scrub of the arterial hub using a Site-Scrub (per facility policy*).
7. Attach an empty 5 cc syringe, open the clamp, and gently withdraw 5 cc of blood (waste). Clamp & discard.
8. Attach a 10 cc NS flush to the arterial port, open the clamp, & flush with a push-pause/pulsatile technique. Clamp with positive pressure, & leave the syringe attached to the port.
9. Repeat steps 5-8 with the venous (blue) port/lumen.
10. Disconnect the access line from the primed CRRT circuit & attach it to the arterial port on the dialysis catheter & ensure that the connection is secure.
11. Disconnect the return line from the primed circuit & attach it to the venous (blue) port on the dialysis catheter & ensure that the connection is secure.
12. Open the clamps on the dialysis catheter & on the access and return blood lines.
13. Perform a final check of the circuit.
14. Initiate CRRT by following the prompts on the machine.
15. Ensure that all alarms are on & parameters are set appropriately.
16. Record the initial transmembrane potential (TMP) & pressure drop (PD) 3-5 minutes after initiating CRRT.

*For more information on TMP & PD, see my "CRRT" cheat sheet!

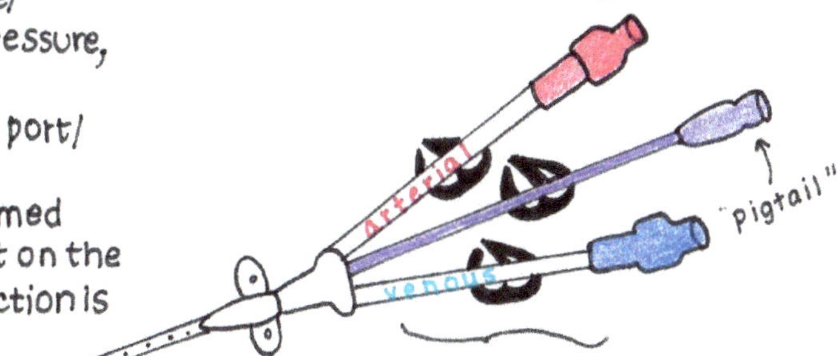

TRIALYSIS CATHETER

@icunursingnotesbycaitlyn

Regional Citrate Anticoagulation In CRRT

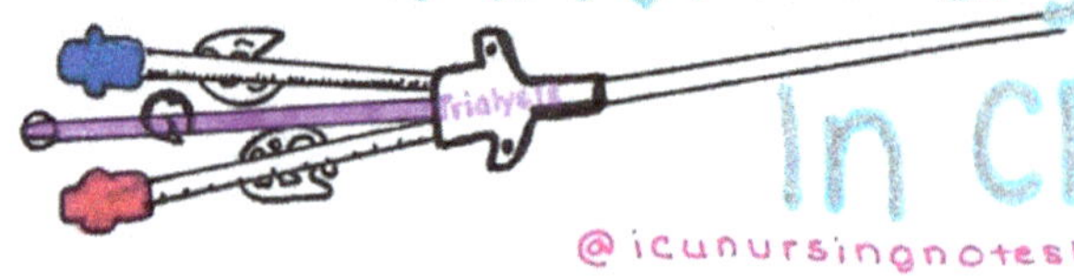

- SCUF
- CVVH
- CVVHD
- CVVHDF

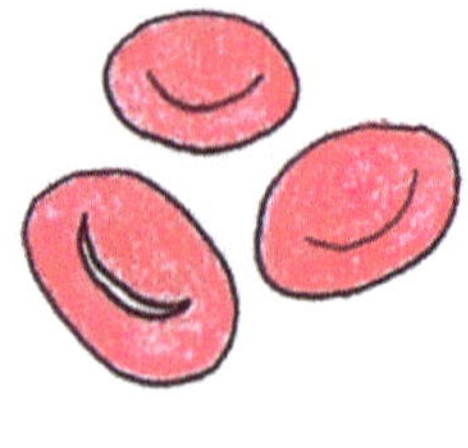

@icunursingnotesbycaitlyn

Indications

For critically ill patients who cannot tolerate conventional anticoagulation c̄ heparin during CRRT for the following reason(s):

1) high risk for bleeding

2) severe coagulopathy

3) heparin-induced thrombocytopenia (HIT)

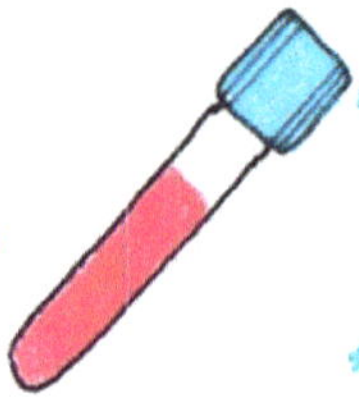

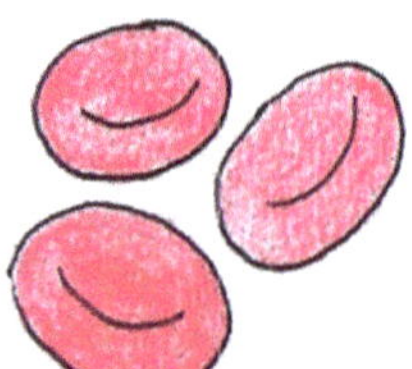

Nursing Care

* Close monitoring of iCa^{2+}, pH, HCO_3^-, and electrolytes (typically Q6 hr labs, but varies - follow your facility's policy).
* Remember that ionized calcium will affect the patient first, so this is a priority if the labs are abnormal.
* Ensure that a calcium-free dialysate solution is used.
* Administer calcium gluconate via the "pigtail" (3rd lumen) of the Trialysis catheter; if CRRT is paused or D/C'd, ensure that the continuous IV calcium infusion is stopped immediately.
* Obtain a baseline iCal and total calcium before initiating CRRT.
* To collect a circuit (post-filter) PTT, aspirate blood from the blue port on the circuit.
* Monitor for complications
  - hypocalcemia, hypomagnesemia
  - metabolic acidosis or alkalosis
  - citrate toxicity*
    - *S/S: persistent or worsening metabolic acidosis, increasing anion gap, and a ↓ in ionized calcium levels c̄ a ↑ in total calcium levels.

Pathophysiology

Citrate is infused via the access line from the pre-blood pump (PBP) where it acts by binding to ionized calcium, which inhibits the clotting cascade at several levels. *It provides regional anticoagulation that is virtually restricted to the extracorporeal circuit* (provides no systemic anticoagulation). Most of the citrate/calcium is cleared through the hemofilter and lost in the effluent, so a continuous IV calcium infusion is required.

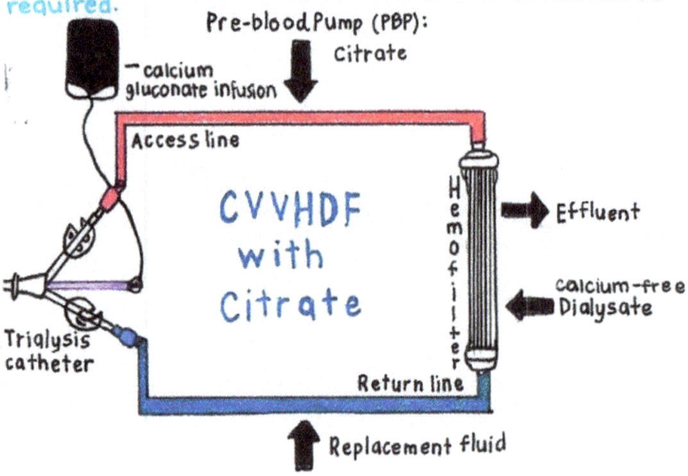

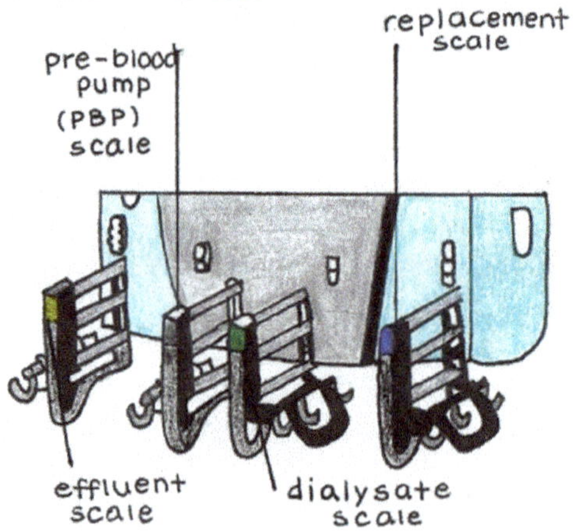

SWAN-GANZ THERMODILUTION CATHETER PORTS

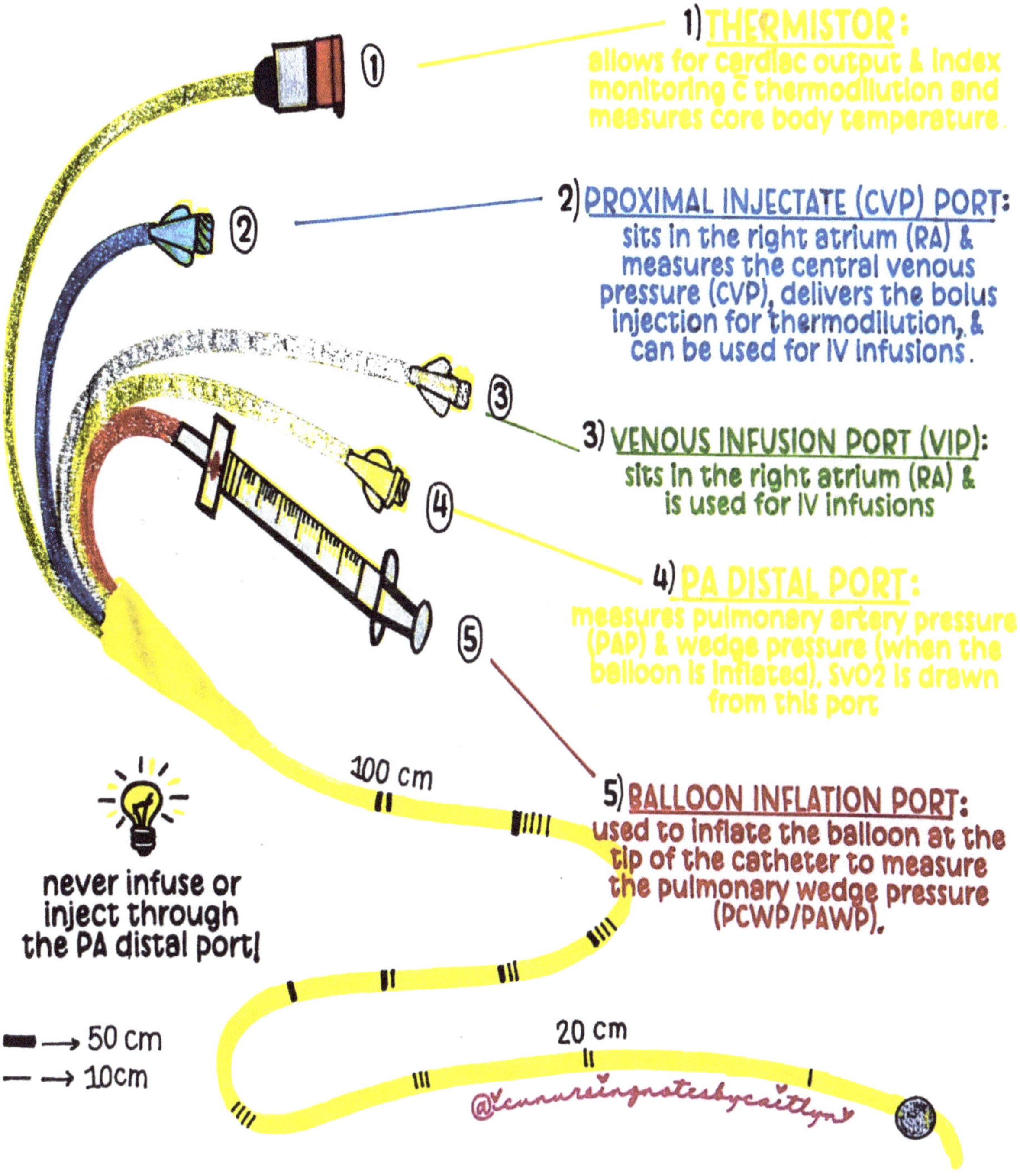

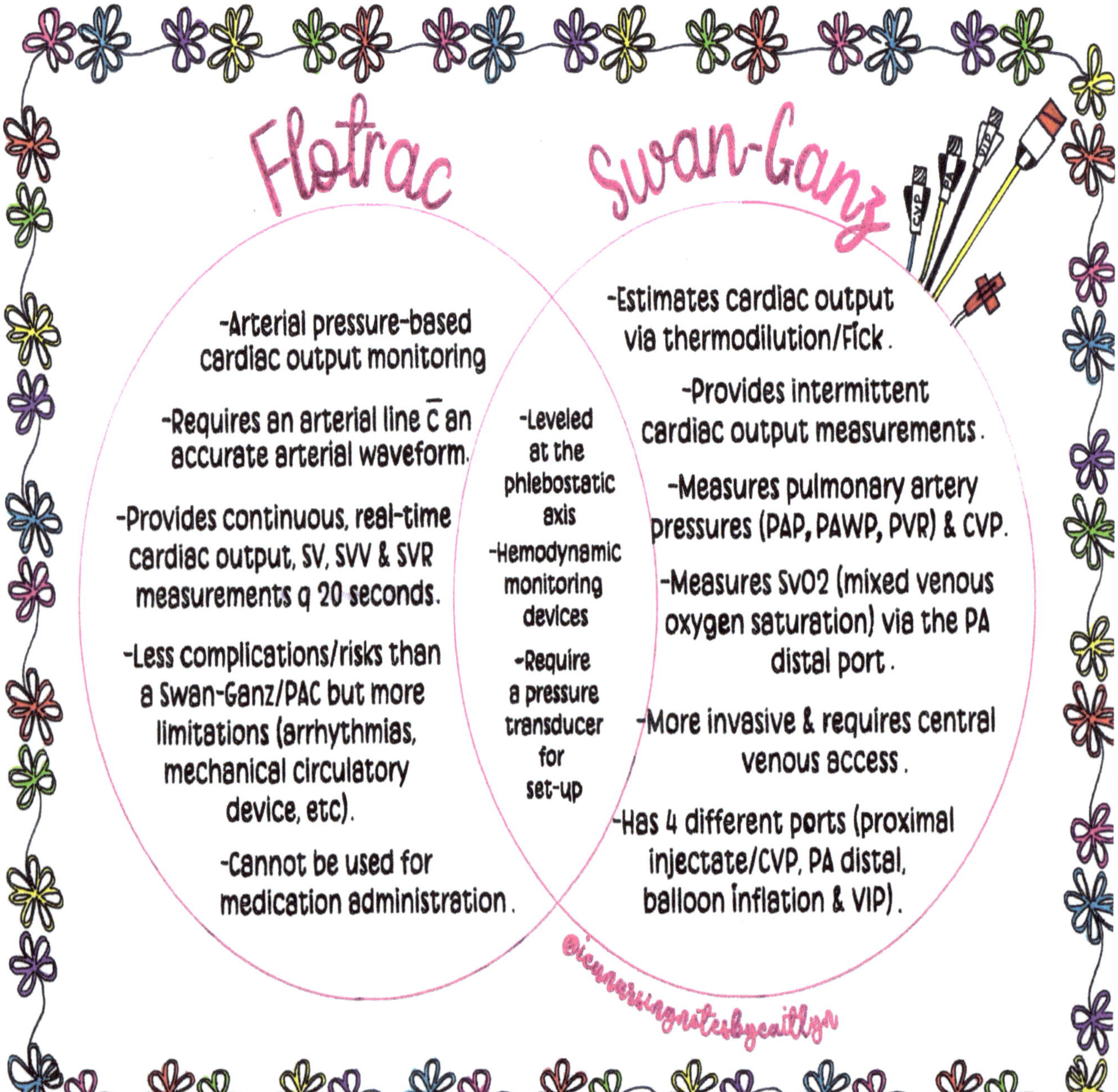
Flotrac
Swan-Ganz
-Arterial pressure-based cardiac output monitoring
-Requires an arterial line c̄ an accurate arterial waveform.
-Provides continuous, real-time cardiac output, SV, SVV & SVR measurements q 20 seconds.
-Less complications/risks than a Swan-Ganz/PAC but more limitations (arrhythmias, mechanical circulatory device, etc).
-Cannot be used for medication administration.
-Leveled at the phlebostatic axis
-Hemodynamic monitoring devices
-Require a pressure transducer for set-up
-Estimates cardiac output via thermodilution/Fick.
-Provides intermittent cardiac output measurements.
-Measures pulmonary artery pressures (PAP, PAWP, PVR) & CVP.
-Measures SvO2 (mixed venous oxygen saturation) via the PA distal port.
-More invasive & requires central venous access.
-Has 4 different ports (proximal injectate/CVP, PA distal, balloon inflation & VIP).
@icunursingnotesbycaitlyn

TRANSVENOUS PACEMAKERS

Part I: Understanding the Pacer Box

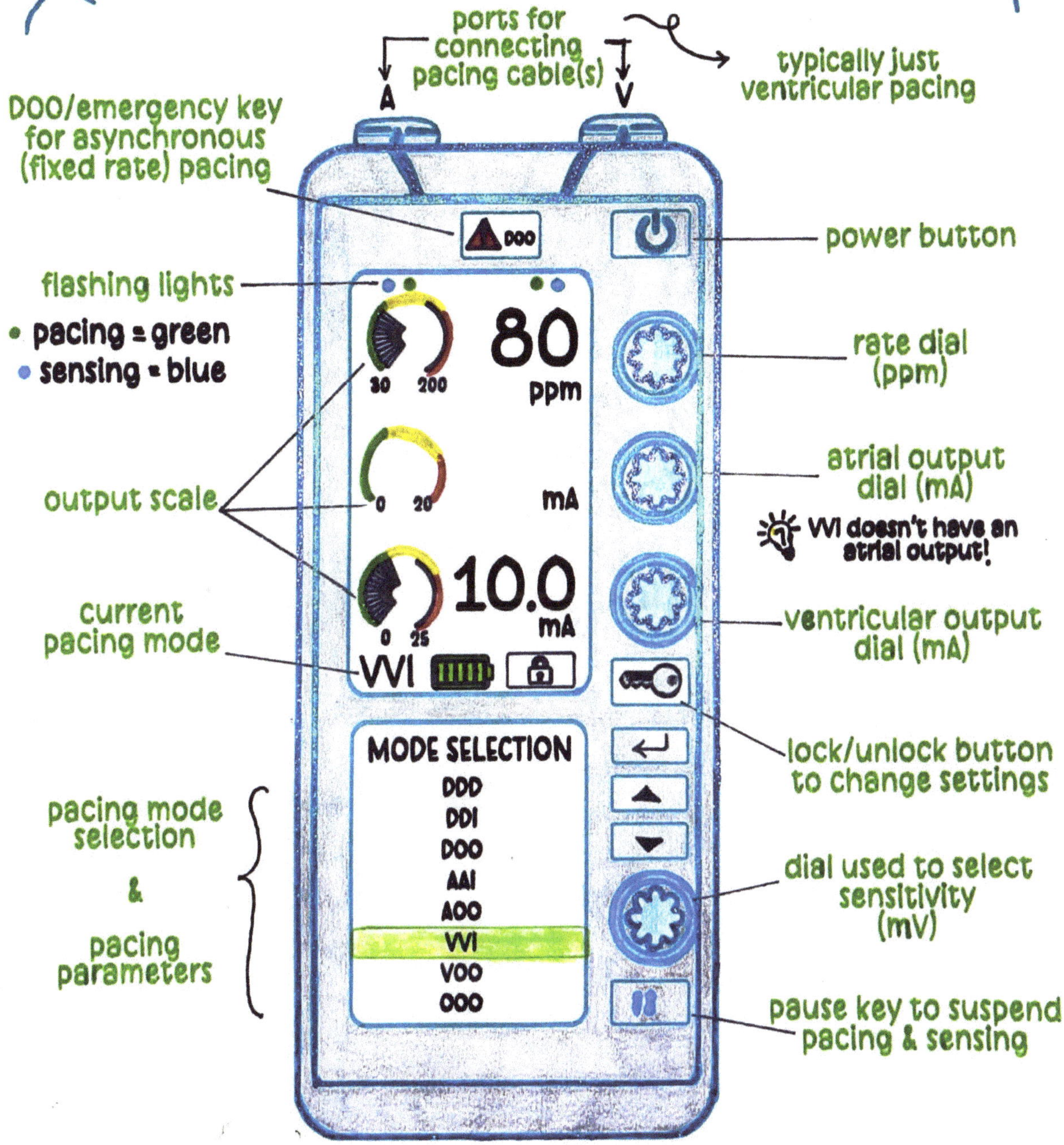

@icunursingnotesbycaitlyn

TRANSVENOUS PACEMAKERS

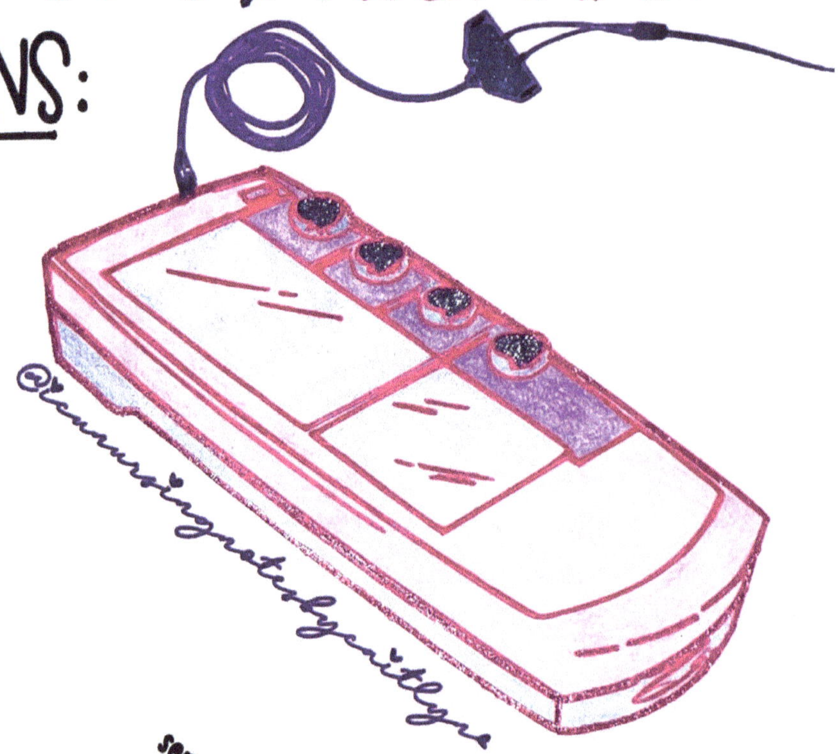

INDICATIONS:

- symptomatic bradycardia
- second degree type II AV block (Mobitz II)
- third degree AV block (complete)
- procedures requiring prophylactic pacing support

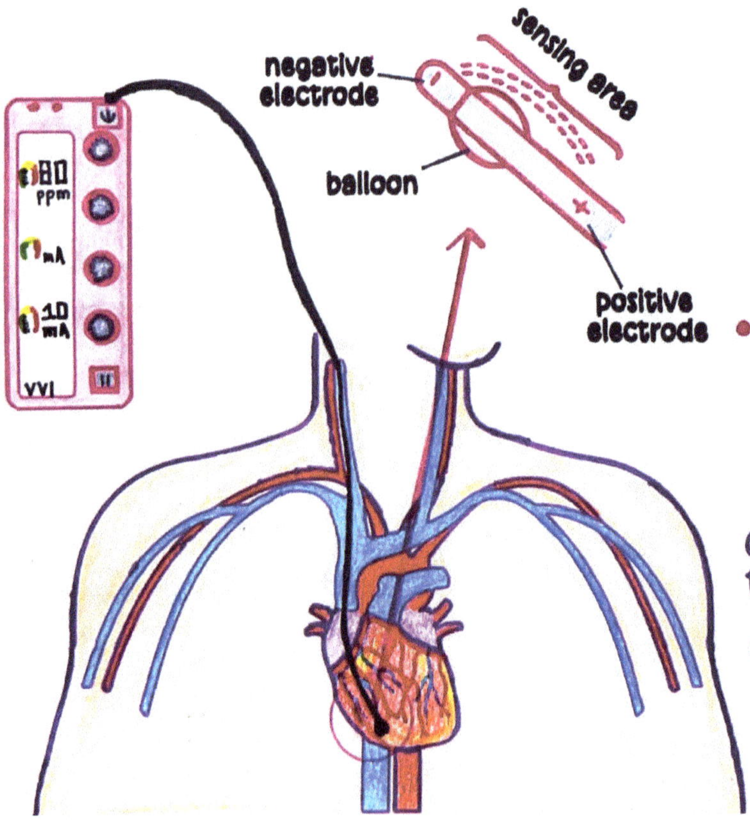

INSERTION:

- requires central venous access c̄ a 6-Fr Cordis sheath
- right internal jugular (RIJ) is preferred
  - left subclavian
  - femoral vein
- pacing electrode catheter is guided into the right ventricle (RV)
- note the position of the temp wire (cm)
  - small dashes - 10 cm
  - 1 big dash - 50 cm

Temporary Pacemakers:

Modes & Basic Settings

The external (temporary) pacemaker has 3 letters that indicate the pacer setting:

VVI

AAI

DDD

AOO/VOO/DOO

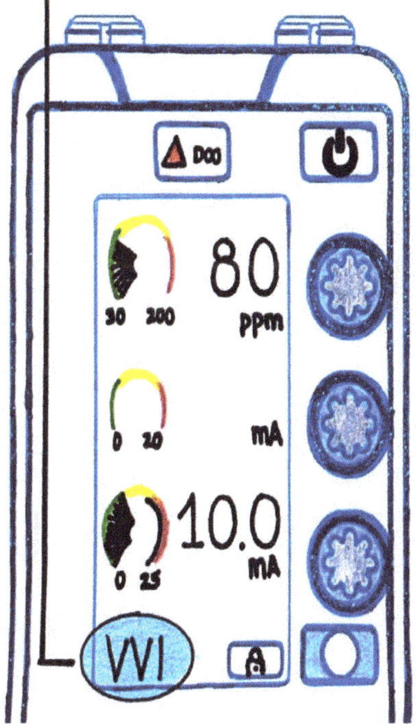

1ST LETTER: CHAMBER(S) PACED

This is the chamber being paced - the atrium (A), ventricle (V), or both (D). The pacer sends the electrical impulse to this chamber.

A = atrium
V = ventricle
D = dual

2ND LETTER: CHAMBER(S) SENSED

This is the chamber that the external pacer is "looking at" (atrium, ventricle, or both) to see if the heart is, in fact, depolarizing or if it needs to be paced.

A = atrium
V = ventricle
D = dual
O = none/nothing

3RD LETTER: RESPONSE TO SENSING

This is what the external pacer does after it senses intrinsic electrical activity (native heartbeat)

T = pacing triggered
I = pacing inhibited
d = dual (T & I)
O = none/nothing

@icunursingnotesbycaitlyn

Nursing Care of Transvenous Pacemakers

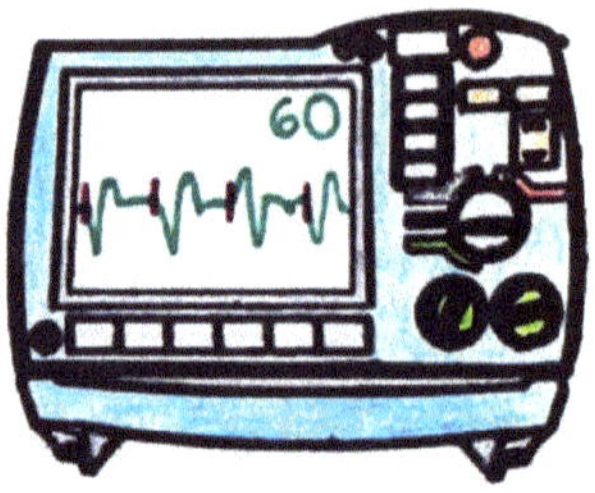

- Keep pads & pacing leads on your patient & have a Zoll/Lifepak at the bedside at all times in the event that your patient requires transcutaneous pacing.
- Verify that the pacemaker mode, rate, & output (mA) is set according to orders, & it's functioning properly. Ensure the screen is locked.

The sensing light (blue) & the pacing light (green) should flash c̄ each sensed & paced beat!

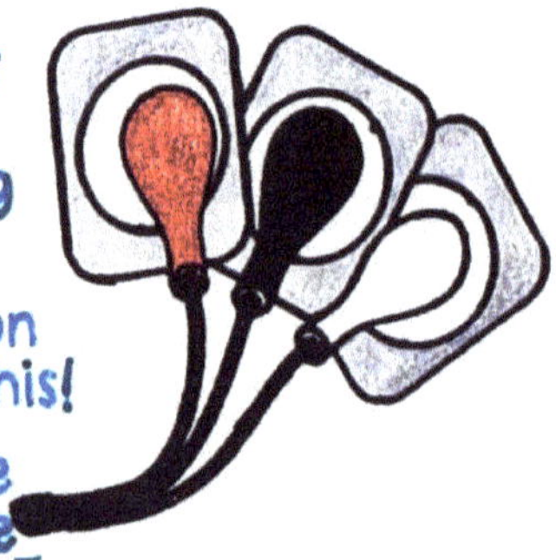

- Monitor rhythm, vital signs & for adequate capture & sensing. Is there a QRS for q ventricular pacing spike? Is the rate appropriate for the pacemaker setting? Does the sensing light flash c̄ q sensed beat? Does the pacing light flash c̄ q paced beat?
- Daily check of the patient's intrinsic rhythm & stimulation threshold (capture mA). Follow your hospital's policy for this!
- If your patient has a balloon-tipped pacing wire, ensure that the balloon port is locked c̄ the empty 3 cc syringe attached. Always make sure that the balloon is deflated ā you remove a TVP!

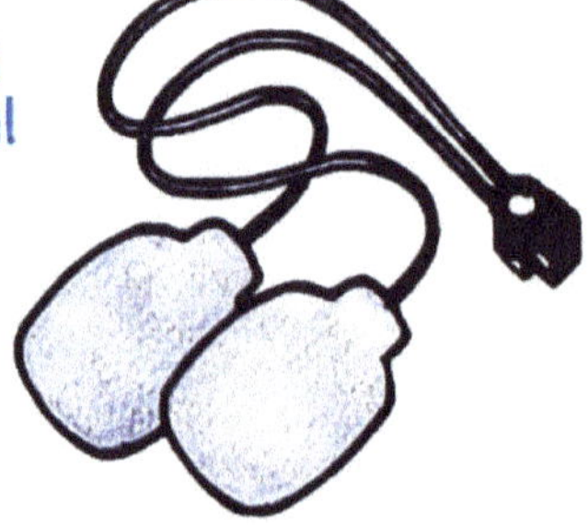

- Hang the pacer box from an IV pole to prevent pulling on wires/cables. Use a Tegaderm to secure the external part of the pacing wire.
- Assess the TVP insertion site (remember that this is a central line) & document the position of the wire.

small dashes = 10 cm
1 big dash = 50 cm

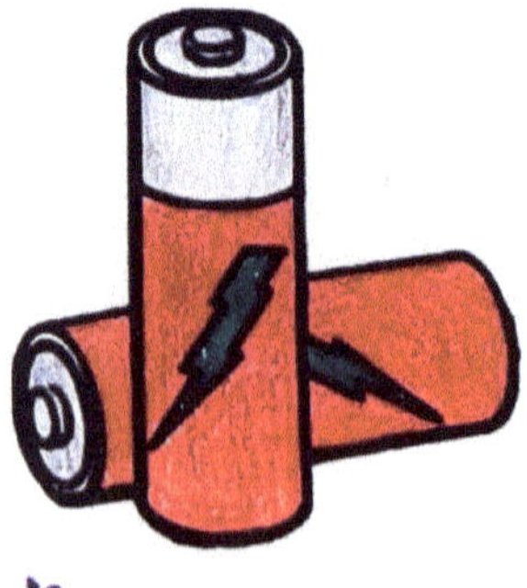

- Continuously monitor the patient's cardiac rhythm & monitor for failure to capture, failure to pace, & failure to sense (see my previous note sheet on troubleshooting).
- Ensure that spare batteries are taped to the back of the pacer box.
- Monitor for complications: lead migration, lead fracture, myocardial perforation/cardiac tamponade, infection, hemothorax, stimulation of the diaphragm, embolus, & thrombosis.

@icunursingnotesbycaitlyn

Troubleshooting Temporary Pacemakers!

Failure to Pace

the pacer fails to send out electrical impulses when it should be

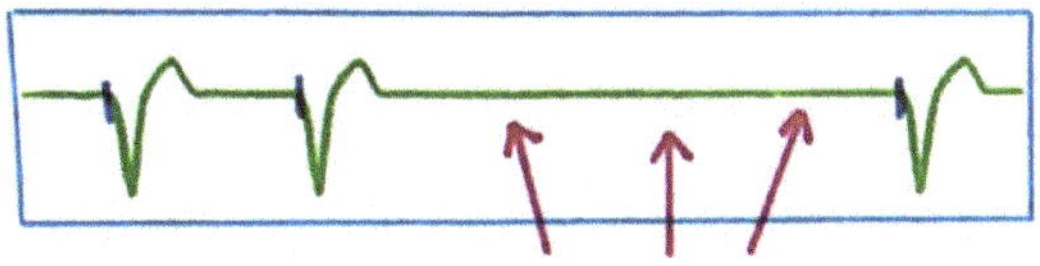

- look for the absence of pacer spikes
- check connections, check the battery, ↓ sensitivity (↑ mV), consider lead fracture
- be prepared to transcutaneously pace (if the patient is pacer-dependent)

@icunursingnotesbycaitlyn

Failure to Capture

the pacemaker delivers a pacing stimulus, but it's unable to initiate depolarization

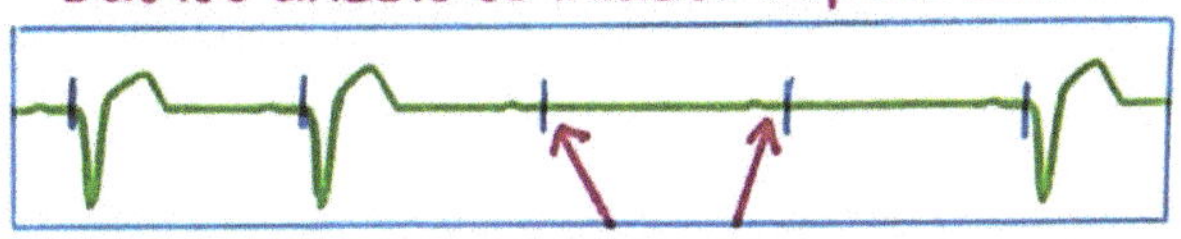

- look for a pacer spike s̄ a P wave or QRS complex after it
- ↑ the output (mA) 10% above capture threshold & check all connections
- r/o lead migration & cardiac perforation
- check labs!
- be prepared to transcutaneously pace!

Undersensing

the pacer fails to sense the patient's underlying rhythm & paces regardless

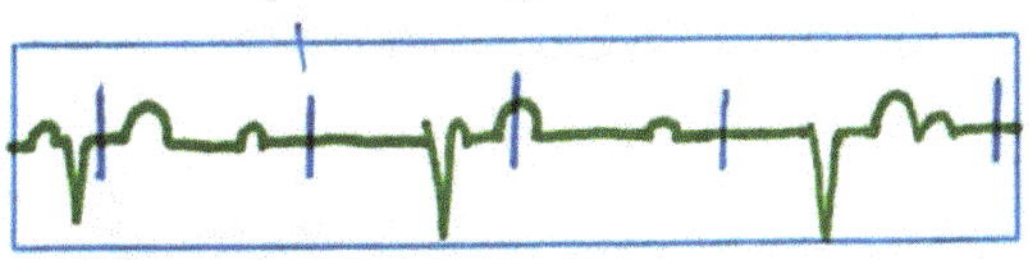

- look for random pacer spikes where they shouldn't be (within the P wave, QRS, or T wave)
- leads to overpacing
- risk of R-on-T phenomenon
- ↑ the sensitivity, check connections, consider lead fracture or migration, & check the battery

Oversensing

the pacer mistakes artifact for intrinsic cardiac activity & inhibits pacing

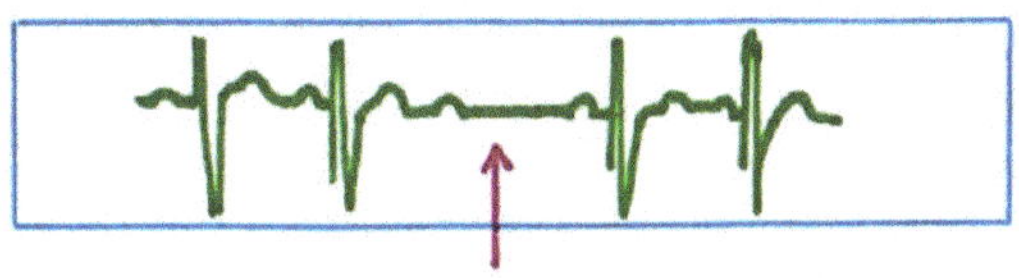

- look for an absent pacer spike
- leads to underpacing
- can be caused by large P & T waves, MRI, electrocautery & muscle movement
- ↓ the sensitivity (↑ mV) to temporarily switch to asynchronous mode

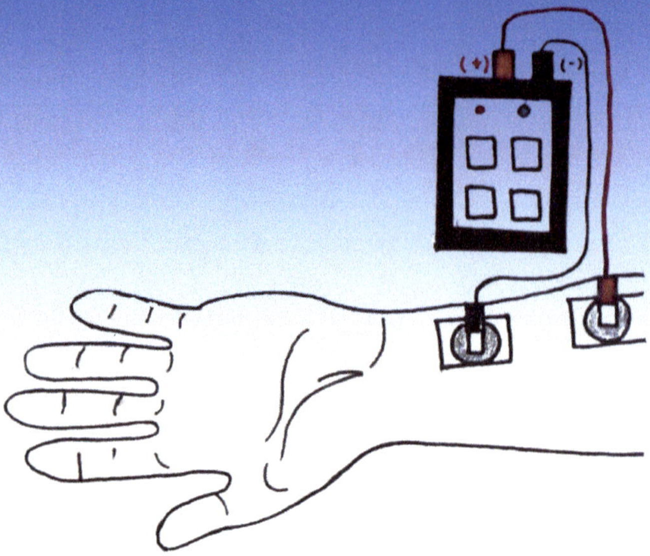

MISCELLANEOUS

miscellaneous

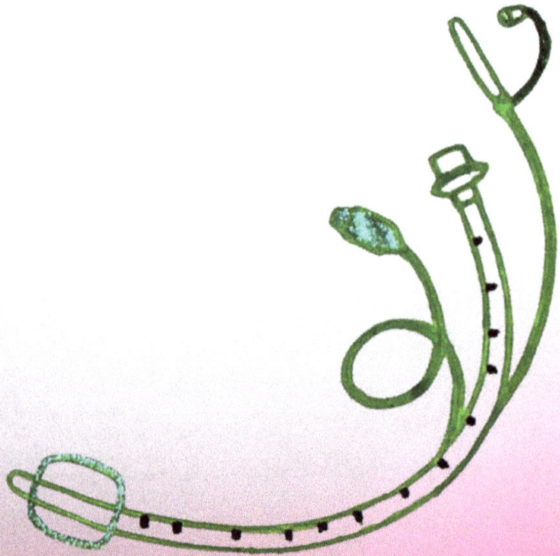

ICU Head-to-Toe Assessment Tips

Bedside Safety Check:

- Are all alarms on the bedside monitor on and set appropriately?
- Is an Ambu-bag and suction readily available and working?
- Are all lines/tubes/drains appropriately secured and draining/infusing?
- Is the patient properly restrained? Or is the bed alarm on PRN?
- Are there any immediate safety concerns?
- Will any drips run dry and need to be replaced soon?
- Is the patient comfortable? Does sedation need to be adjusted?
- Do you have emergency IV access available? Ask yourself, "In the event of an emergency, where can I push code medications?"
- Is the ETT secure?
- Does the gtt concentration and rate on the pump match the order?
- Did you level, zero, and flush the transducers and note waveforms?

* tip: This is critically important when titrating vasoactive gtts. Abnormal waveforms can also indicate catheter migration (ex: Swan-Ganz).

Neuro:

- orientation status / LOC
- pain assessment: 0-10, CPOT
- pupil assessment
- assess for ability to follow commands and move all extremities
- RASS score - does sedation need to be ↑ or ↓? or is the patient comfortable?
- basic reflexes (cough, gag, corneals) - important for intubated/sedated patients.

* tip: pause sedation for an accurate and thorough neuro assessment (exception: TTM post-cardiac arrest).

Cardiac:

- rate/rhythm
- pacemaker/ICD
  - → if the pt has a pacemaker, ensure that you select the "paced" mode on the bedside monitor
- heart sounds, murmurs
- perfusion (CRT, pulses, SvO_2, skin color/temp).
- check if the patient has had a recent echo - it's important to know your patient's EF!
- level and zero all hemodynamic monitoring systems (Swan-Ganz, art line, CVP, etc).
- DVT prophylaxis

Respiratory:

- lung sounds
- oral care
- WOB
- O_2 devices
- ETT: location, vent settings, skin breakdown, secure?, need for suctioning, synchrony.
- ABGs
- Chest tubes: presence of an air leak?, tidaling, correct level of H_2O in the suction chamber.

GI/GU:

- nutrition: tube feeds (goal rate? residuals?), NPO? Diet order?
- bowel sounds, last BM
- OGT placement/securement/residuals, PUD prophylaxis
- abdomen: soft? firm? tender?
- hourly UOP, strict I/O
- Foley care + maintenance
- most recent labs?

Skin:

- color/temperature
- assess for wounds

* tip: Time your skin assessment c̄ a turn; look at the patient's back/do your skin assessment, and listen to posterior lung sounds at the same time!

- assess incision sites
- pressure injury prevention strategies
- daily CHG bath
- wound care

Lines/Tubes/Drains:

- access site assessments
- document insertion length for a Swan-Ganz catheter
- flush all peripheral IVs + central line lumens to ensure patency
- tubing and CVC dressings are labeled + CDI.
  - ← Check for compatibility before Y-siting IV meds.
- Check the settings on any device + the insertion site for any complications: IABP, Impella, TVP, Swan-Ganz, CRRT, etc!

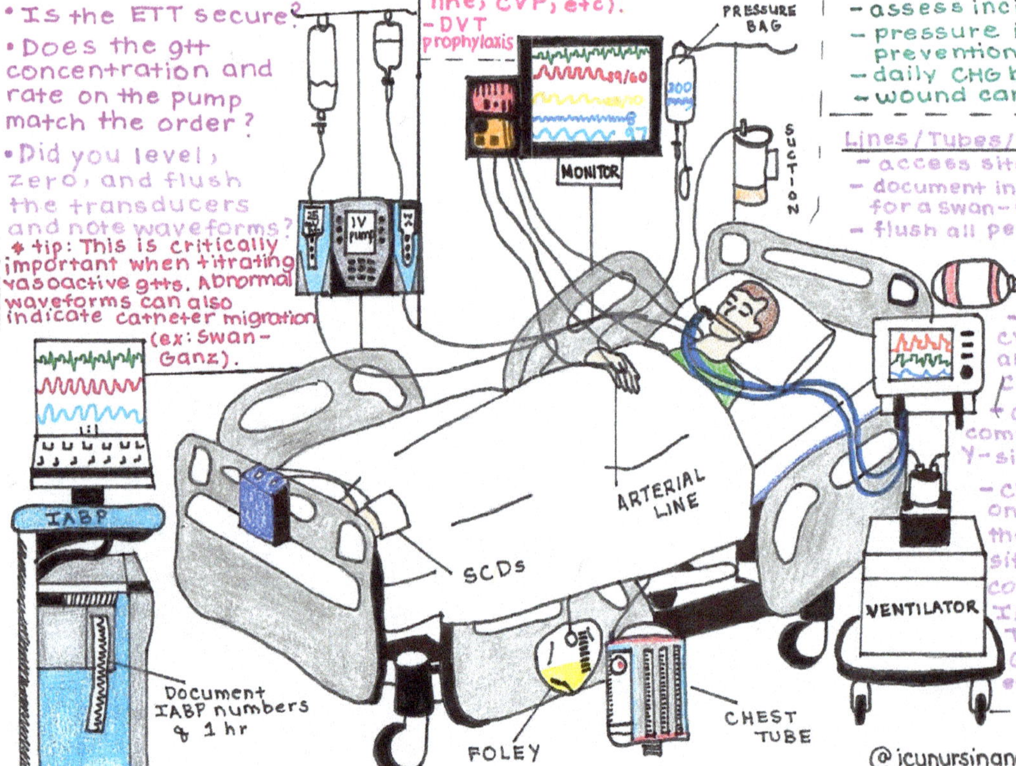

@icunursingnotesbycaitlyn

VASCULAR ACCESS DEVICES

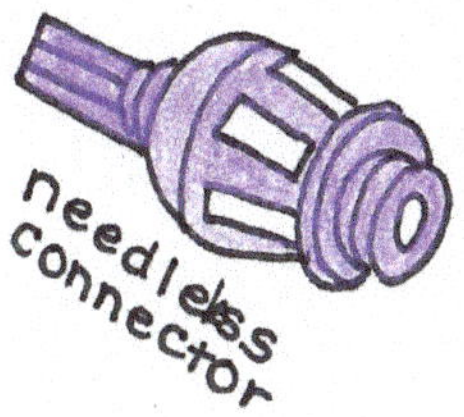

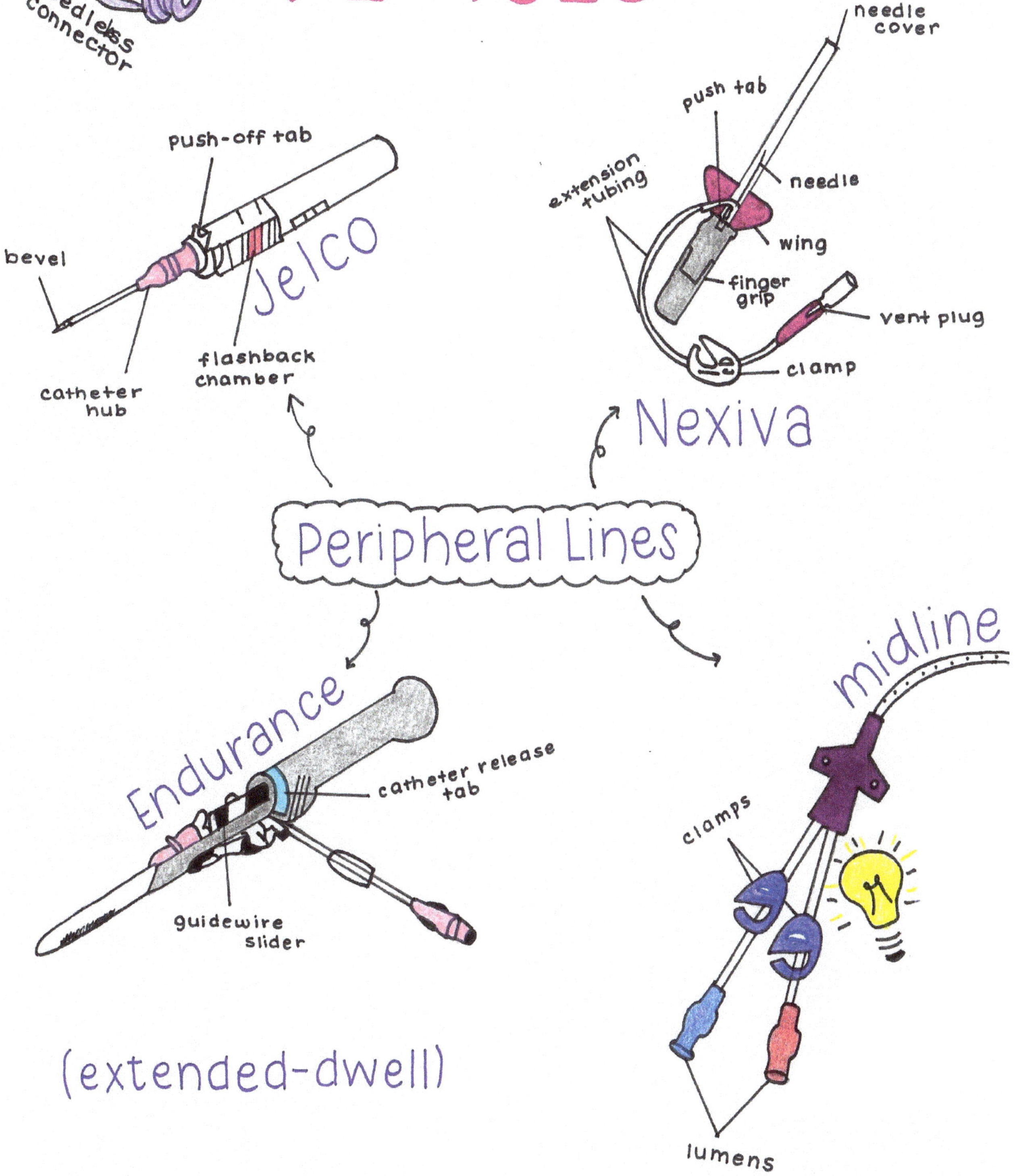

Central Lines

Cordis

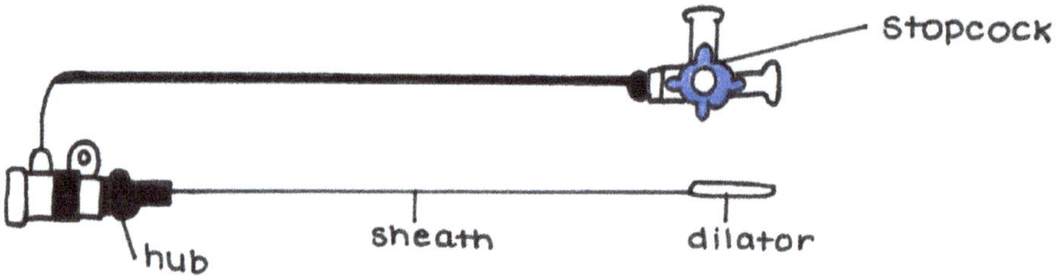

- essentially a sheath introducer c̄ a side port.
- a transvenous pacer (TVP), Swan-Ganz catheter (SGC), or a triple lumen can be floated through a Cordis.
- typically inserted in the internal jugular (IJ).

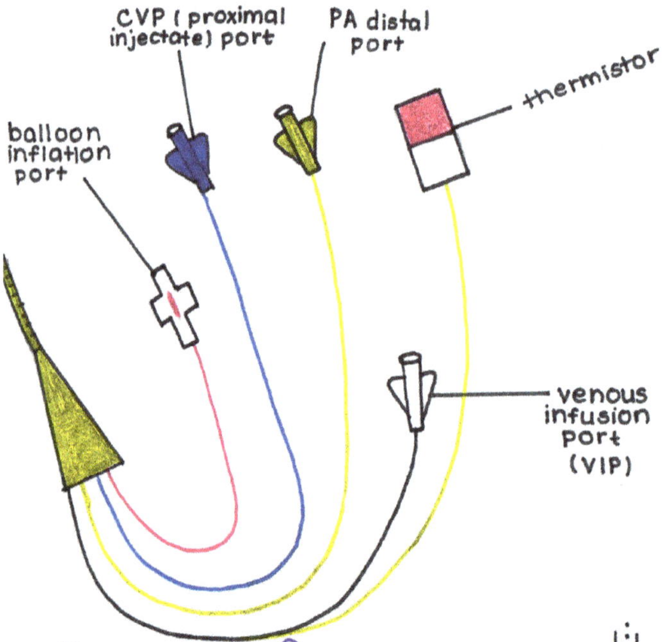

Swan-Ganz

- also known as a pulmonary artery catheter (PAC)/ thermodilution.
- used to perform thermodilution/determine cardiac output and to monitor a patient's hemodynamics.
- tip terminates in the pulmonary artery (PA).

triple lumen

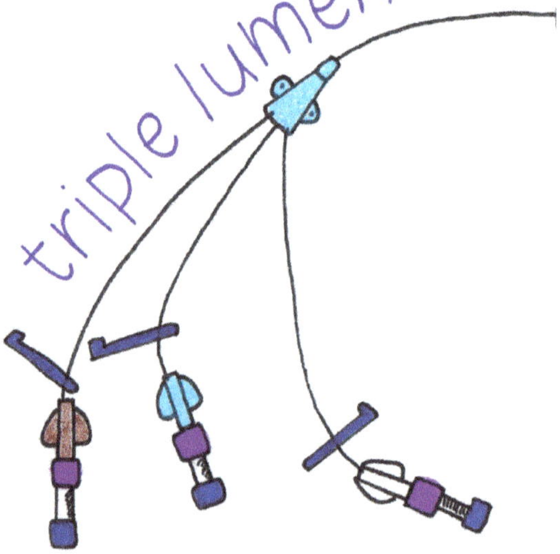

- typically inserted in the IJ (or fem)
- more lumens = ↑ risk of infection
- distal port can be used to transduce CVP.

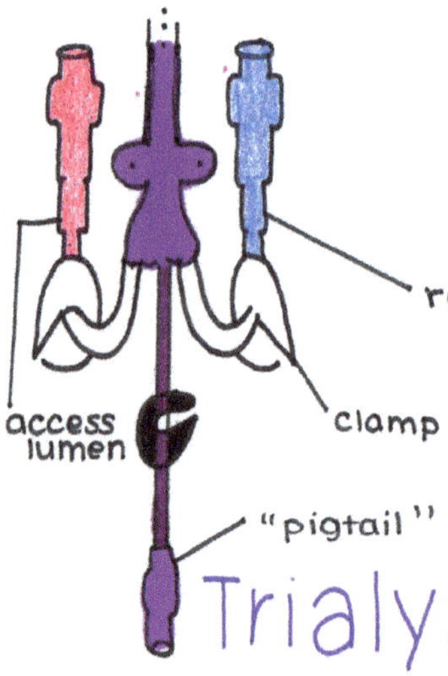

Trialysis

temporary HD catheter

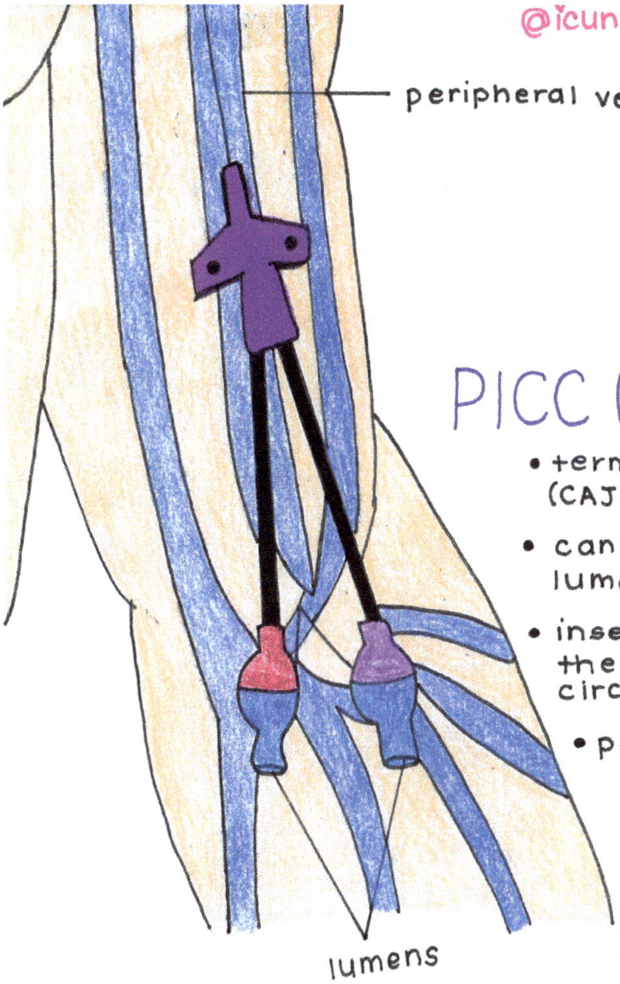

PICC (double lumen)

- terminates in the cavo-atrial junction (CAJ) - lower 1/3 of the SVC.
- can be a single, double, or triple lumen.
- inserted in a peripheral vein, but the catheter tip terminates in central circulation.
- patients can be discharged c̄ PICCs.

Port-a-Cath

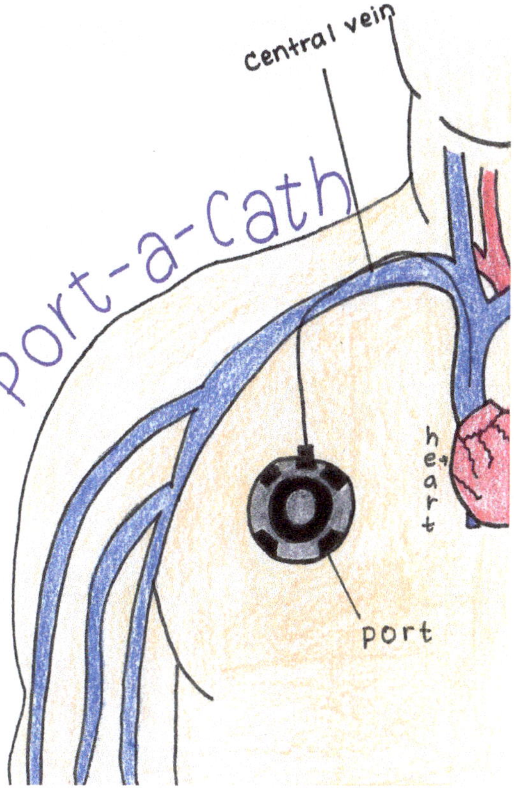

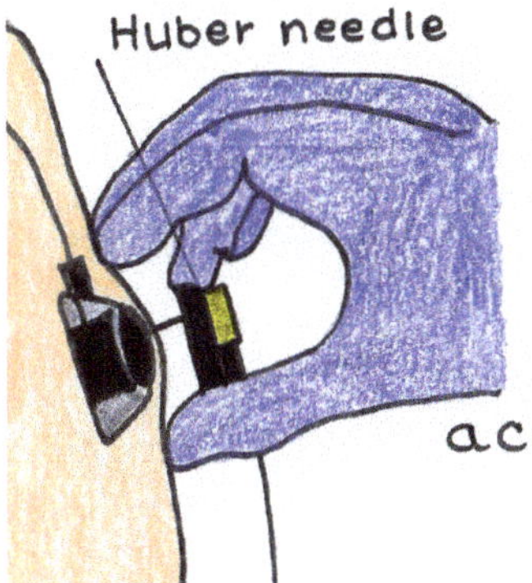

Always use a Huber needle to access a port!

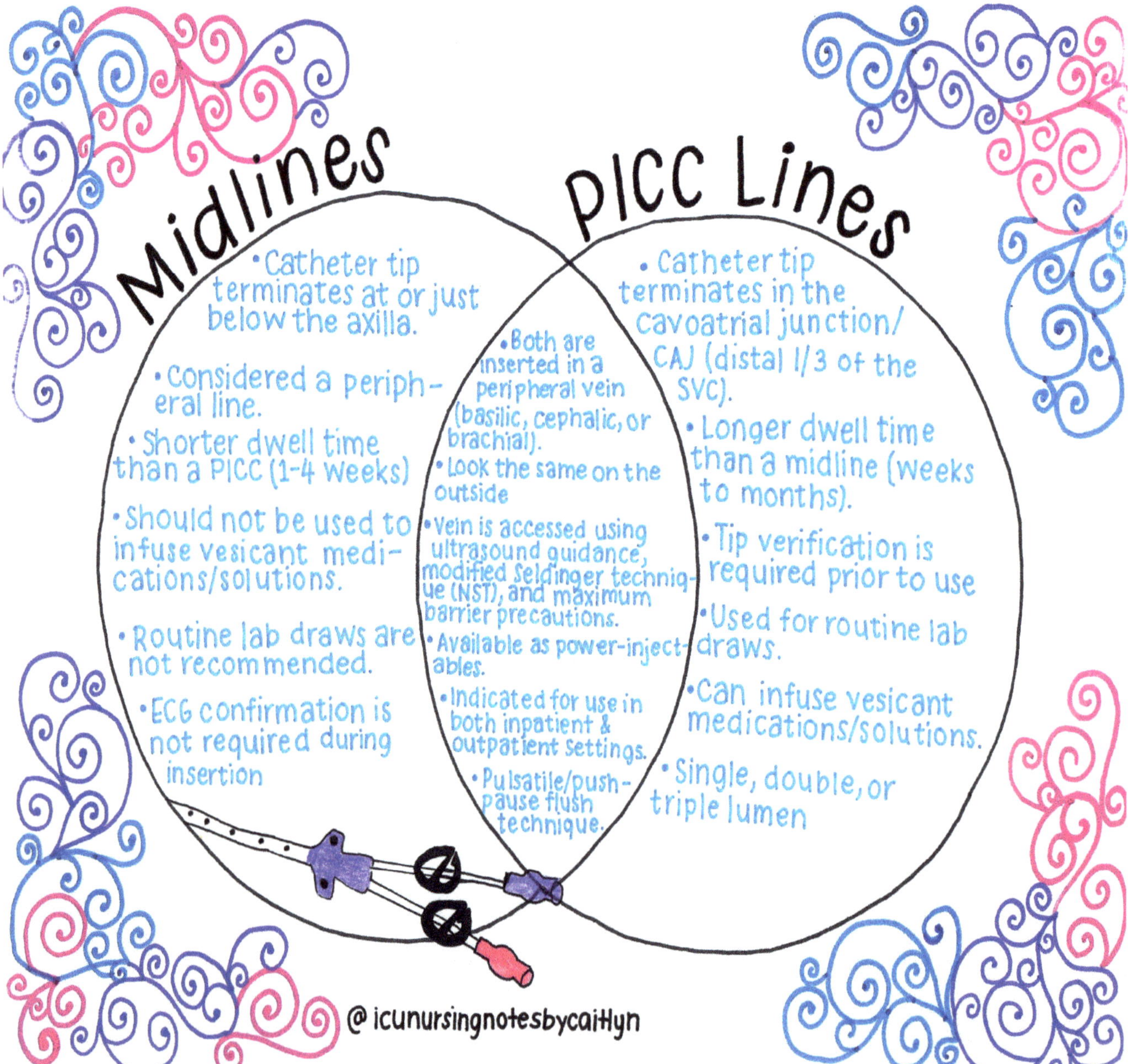
Midlines
PICC Lines
•Catheter tip terminates at or just below the axilla.
•Considered a peripheral line.
•Shorter dwell time than a PICC (1-4 weeks)
•Should not be used to infuse vesicant medications/solutions.
•Routine lab draws are not recommended.
•ECG confirmation is not required during insertion
•Both are inserted in a peripheral vein (basilic, cephalic, or brachial).
•Look the same on the outside
•Vein is accessed using ultrasound guidance, modified Seldinger technique (NST), and maximum barrier precautions.
•Available as power-injectables.
•Indicated for use in both inpatient & outpatient settings.
•Pulsatile/push-pause flush technique.
•Catheter tip terminates in the cavoatrial junction/ CAJ (distal 1/3 of the SVC).
•Longer dwell time than a midline (weeks to months).
•Tip verification is required prior to use
•Used for routine lab draws.
•Can infuse vesicant medications/solutions.
•Single, double, or triple lumen
@icunursingnotesbycaitlyn

INTRAOSSEOUS (IO) ACCESS

Using the Bones When the Veins Won't Do!

INDICATIONS

In patients requiring emergent vascular access & peripheral or central venous access is not possible/feasible in a timely manner (i.e. cardiac arrest c̄ poor access, traumas, rapid sequence intubation/RSI, etc).

ACCESS SITES:

* Proximal humerus
* Proximal tibia
* Distal tibia

PATHOPHYS

The IO route provides access to the systemic venous circulation via the medullary cavity, which provides a non-collapsible entry point to central venous circulation. Infused medications or fluids enter the small vessels (venous sinusoids) within the medullary cavity, drain into the central venous channel, and exit the bone via the nutrient or emissary veins. The major vessels into which the emissary veins drain depends on the insertion site:

- proximal humerus: axillary vein
- proximal tibia: popliteal vein
- distal tibia: great saphenous vein

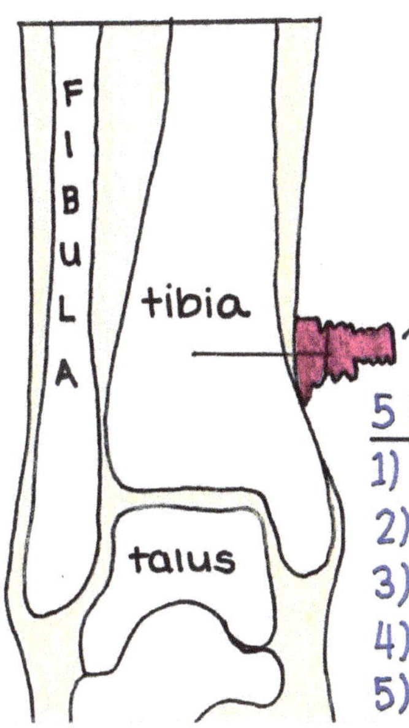

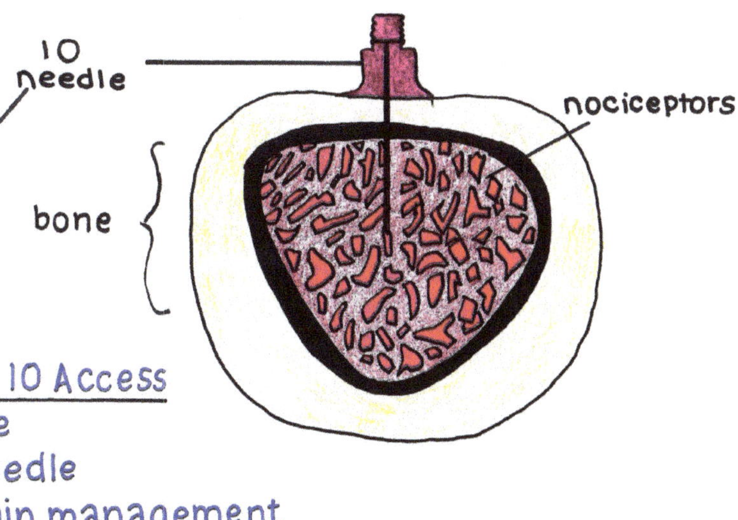

5 Rights of IO Access

1) Right site
2) Right needle
3) Right pain management
4) Right flush
5) Right amount of pressure

EZ-IO

- EZ-IO power driver
- Needle sets (15 mm, 25 mm & 45 mm)
- Extension set (Luer-Lock that twists onto the catheter hub once the stylet has been removed; it must be primed beforehand)
- Stabilizer dressing

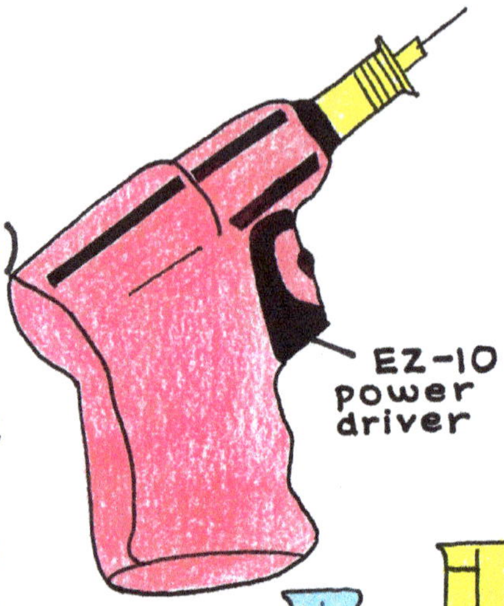

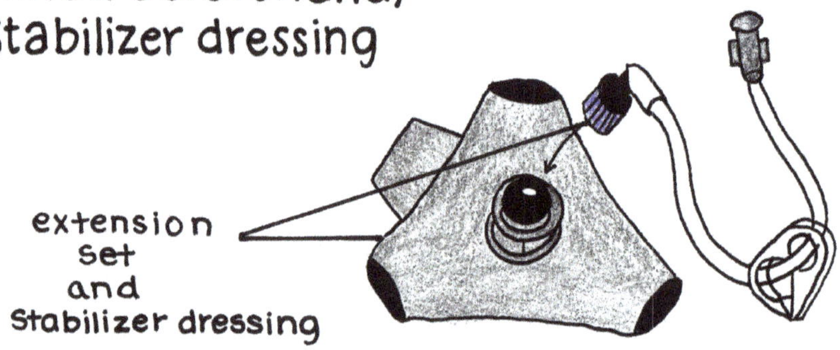

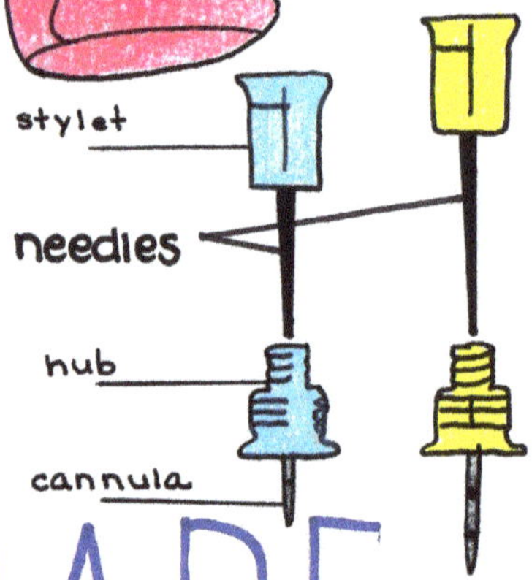

NURSING CARE

- Remember that IO access is meant to be temporary; an IO line should be removed as soon as other venous access is obtained or within 24 hours of insertion (general guideline).
- Consider the need for analgesics; infusion through an IO is often more painful than the insertion itself.
- A pressure bag will likely be needed to infuse fluids because the pressure needed to push the fluid into the bone marrow may exceed that of an IV pump.
- Monitor for complications: compartment syndrome, extravasation, osteomyelitis, necrosis, & infection).
- Like any other vascular access device, assess for patency & flush before and after medication administration through an IO line.
- To remove an IO, remove the extension set & the dressing, stabilize the catheter hub & attach a Luer-Lock syringe, twist clockwise & pull straight out, and apply pressure to the site & cover the site with sterile gauze and a Tegaderm.

implanted ports

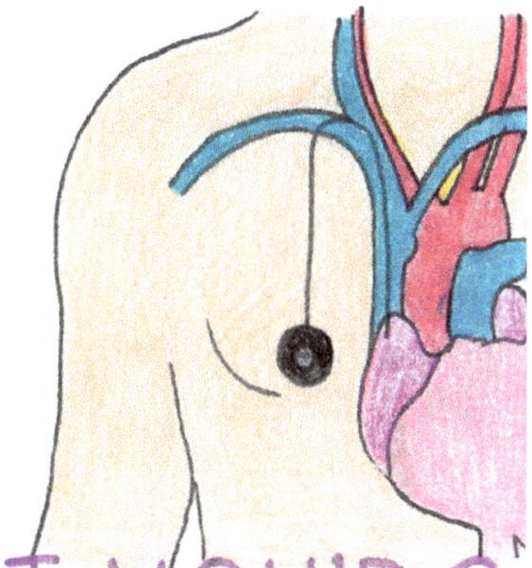

INDICATIONS

- long-term intermittent venous access (months to years)
- chemotherapy
- chronic illness (i.e. CF)

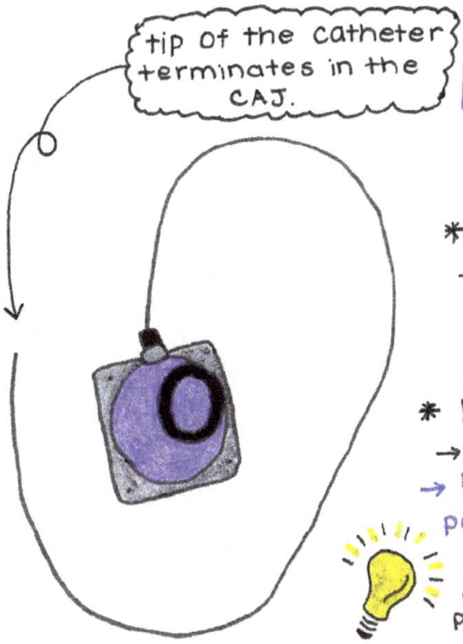

KNOW WHAT YOU'RE ACCESSING!

* single lumen or double lumen port
→ double lumen ports are helpful if two medications need to be infused simultaneously.

* power injectable or non-power injectable
→ power injectable ports are CT compatible.
→ If you're accessing a power injectable port, then use a power injectable needle

To check if a patient has a power port, look at the CXR; if it's a power port, then it will have the letters "CT" on it!

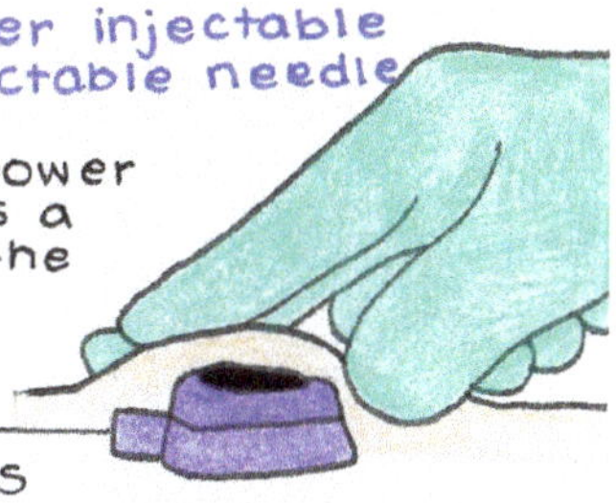

NURSING CARE

- Use only a non-coring Huber needle to access a port; change the needle and dressing q 7 days while accessed.
- Do not use a regular Huber needle to access a power port; use a power injectable needle.
- Use aseptic technique when accessing a port.
- Although it varies by facility, ports are typically heparin locked c̄ 5cc of heparin (100 units/mL).
- Patient education
- Always verify the type of port (single lumen vs. double lumen, power injectable vs. non-power injectable) prior to accessing.

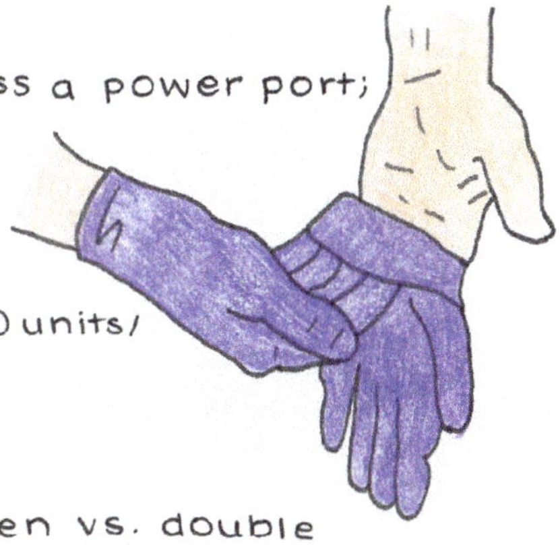

@icunursingnotesbycaitlyn

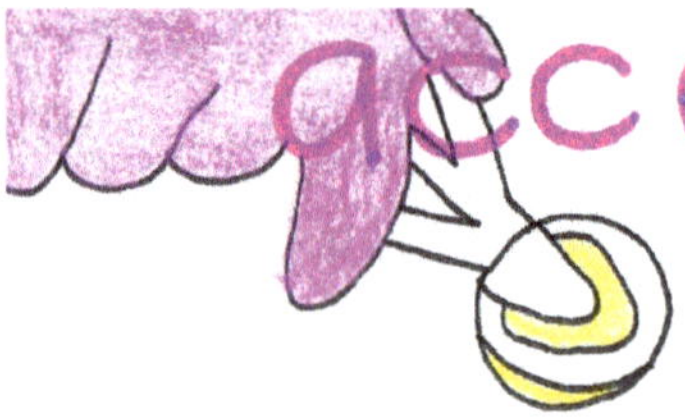

accessing a port

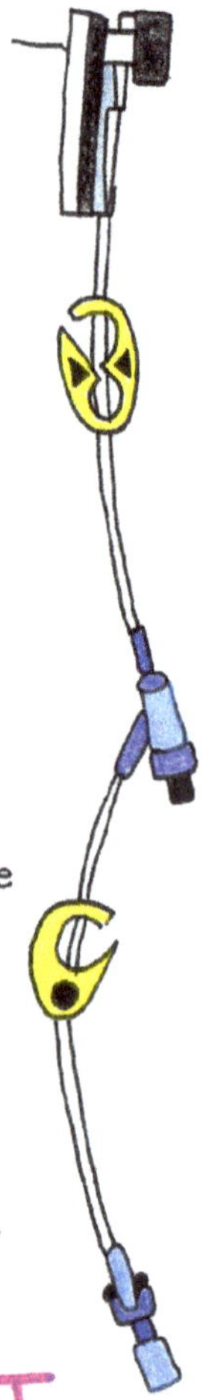

Supplies:

- CVC dressing kit
- 10 cc sterile flush
- Huber needle
- IV connector
- mask (for the patient)

1) Determine the location and the type of port.
2) Open the central line dressing kit, and drop the sterile flush, IV connector, and Huber needle on to the sterile field.
3) Don sterile gloves.
4) Use the Chloraprep to clean the site (30 second friction rub), and allow it to dry.
5) Prep the Huber needle and needleless connector (prime c̄ saline flush).
6) Leave the syringe attached to the primed Huber needle, and place it back on the sterile field.
7) Now that the site is dry, use your non-dominant hand to stabilize the port (this hand is no longer sterile).
8) With your dominant hand, insert the primed Huber needle just perpendicular to the port septum until the tip of the needle contacts the back of the port.
9) Aspirate for blood return to confirm patency, and flush c̄ 10 cc of saline.
10) If the port is to remain accessed, then flush per protocol, cover the site c̄ a sterile occlusive dressing, and maintain a closed system at all times.

Deaccessing a port

1) Don clean gloves. (after washing hands).
2) Confirm blood return, and flush c̄ 10cc normal saline.
3) Heparin lock c̄ 5 cc (100 units/mL) per policy.
4) Remove the dressing.
5) Using your non-dominant hand to stabilize the port, remove the Huber needle and discard in the sharps.
6) Cover the site c̄ a dry sterile gauze dressing or a band-aid.

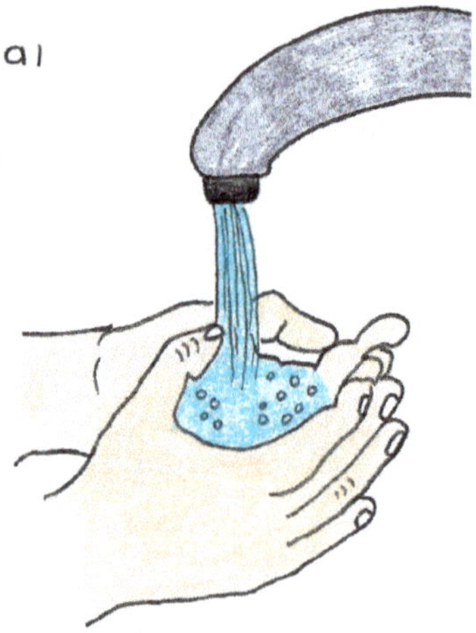

The Art of the IV Start

Supplies

- IV start kit
- IV catheter (Nexiva, Jelco)
- extension tubing
- flushes (0.9% NaCl)
- gloves
- alcohol wipes or CHG

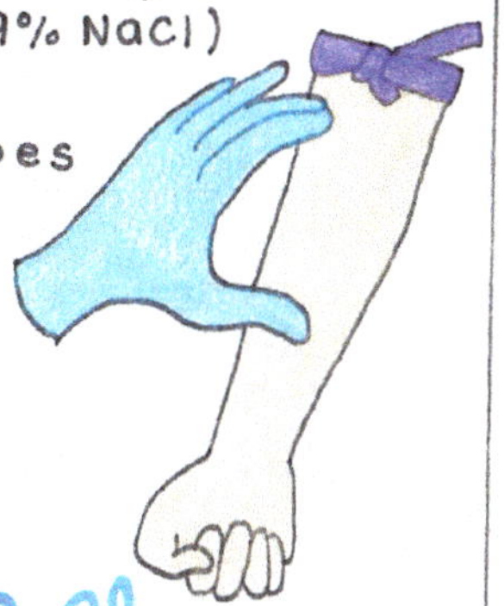

General Insertion Technique

1) Prepare your supplies, and prime the extension tubing.
2) Apply the tourniquet above the selected site.
3) Attempt to visualize the vein (not always possible if it's deep) and palpate – ideal: (smooth + straight, bounce + spring).
4) Clean the site; let it dry.
5) Stabilize by anchoring the vein.
6) Insert the needle (bevel up).
7) Lower the angle, and advance slightly once a flash is visible in the flashback chamber.
8) Release the tourniquet.
9) Thread the catheter (not the needle) into the vein.
10) Retract the needle while stabilizing the hub.
11) Hold pressure above the site, and attach the primed extension set.
12) Aspirate for blood return, and ensure that the IV flushes $\bar{s}$ resistance.
13) Apply a Tegaderm, and secure tubing $\bar{c}$ tape. Date/time/initial it.

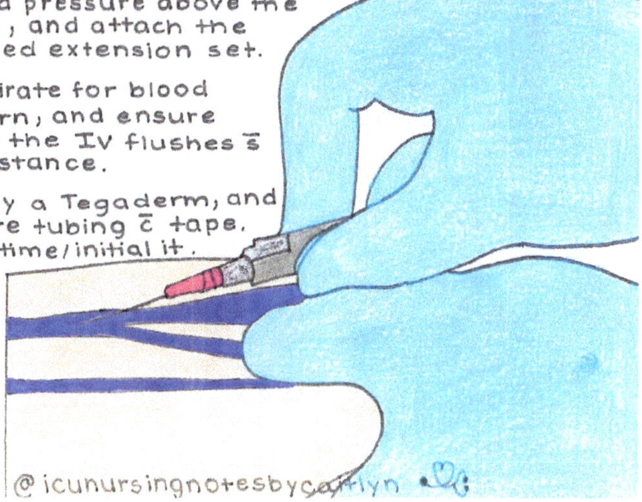

IV Gauges

18G 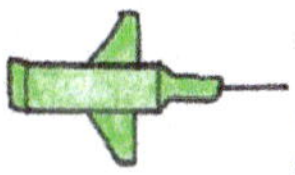
- blood administration
- rapid infusions
- trauma

20G 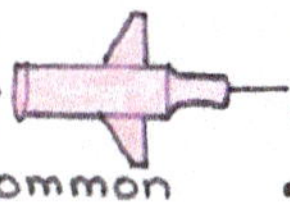
* most common
- blood administration
- routine IV therapy
- can accommodate CT contrast

22G 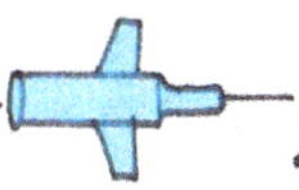
- IV fluids/medications
- poor venous access/small veins

24G 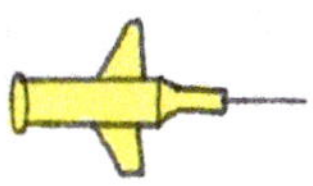
- generally used in pediatrics
- can be used $\bar{c}$ poor venous access.

When Good IVs Go Bad

Infiltration

- Occurs when a non-vesicant/non-irritating solution or medication inadvertently leaks into the surrounding tissue.
- Although the solution itself may not cause damage (unlike extravasation), excessive fluid build-up into a confined space may cause ↓ perfusion and, ultimately, tissue ischemia (if left untreated).
- S/S: edema, discomfort, coolness and blanching around the site, fluid leakage from the IV site.
- Tx: Stop the infusion, D/C the IV, elevate the extremity, apply a warm or cool compress, re-establish IV access in the opposite extremity.

Remember that infiltration and extravasation can happen to any patient, including those who are unable to report pain, so keep an eye on those lines!

Extravasation

- Occurs when a vesicant inadvertently infuses into the surrounding tissue with the potential to cause blistering, severe tissue injury + necrosis, and tendon/nerve/joint damage.
- Common vesicants: KCl, phenytoin (Dilantin), antineoplastics, hypertonic solutions, vanco, milrinone, dobutamine, vasopressors (should be infused centrally)
- S/S: pain, swelling, erythema, change in sensation, circulatory impairment, induration, blistering + sloughing, & vesicle formation
- Tx: immediately stop the infusion, attempt to aspirate residual drug, D/C the IV, elevate the extremity, apply a cool compress (aids in vasoconstriction), administer an antidote subcutaneously (typically phentolamine or hydluronidase, depending on extravasated medication), wound care, and administer an analgesic.

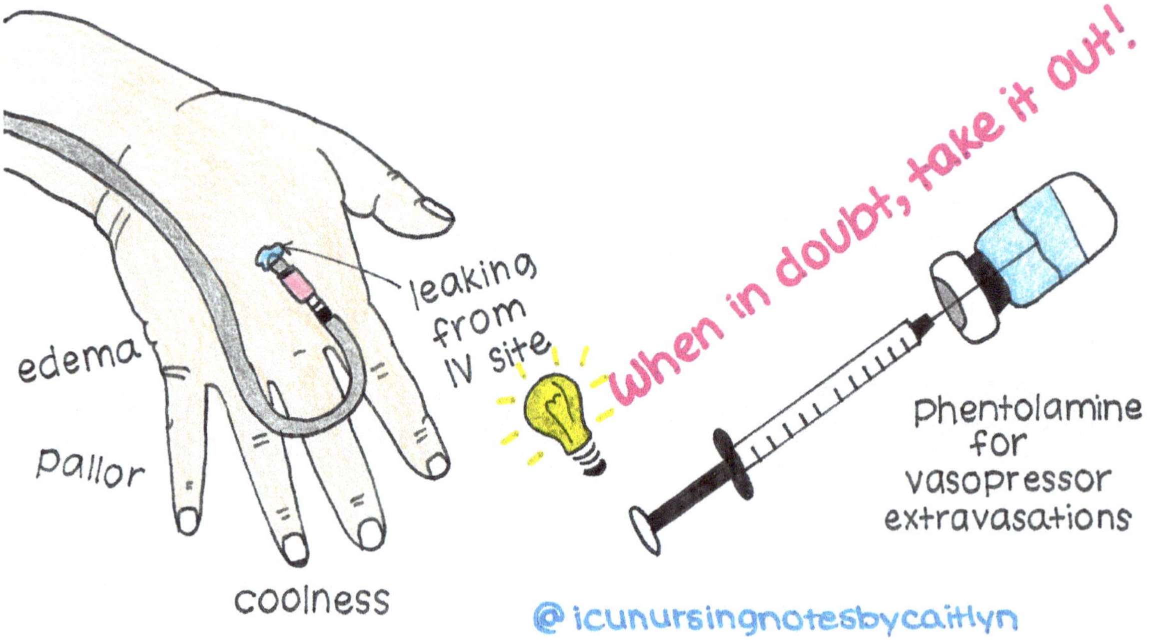
leaking from IV site
edema
pallor
coolness
When in doubt, take it out!
phentolamine for vasopressor extravasations

@icunursingnotesbycaitlyn

Phlebitis

Inflammation of the vein

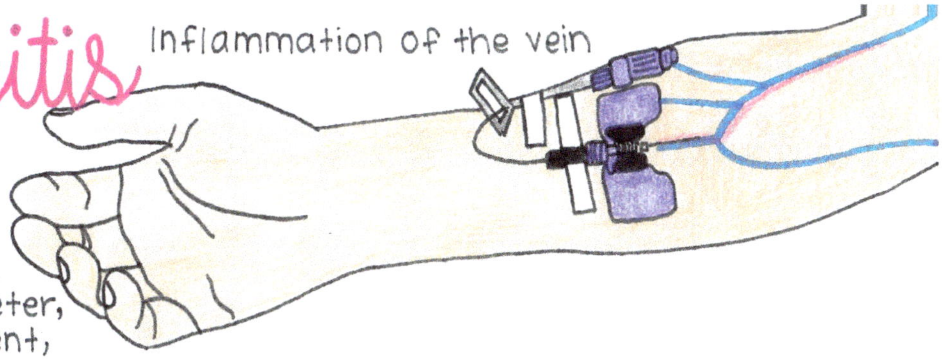

- Three primary causes:

1) mechanical (irritation of the vein by the catheter, excessive movement, etc).
2) chemical (solution is infused too rapidly or at a volume that is too large for the vein, solution is irritating to the vein, etc).
3) bacterial (infection caused by improper aseptic technique)

- S/S: erythema, warmth, tenderness, pain/burning along the course of the vein, palpable venous cord, streak formation along the vein
- Tx: stop the infusion, D/C the IV, elevate the affected extremity, apply a warm compress, NSAIDs, abx (presence of an infection), re-establish IV access in the opposite extremity.

Be alarmed even when your infusion pump isn't! Occlusion alarms do not detect nor prevent infiltration or extravasation, so assessment skills are key!

Nursing Care

- Frequent IV site assessments, especially for vesicant medications.
- Prevention is key!
- Avoid areas of joint flexion (wrist, AC) when inserting an IV, if possible
- Use the smallest gauge catheter possible for delivering the prescribed therapy
- Advocate for a CVC for vesicant medications (i.e. vasopressors)
- Ensure that the catheter is secure and stabilized properly.
- Use an in-line filter when administering amiodarone to help prevent phlebitis.
- Y-site the vesicant medication (i.e. KCl) to the primary line (NaCl) to dilute the drug.
- Know your facility's policy for infiltration and extravasation.
- Educate the patient to report pain, burning, stinging, or temperature changes at the IV site.

@icunursingnotesbycaitlyn

IV FLUIDS

Physiology Review

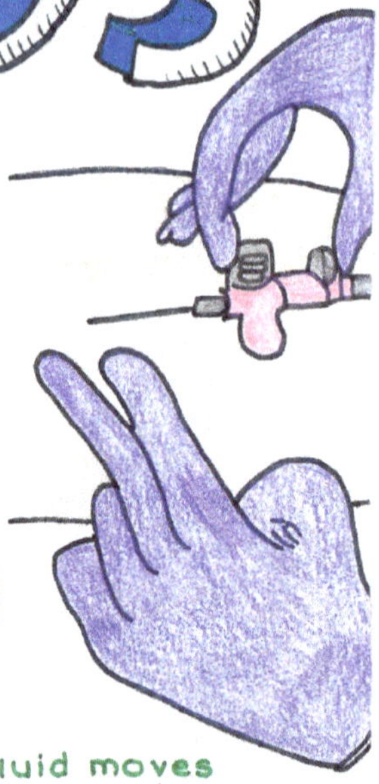

Hypertonic

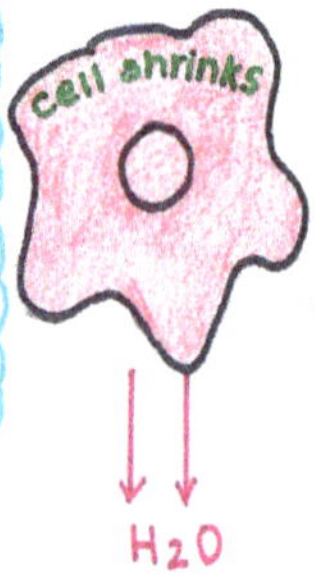

- Fluid moves out of the cells/ICF and into the intravascular space.
- Typically used to treat hypovolemia and hyponatremia.
- Vesicants

Remember: Where sodium goes, water will follow.

Isotonic

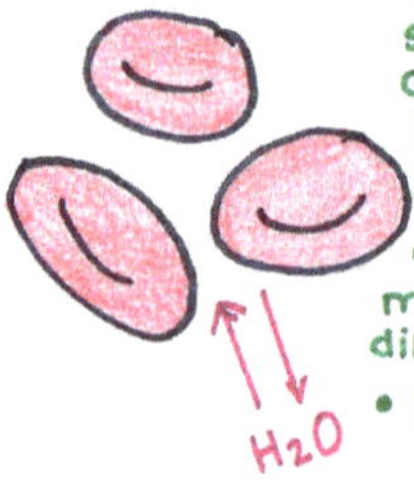

- No fluid movement in/out of the vasculature (isotonic solutions don't alter serum osmolarity, so it stays where it's infused – the intravascular space).
- Used for fluid resuscitation, maintenance IV fluids, KVOs, diluting IV meds, etc.
- Most common

Hypotonic

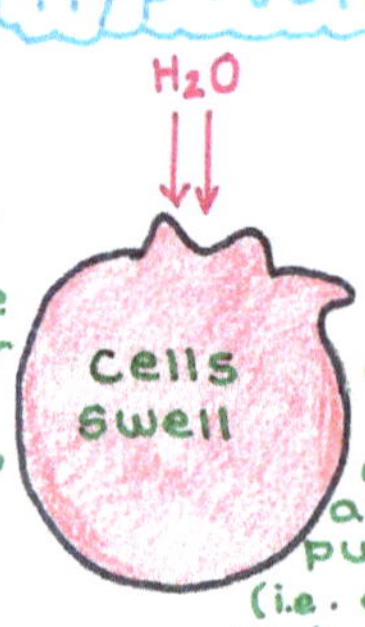

- Fluid moves out of the intravascular space and into the cells/ICF.
- Used when the cells are dehydrated, and fluids need to be put back intracellularly (i.e. diuretic therapy, DKA, HHS).

Classification

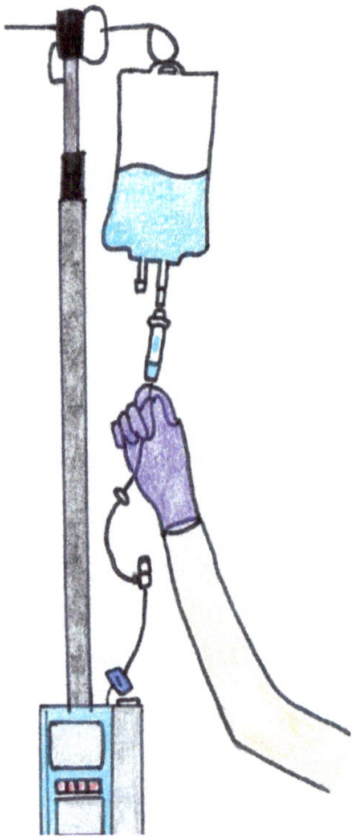

IV fluids

- colloids
  - albumin
  - dextran
- crystalloids
  - hypotonic
    - 0.45% NaCl (1/2 NS)
    - 0.33% NaCl
  - isotonic
    - NS
    - LR
    - D5W*
  - hypertonic
    - D5NS
    - D5 1/2 NS
    - D5LR
    - 3% NaCl

This is important to know because, depending on what kind of IV fluid is given (hypotonic, isotonic, or hypertonic), fluid will shift in and out of different compartments, which has the potential to yield detrimental effects in a critically ill patient.

IV Fluids Made Easy!

0.9% NaCl (normal saline): an isotonic fluid that is typically used in the setting of hypovolemia, GI tract fluid losses, and mild hyponatremia.

- nursing considerations - use caution in patients c̄ cardiac and/or renal disease, monitor for s/s of fluid overload, and use NS when administering blood.

Lactated Ringer's (LR): an isotonic solution used for fluid resuscitation c̄ burns/trauma and for surgical patients.

- nursing considerations: do not use in patients c̄ liver disease (impaired ability to metabolize lactate), and caution c̄ lactic acidosis and alkalotic states.

D5W: an isotonic solution (initially) that becomes a hypotonic solution once the body metabolizes the dextrose ("isotonic in the bag but hypotonic in the body"); it's typically used to treat hypoglycemia.

- nursing considerations: avoid using in patients at risk for ↑ ICP (cerebral edema risk), use c̄ caution in the early post-op period, and it's not used as a resuscitation fluid (dilutes plasma electrolyte concentrations).

0.45% NaCl (1/2 NS): a hypotonic solution used to treat hypovolemia c̄ hypernatremia and for hyperosmolar conditions (DKA and HHS).

- nursing considerations: monitor for worsening hypovolemia and hypotension, never administer to patients at risk for ↑ ICP, and avoid using in patients c̄ liver disease, trauma, or burns.

3% NaCl: a hypertonic solution used to treat severe hyponatremia.

- nursing considerations: administer slowly, administer via a central line, monitor for s/s of fluid overload (remember that hypertonic fluids draw fluid into the intravascular space).

D5 1/2 NS: a hypertonic solution used to treat hypovolemia

- nursing considerations: monitor for s/s of fluid overload

D5LR: a hypertonic solution that provides calories/water/electrolytes and acts as an alkalizing agent.

Nursing Considerations

- Remember that critically ill patients have dynamic fluid requirements.
- Ask yourself, "Will my patient benefit from IV fluids? Can my patient tolerate IV fluids? When should I stop IV fluids? Should I be removing fluid instead?"
- Remember that D5W is isotonic in the bag but hypotonic in the body.
- Administer hypertonic IV fluids via a central line.
- Be cautious to use fluids in cardiac and renal patients (that is why it's important to know your patient's EF!).
- As a general tip, monitor for s/s of hypovolemia c̄ hypotonic IV fluids, and monitor for s/s of hypervolemia c̄ hypertonic IV fluids.

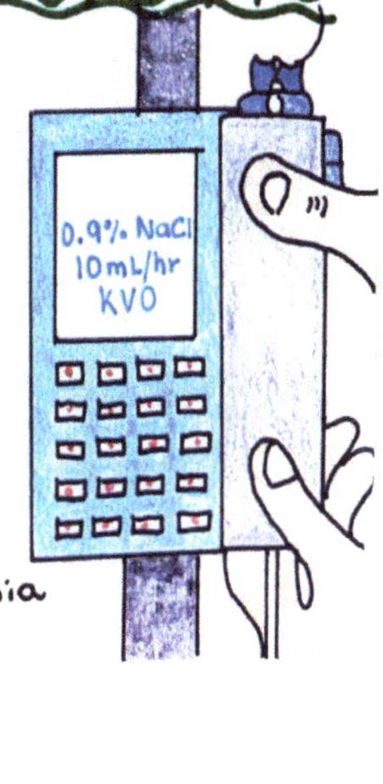

@icunursingnotesbycaitlyn

GOT PATENCY??

THE PULSATILE (PUSH-PAUSE) FLUSHING TECHNIQUE

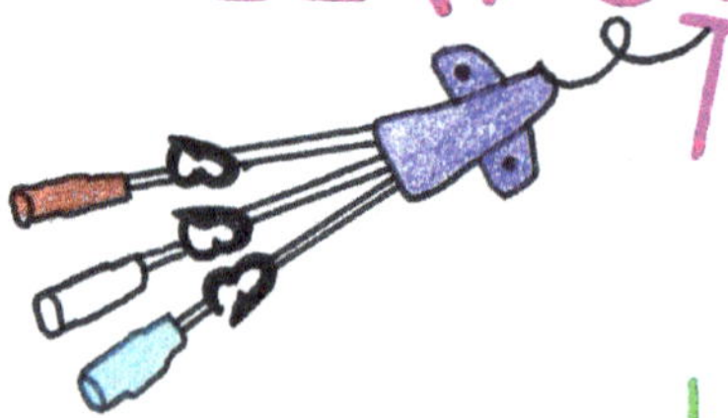

WHO?

Any patient c̄ a central line (triple lumen/IJ, PICC, port, Cordis, dialysis catheter, etc).

* Exception: midlines

HOW?

Quick, forceful & repeated pressure is applied to the syringe barrel to generate turbulence within the catheter lumen. Inject 1-3 cc of NS per push with brief pauses in between each push. Then, simultaneously flush & clamp the line to maintain positive pressure.

It's a simple, easy, inexpensive, & evidence-based nursing intervention!

WHAT?

A special technique used to flush central lines that involves a "push-pause" or "start-stop-start" motion to ↓ the risk of catheter occlusion.

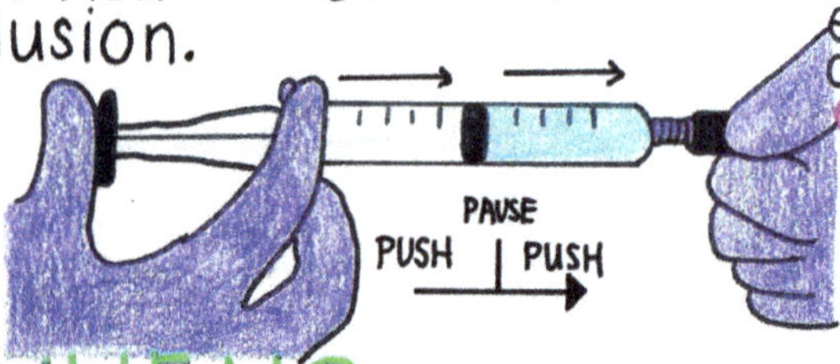

WHY?

The push-pause flushing method generates turbulence within the catheter lumen, which helps to dislodge fibrin & medication residue, thereby reducing the incidence of catheter occlusion. It's more effective than the traditional continuous flushing technique & it's evidence-based!

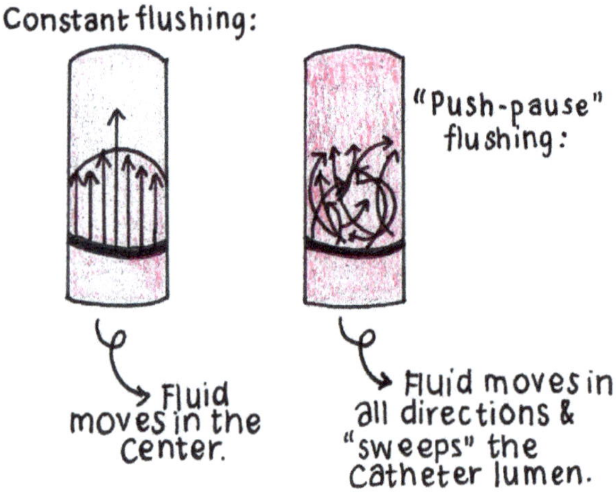

WHEN?

- Before & after medication administration.
- Accessing/deaccessing a line
- Before & after blood draws

WHO?

Patients c̄ peripheral or central lines

WHEN?

Before accessing <u>ANY</u> kind of vascular access device (VAD)

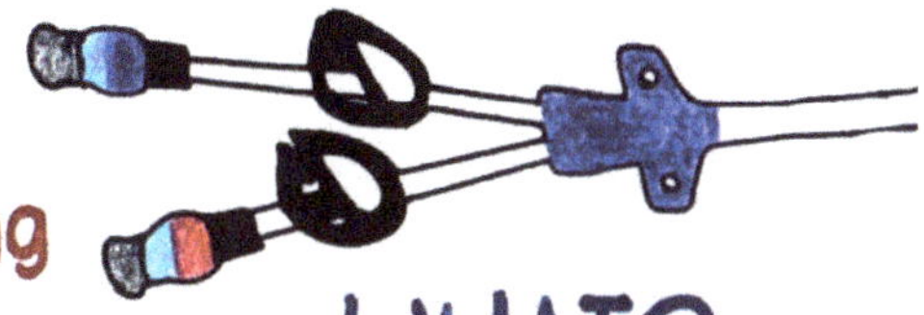

WHAT?

Best practice for nursing care of peripheral & central lines.

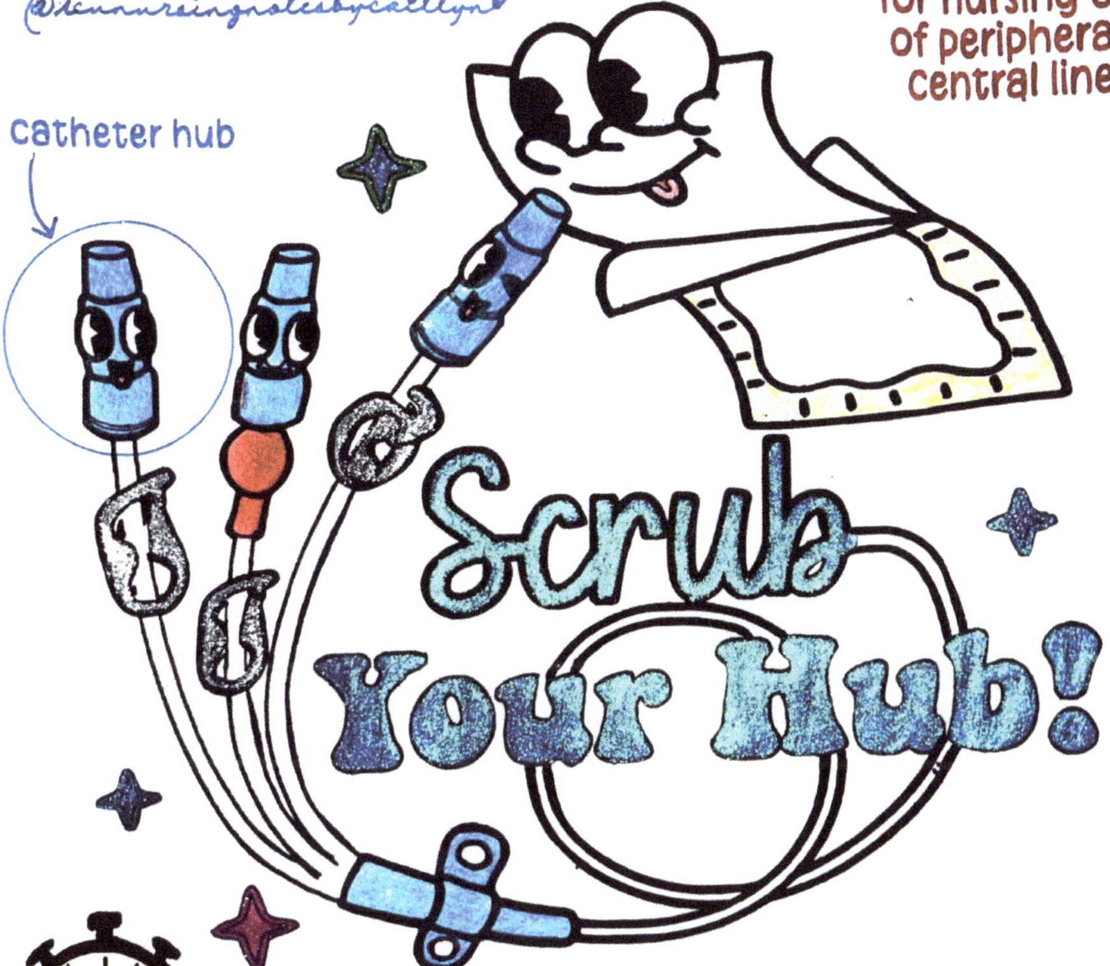

HOW?

Clean the injection port (hub) using alcohol/CHG c̄ friction & in a twisting motion (almost as if you were juicing an orange)!

WHY?

The external surface of the catheter hub is contaminated c̄ bacteria & is a known source for CLABSI. <u>71%</u> of CLABSIs occur 2/2 catheter hub contamination (Joint Commission).

RAPID SEQUENCE INTUBATION (RSI)

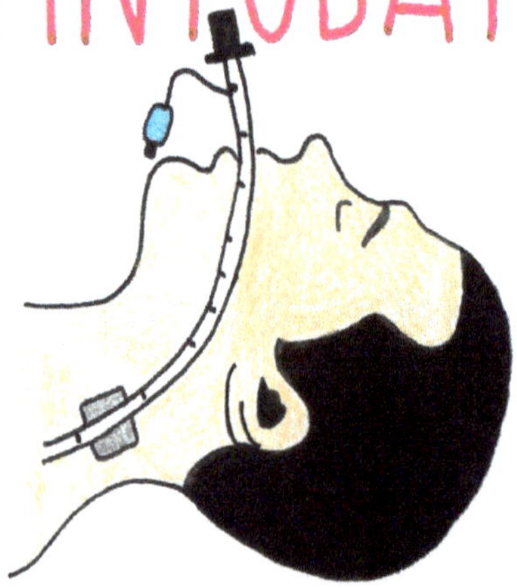

INDICATIONS

RSI, the cornerstone of emergency airway management, is a method of induction that involves the near simultaneous administration of an induction agent (sedative) followed immediately by a rapid-onset paralytic to render immediate unconsciousness & motor paralysis for emergent endotracheal intubation. The patient is then intubated s̄ interposed positive-pressure ventilation via a bag-valve-mask to reduce the risk of aspiration. The goal is to minimize the time between the administration of the induction agent and endotracheal intubation & to avoid positive-pressure ventilation until the ET tube has been placed correctly in the trachea, because the patient is a high aspiration risk.

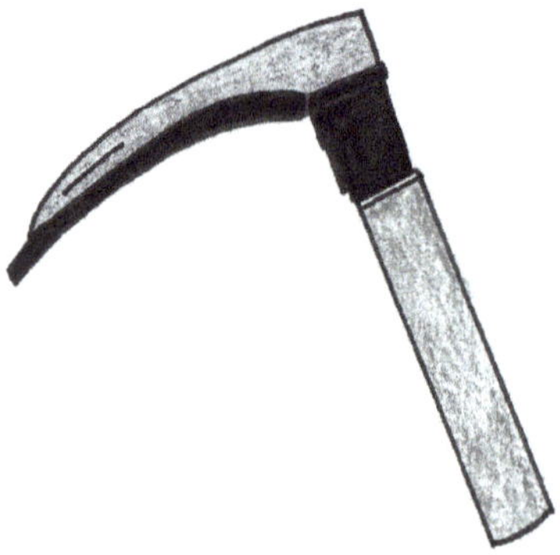

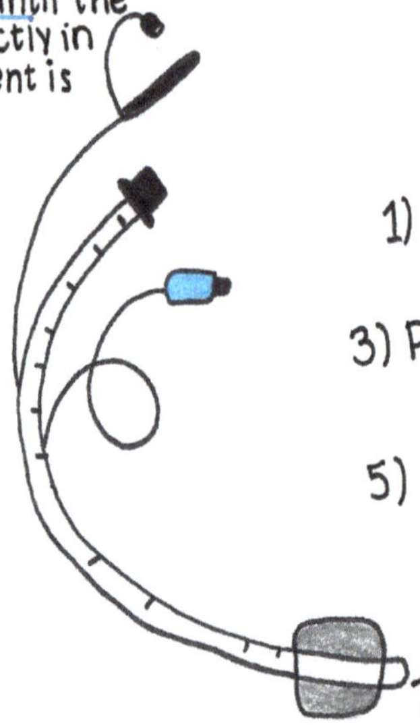

THE "7 Ps" OF RSI:

1) Preparation
2) Preoxygenation
3) Pretreatment
4) Paralysis c̄ induction
5) Positioning
6) Placement of the tube
7) Post-intubation management

RSI vs. ELECTIVE INTUBATION

- The patient is intubated s̄ any positive-pressure ventilation via a BVM c̄ RSI. In a routine/elective intubation, the patient is manually ventilated before intubating.

- RSI is emergent; there is no time to wait or prep the patient's airway, whereas a routine intubation is less emergent/elective.

- RSI often requires ↑ doses of paralytics compared to a routine intubation. Succinylcholine is the ideal paralytic for RSI because of its rapid onset. Other paralytics (i.e. cisatracurium & vecuronium) do not work fast enough.

PHARMACOLOGY

#1: INDUCTION AGENTS

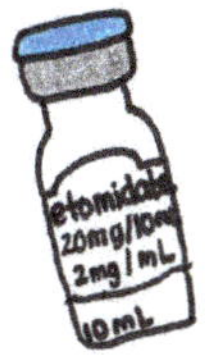

USE: SEDATION

	ETOMIDATE	KETAMINE	PROPOFOL	MIDAZOLAM
DOSE	0.2 - 0.3 mg/kg	1-2 mg/kg	2-3 mg/kg	0.2 mg/kg
ONSET	30 seconds	1 minute	15-30 seconds	60-90 seconds
DURATION	3-5 minutes	10-15 minutes	3-5 minutes	30-60 minutes (dose-dependent)
SIDE EFFECTS	minimal effect on BP, muscle twitching, potential adrenal suppression in septic patients	HTN, tachycardia, caution in cardiovascular disease*	hypotension best for hemodynamically stable patients*	hypotension, reduced dose for hemodynamic instability*

#2: PARALYTICS (NMBAS)

THESE WORK BY BLOCKING ACETYLCHOLINE AT THE NEUROMUSCULAR JUNCTION, PREVENTING MUSCLE CONTRACTION.

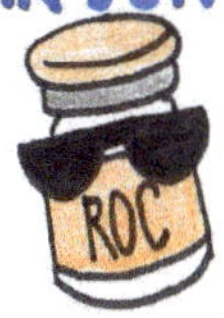

	SUCCINYLCHOLINE ("SUX")	ROCURONIUM ("ROC")	VECURONIUM ("VEC")
DOSE	1.5 mg/kg	0.6-1 mg/kg	0.1-0.2 mg/kg
ONSET	within 30 seconds	1-2 minutes	2-4 minutes
DURATION	10 minutes	45-60 minutes	30 - 40 minutes
SIDE EFFECTS	↑ ICP, bradycardia, fasiculations, hyperkalemia, trigger for malignant hyperthermia.	typically used if succ is contraindicated, can be reversed with sugammadex.	slow onset, long duration of action.

When your patient needs to be intubated:

NURSING TIPS 101

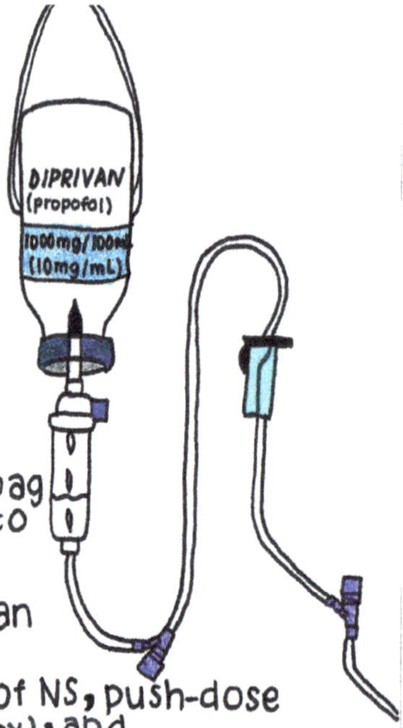

- Confirm your patient's code status.
- Make sure the room is set up: intubation box, BVM/Ambu bag (have it ready by attaching it to O_2), & suction x 2 (test it to make sure it works!).
- Call RT.
- Move the bed away from the wall so that the provider can stand at the H.O.B.
- Supplies that you may need to anticipate: prepped bolus of NS, push-dose pressors, crash cart/defibrillator (nearby), ACLS meds (nearby), and restraints.

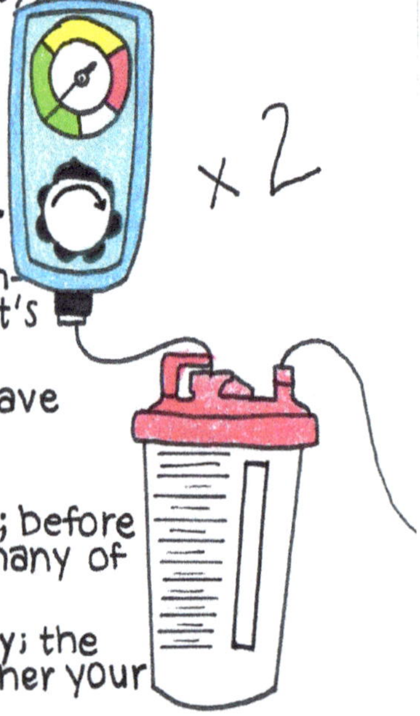

- Make sure your patient doesn't have dentures in (this is easy to forget)!
- Reassure your patient & explain what to expect.
- Ensure that you have patent IV access & remember that not all medications are compatible through the same line.
- Know your patient's K^+ level because the CRNA/anesthesiologist may ask you this; succinylcholine can cause a transient hyperkalemia, so a different paralytic will be used if it's high.
- Have your post-intubation gtts primed & ready to go & have restraints on hand (ensure that you have an order!).
- The sedative is always given before the paralytic!
- Monitor your patient's vitals throughout the intubation; before the provider intubates, change the BP to cycle q 5 min (many of the drugs given for intubation cause hypotension).
- Post-intubation care is important & it's very nursing heavy; the more that you have set up prior to intubation, the smoother your post-intubation care will be.
- Once your patient is intubated, make sure that you get orders for sedation & pain control.
- Ensure that placement of the tube is verified with a CXR.

Tip: Insert the OGT before X-ray comes so that you can verify your OGT placement, too!

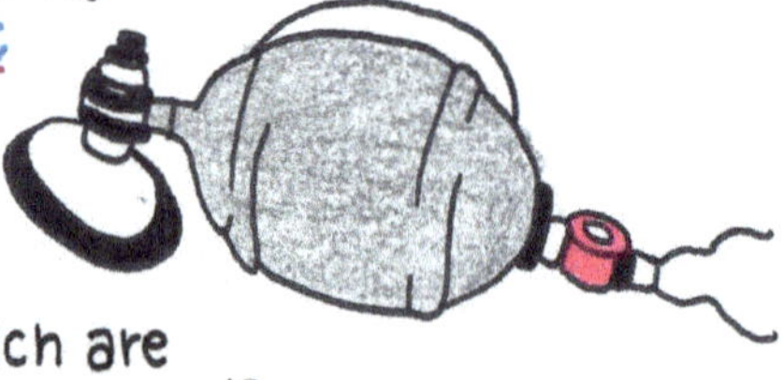

- An ABG will be checked ≈30 min after intubation.

Learn your medications! Which are sedatives? Which are paralytics? Which are short-acting? Which can be reversed? Although nurses aren't the ones placing the ETT, it's still important to understand the intubation process; it takes a team of nurses, RTs, & providers to have a successful intubation $\bar{s}$ any complications!

TRAIN-OF-FOUR monitoring

TERMS

- neuromuscular blockade (NMB): skeletal muscle paralysis induced pharmacologically or by neuromuscular disorders
- neuromuscular blocking agents (NMBAs): medications that induce paralysis by blocking the transmission of nerve impulses at the neuromuscular junction
  - → examples: succinylcholine (used for RSI), rocuronium, cisatracurium (Nimbex), atracurium, etc.
- train-of-four (TOF): a type of peripheral nerve stimulation monitor that delivers a small electrical current to a superficial nerve (ulnar), which causes muscle movement evidenced by a "twitch." It's used to assess/estimate the level of blockade and to titrate continuous NMBA infusions.
  - → TOF indicates the degree of NMB.
  - → ranges from 0/4 to 4/4 twitches.

INDICATIONS

A neuromuscular blockade [NMB] in the setting of:

- Acute respiratory distress syndrome (ARDS)
- significant patient-ventilator asynchrony
- ↑ intracranial pressure (i.e. TBI)
- persistent shivering during targeted temperature management post-cardiac arrest

RESPONSES

TOF Suppression	% of Blockade
4 responses (4/4)	< 75%
3 responses (3/4)	75 – 80%
2 responses (2/4)	80 – 90% (* Goal TOF)
1 response (1/4)	90%
No response (0/4)	100%

↑ degree of NMB

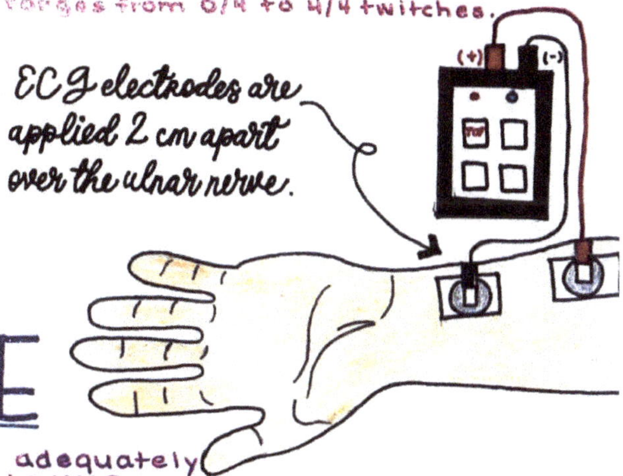
ECG electrodes are applied 2 cm apart over the ulnar nerve.
(+)
(-)
TOF

NURSING CARE

- Always ensure that the patient is adequately sedated (CPOT < 3, RASS -4 to -5) prior to NMB and TOF initiation (NMBAs do not provide sedation, analgesia or amnesia).
- Titrate the continuous NMBA infusion to orders (target of 80% to 90% blockade or 2/4 twitches.
- Obtain a baseline threshold current prior to the initiation of a NMBA.
- Test the T.O.F. 10-15 minutes after a bolus dose and when a continuous IV infusion of a NMBA is initiated or changed/adjusted.
- Ensure adequate eye lubrication (corneal abrasions), DVT prophylaxis, passive ROM exercises, sedation/analgesia.
- Frequent CPOT and RASS assessments
- Frequent pupillary assessments
- Implement pressure injury prevention and ventilator-associated PNA (VAP) prevention strategies.
- Assess the patient's oxygenation and ventilation status, neurological function, and tissue perfusion before ↑ the rate of a NMBA infusion.

Adequate sedation/analgesia is key!

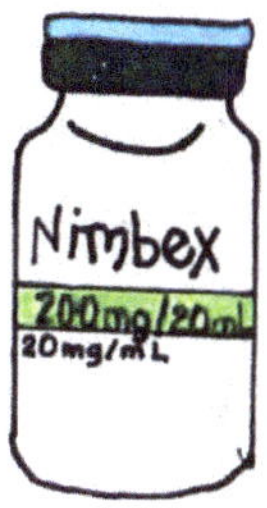

aortic arch anatomy

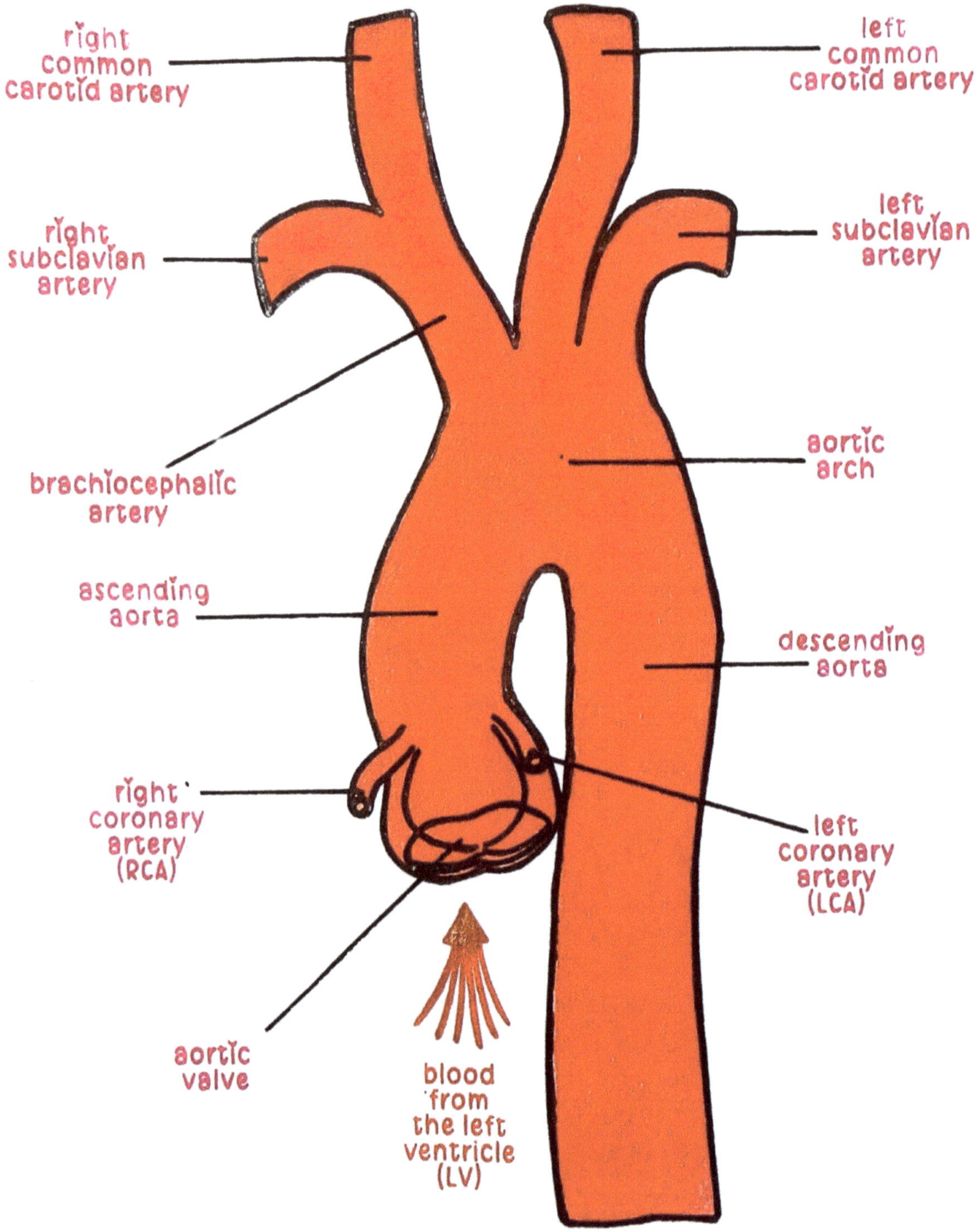

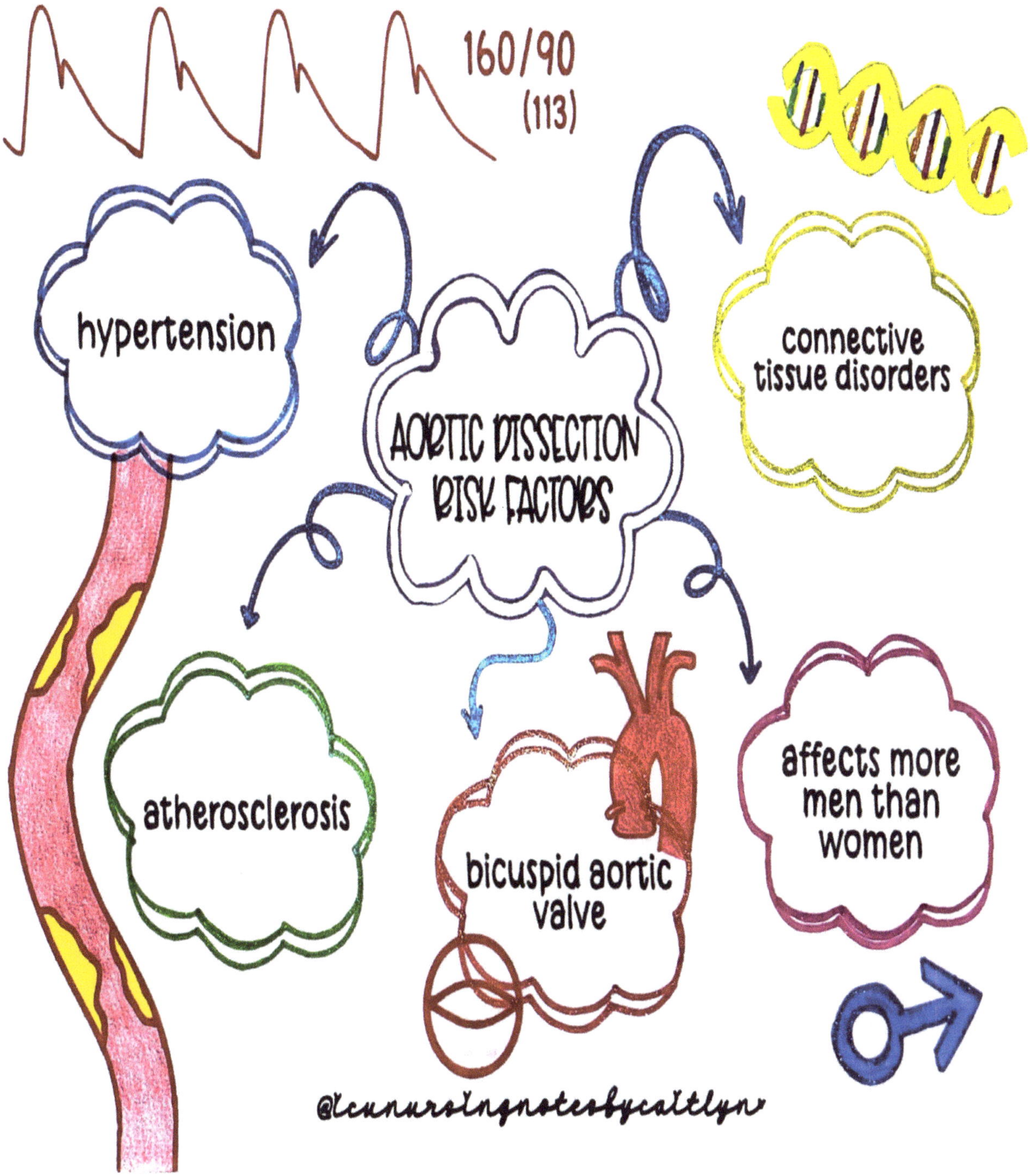
160/90
(113)
hypertension
AORTIC DISSECTION
RISK FACTORS
connective
tissue disorders
atherosclerosis
bicuspid aortic
valve
affects more
men than
women
@icunursingnotesbycaitlyn

AORTIC DISSECTION

Blood surges through a tear in the innermost layer of the aortic wall, causing the inner & middle layers of the aorta to separate (dissect), creating another pathway (false lumen) for blood flow.

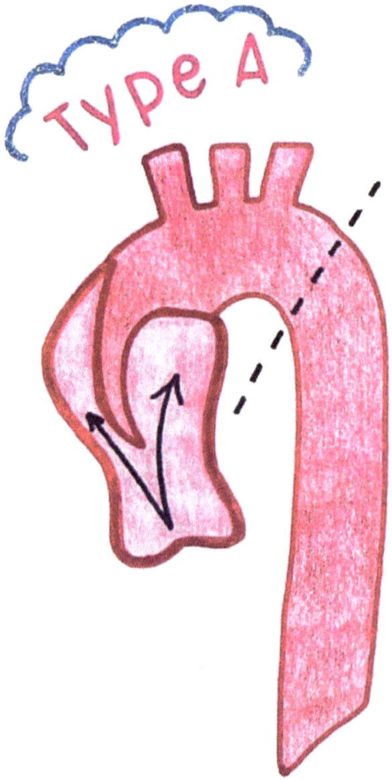

Type A affects the ascending aorta (proximal to the brachiocephalic artery). Type B affects the descending aorta (past the left subclavian artery), & it propagates distally!!

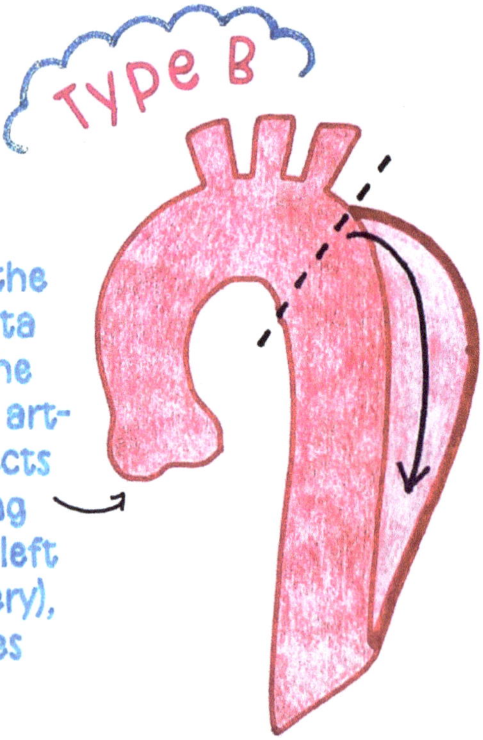

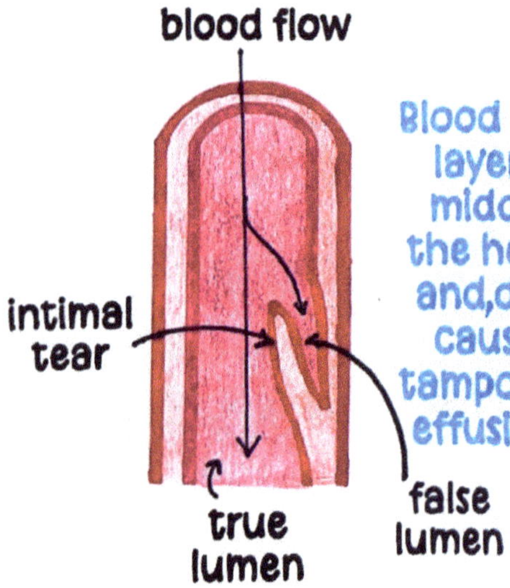

PATHOPHYSIOLOGY

Blood passes through the tear separating the inner layer (tunica intima) of the aortic wall from the middle layer (media), creating a "false lumen." As the heart contracts, the dissection can propagate and,depending on its location, the dissection can cause an acute MI, acute aortic regurg, cardiac tamponade, stroke, renal failure, paraplegia, pleural effusion, mesenteric ischemia, &, ultimately, aortic rupture.

@icunursingnotesbycaitlyn

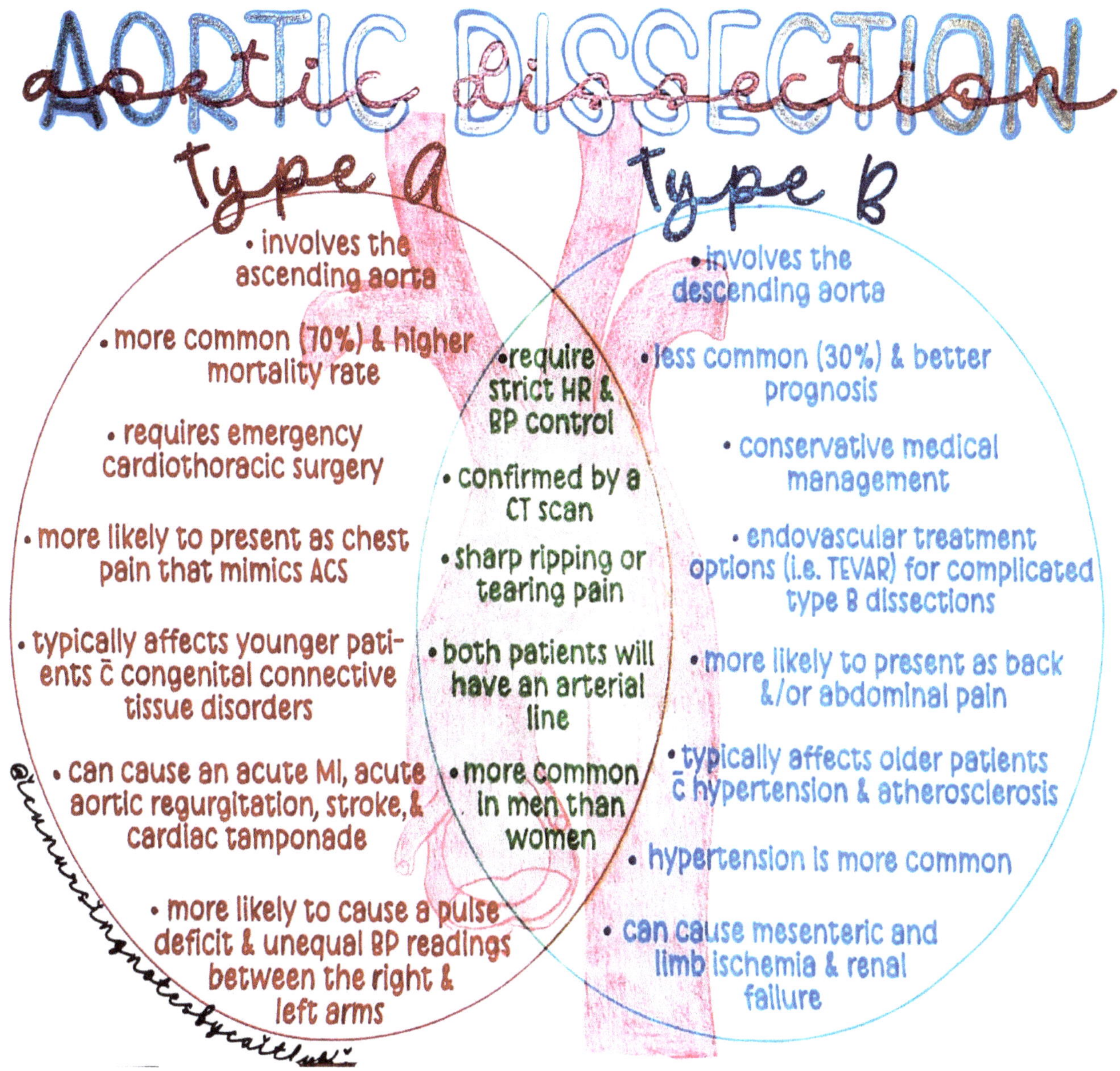
AORTIC DISSECTION
aortic dissection
Type A
Type B
• involves the ascending aorta
• more common (70%) & higher mortality rate
• requires emergency cardiothoracic surgery
• more likely to present as chest pain that mimics ACS
• typically affects younger patients c̄ congenital connective tissue disorders
• can cause an acute MI, acute aortic regurgitation, stroke, & cardiac tamponade
• more likely to cause a pulse deficit & unequal BP readings between the right & left arms
• require strict HR & BP control
• confirmed by a CT scan
• sharp ripping or tearing pain
• both patients will have an arterial line
• more common in men than women
• involves the descending aorta
• less common (30%) & better prognosis
• conservative medical management
• endovascular treatment options (i.e. TEVAR) for complicated type B dissections
• more likely to present as back &/or abdominal pain
• typically affects older patients c̄ hypertension & atherosclerosis
• hypertension is more common
• can cause mesenteric and limb ischemia & renal failure
@icunursingnotesbycaitlyn

Management of Aortic Dissections

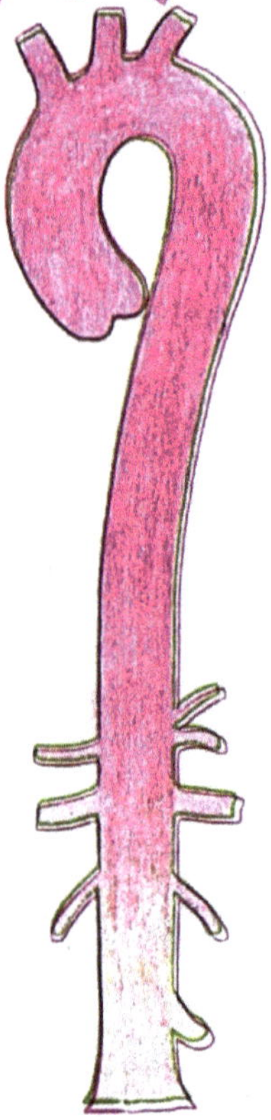

Type A

emergent cardiac surgery

- aortic resection & graft
- possible CABG & AVR if there is coronary involvement

temporizing measures for shock

- blood, IV fluids, vasopressors, etc

Type B

medical management

- beta blockers +/- vasodilators

endovascular repair for complicated dissections

- TEVAR

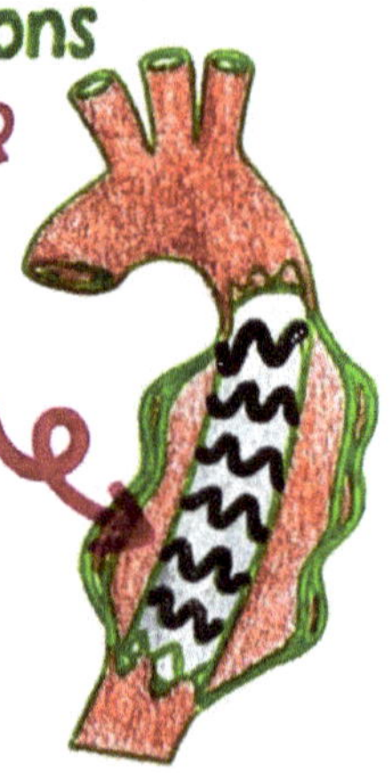

Both A & B

heart rate & blood pressure control + pain control + secondary pressure control

heart rate & blood pressure control	pain control	secondary pressure control
IV beta-blocker	IV opioids	IV vasodilator
labetalol	fentanyl	nicardipine
esmolol	morphine	sodium nitroprusside (Nipride)
metoprolol		

AORTIC DISSECTIONS: NURSING CARE

- These patients often report a sudden "tearing" c/p radiating to the back, but know that not all patients c̄ a dissection will present like this.
- Anticipate bringing your patient to CT to r/o a dissection. TEE is another option, but a CT is ideal!
- The #1 priority is to ↓ the heart rate (<60 bpm) & blood pressure (<120 mmHg) to prevent worsening of the dissection & ↓ the risk of rupture.
- If the patient's systolic BP goal isn't met c̄ heart rate control, then consider advocating for a vasodilator infusion (nicardipine, clevidipine, or nitroprusside) to reduce afterload & BP.
- Know that a patient c̄ an aortic dissection may have different blood pressure readings in each arm.
- Anticipate arterial line insertion.
- Assess all peripheral pulses.
- Aortic dissections are painful! IV fentanyl is a good option for pain control & to help ↓ the sympathetic surge that further increases the BP & HR.
- If your patient becomes hypotensive, consider the possibility of cardiac tamponade, aortic rupture, or acute aortic insufficiency. Anticipate a bedside echo.
- Don't attribute hypotension solely to starting/titrating the beta blocker &/or vasodilator infusion. Consider what else could be causing the hypotension.
- In the setting of aortic insufficiency (AI), the heart tries to maintain its cardiac output, so you may see a refractory tachycardia. It's important to remember to avoid giving these patients beta blockers!
- Start the beta blocker infusion prior to the vasodilator to avoid a reflex tachycardia & ↓ in aortic wall stress.
- Listen to your patient's heart sounds! A diastolic murmur can indicate acute aortic insufficiency, & muffled heart sounds are characteristic of cardiac tamponade.
- Monitor for S/S of heart failure, which may indicate that the dissection involves the aortic valve.
- Monitor for S/S of end-organ perfusion. Maintain adequate MAP.
- Strict I&O. A ↓ in UOP may indicate renal artery involvement.
- Make sure that a type & screen has been drawn.
- Neuro checks are important! An aortic dissection can affect the carotids and cause an ischemic stroke.

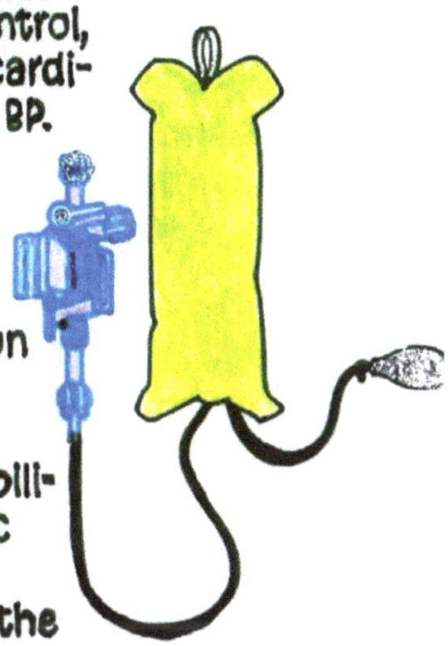

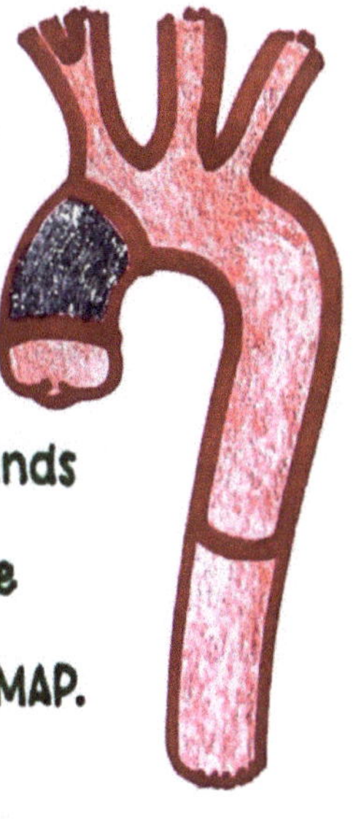

HEPARIN-INDUCED THROMBOCYTOPENIA

@icunursing (TYPE II) notesbycaitlyn

An adverse drug reaction & immune response to heparin therapy that is characterized by a ↓in platelet count (≥ 50% from baseline) and hypercoagulability that can result in end-organ damage.

PATHOPHYSIOLOGY:

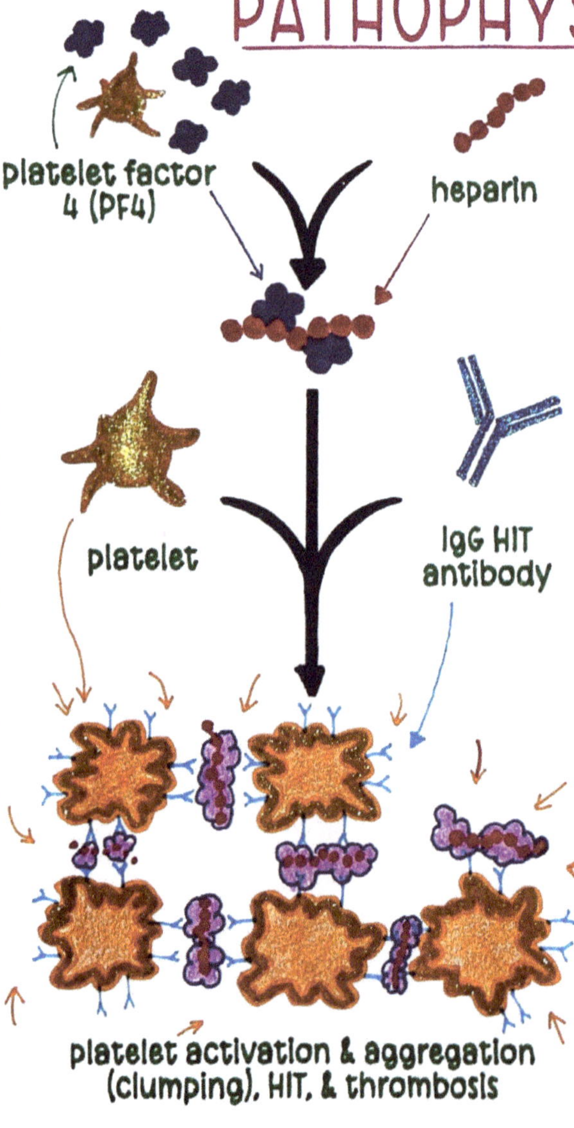

Lo, M. (2019). Five Pearls on HIT. Core IM.

Heparin binds to platelet factor 4 (PF4) – a protein released by activated platelets.

↓

The body identifies the heparin-PF4 complex as "foreign" & produces IgG antibodies against it (typically 5 to 10 days p̄ heparin exposure).

↓

These antibodies bind to the heparin-PF4 complex & activate platelets.

↓

↓platelet count (thrombocytopenia), thrombin release, further release of PF4, & clotting (platelet aggregation).

↓

Clots can wedge in the veins & arteries, causing venous &/or arterial thrombosis (DVT, PE, limb ischemia, stroke, MI, etc).

Heparin - Induced Thrombocytopenia Complications

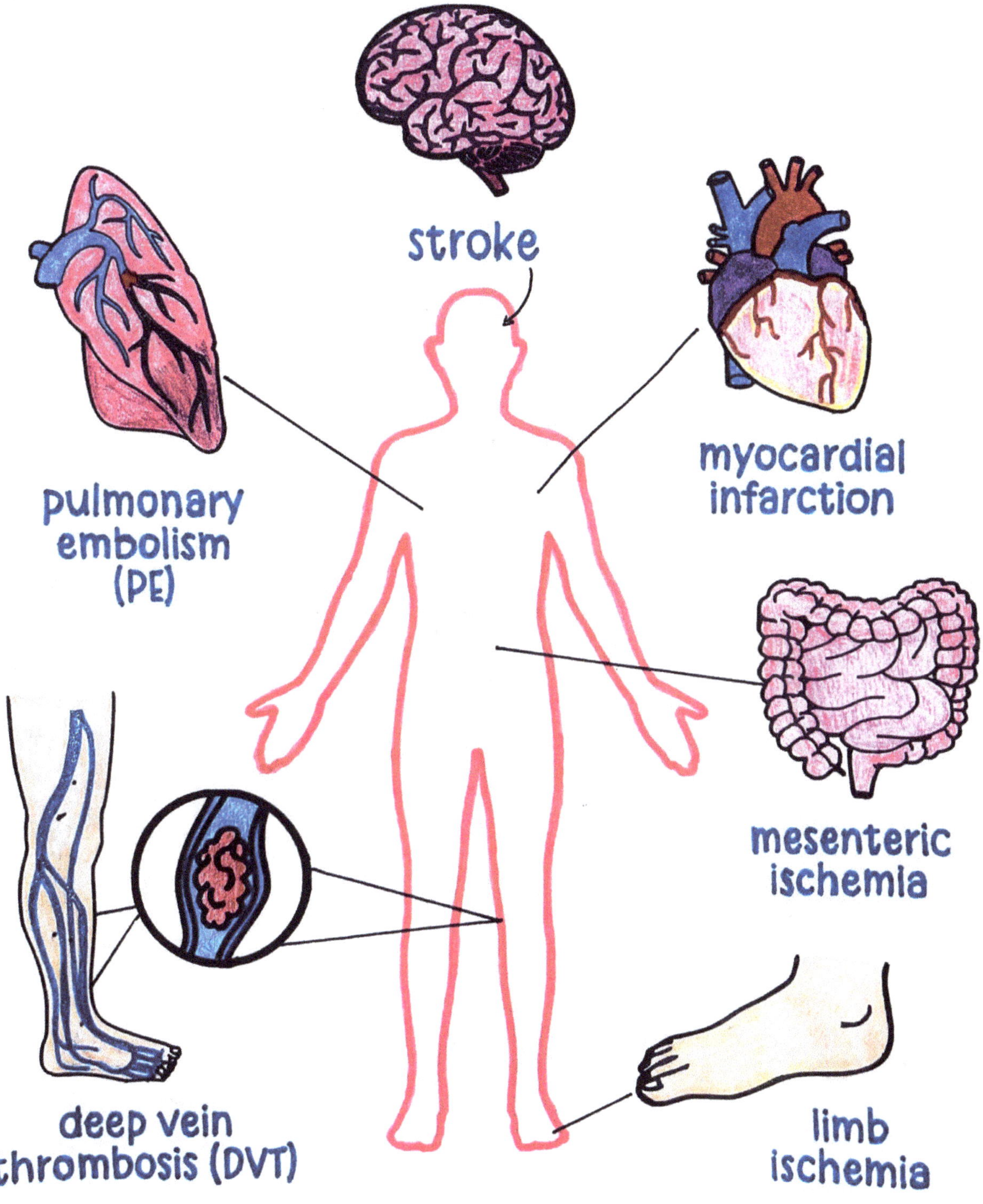

FLASH PULMONARY EDEMA

A severe form of acute pulmonary edema occurring in patients c̄ hypertensive acute heart failure that develops within minutes to hours, resulting in respiratory distress & hypoxia that isn't optimally managed by IV diuresis.

norepi

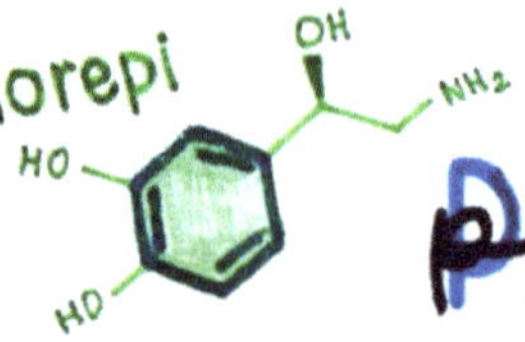

PATHOPHYSIOLOGY

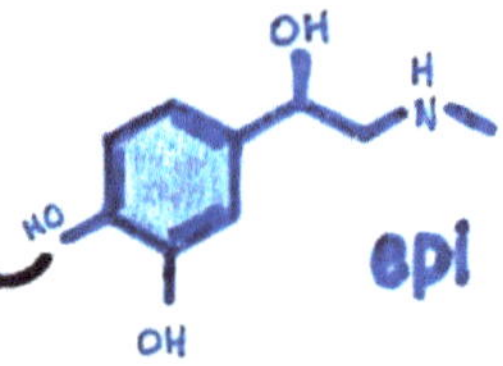

epi

A trigger sends the body's sympathetic (fight-or-flight) nervous system into overdrive. The catecholamine surge (i.e. release of norepinephrine, epinephrine, etc) induces systemic vasoconstriction, & ↑s afterload (SVR) & BP. It also ↑s the heart rate, ↓cardiac diastolic filling time. If the LV is failing, it can't adequately pump against a high afterload, so pressure backs up into the pulmonary system: this pressure forces fluid into the alveoli, causing pulmonary edema.

This is typically an afterload problem, not a fluid problem! Think afterload reduction rather than diuresis!

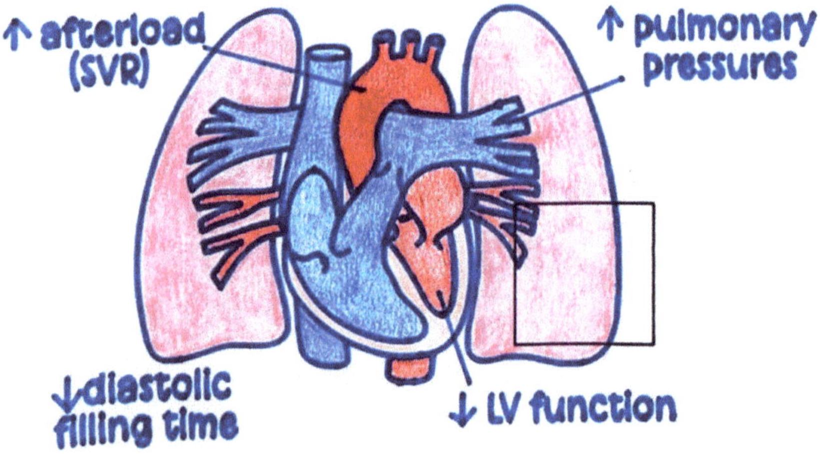

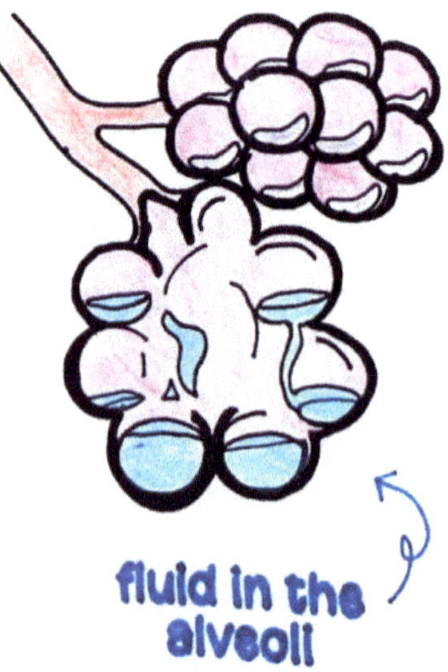

Management of Flash Pulmonary Edema

@icunursingnotesbycaitlyn

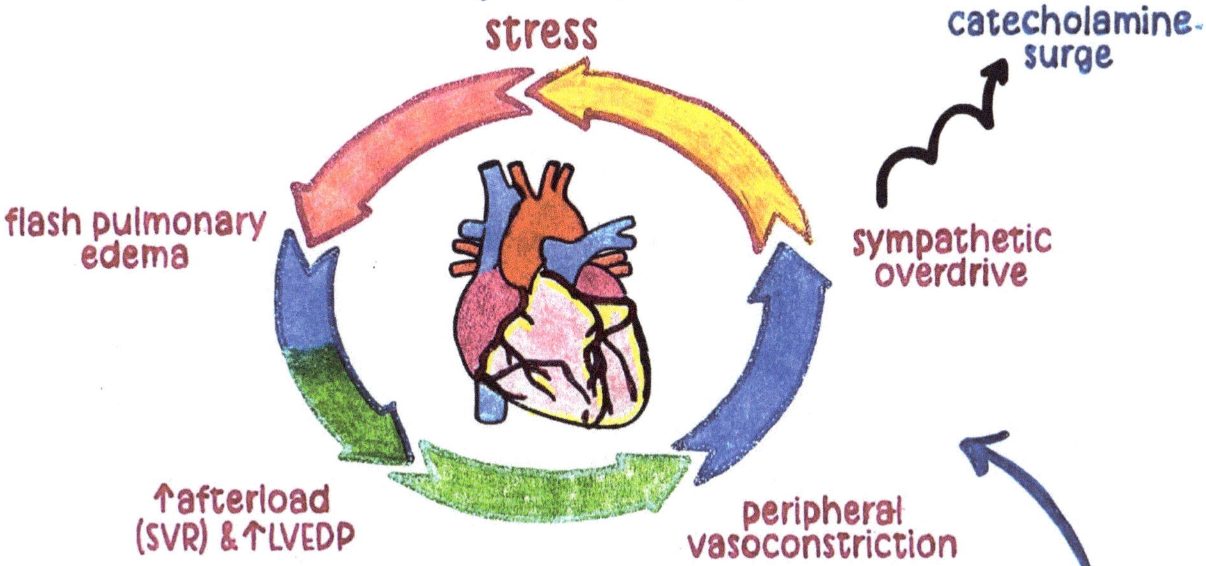

Management focuses on interrupting this cycle

Goals: preload & afterload reduction, improve work of breathing, & ↑ oxygenation!

BiPAP/CPAP (intubation if NIPPV fails)

↑ low-dose fentanyl can help c̄ patient comfort here!

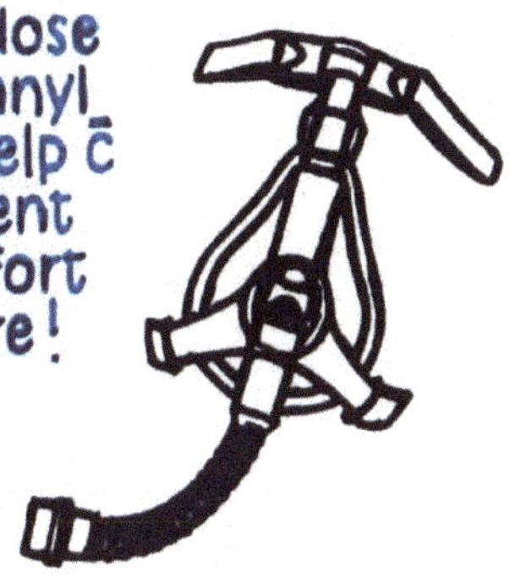

high-dose IV nitro

↑ depends on BP, but most of these patients are hypertensive

↓ do NOT use in patients who are preload-dependent (i.e. severe AS)!

IV diuretics

↑ only if the patient is volume overloaded; most of these patients are dry!

↓ Remember that this is usually a problem c̄ fluid distribution, not amount.

LV THROMBUS

A blood clot in the left ventricle (apex) of the heart that ↑s the risk of systemic embolization & forms in the setting of severe LV systolic dysfunction 2/2 an anterior wall MI (AWMI), heart failure c̄ a reduced EF (HFrEF), & dilated cardiomyopathy.

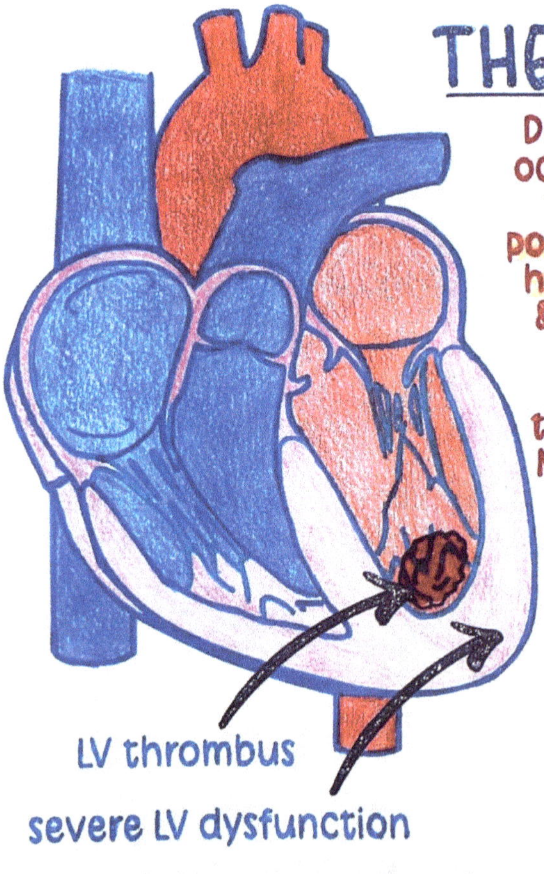

THE PATHOPHYSIOLOGY:

Development of a LV thrombus primarily occurs as a result of endothelial damage 2/2 ischemic insult, blood stasis 2/2 a poorly contracting LV (LV dysfunction), & a hypercoagulable state 2/2 inflammation & clotting factor activation. If the clot dislodges from the ventricular wall & embolizes, it can cause a number of thromboembolic complications (stroke, MI, brain/spleen/renal/mesenteric/limb ischemia, etc).

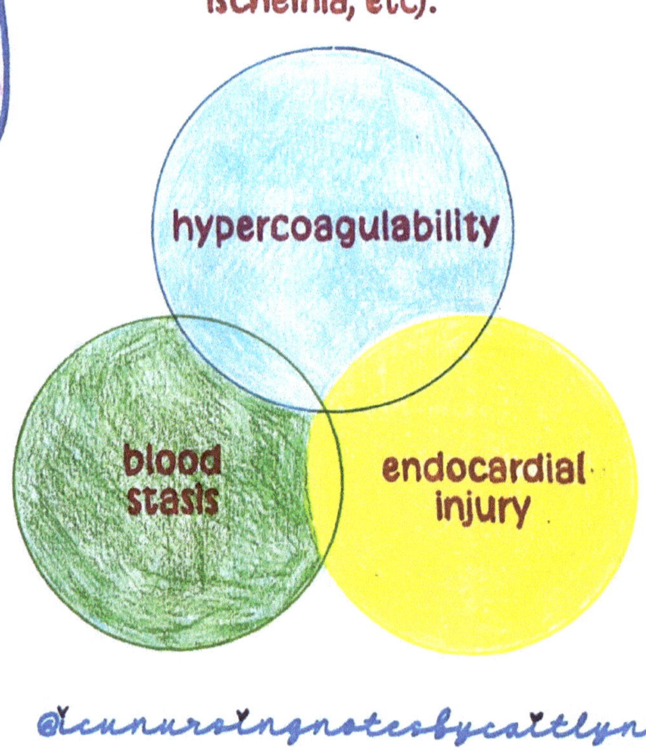

MANAGEMENT:

- anticoagulation c̄ a heparin bridge to warfarin (Coumadin)
- treatment of the underlying cardiomyopathy
- surgical removal (rare)

Dilated Cardiomyopathy

PATHOPHYSIOLOGY

Extensive damage to the cardiac muscle cells ↓ contractility of the left ventricle (LV). As systolic function declines, the cardiac output (CO) ↓ & end-diastolic volumes ↑!
The body attempts to compensate by activating the sympathetic nervous system to ↑ HR & contractility. When the body's compensatory mechanisms can no longer maintain an adequte cardiac output (CO), the heart begins to fail.

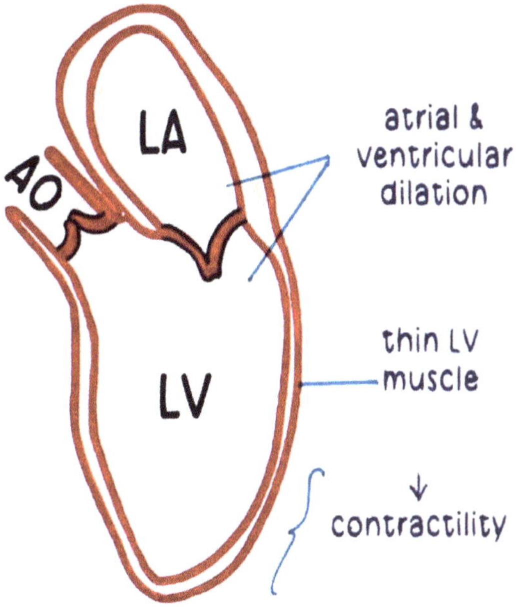

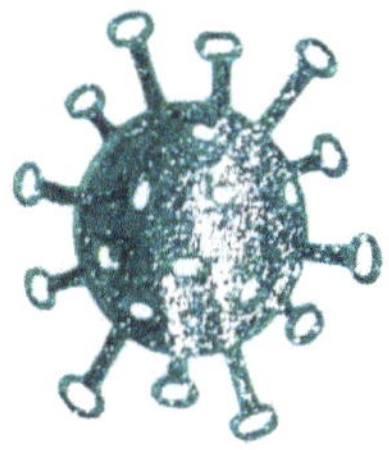

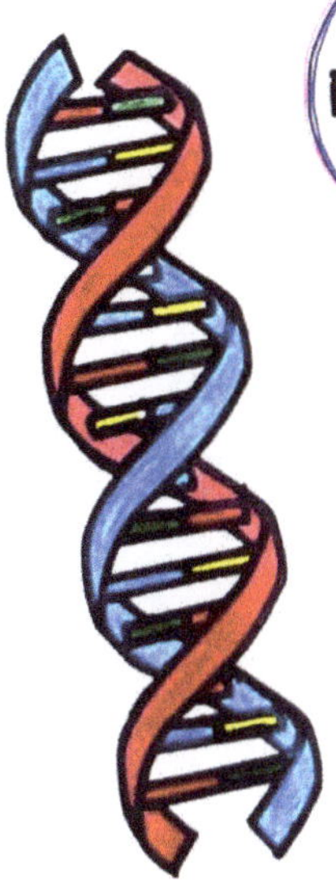

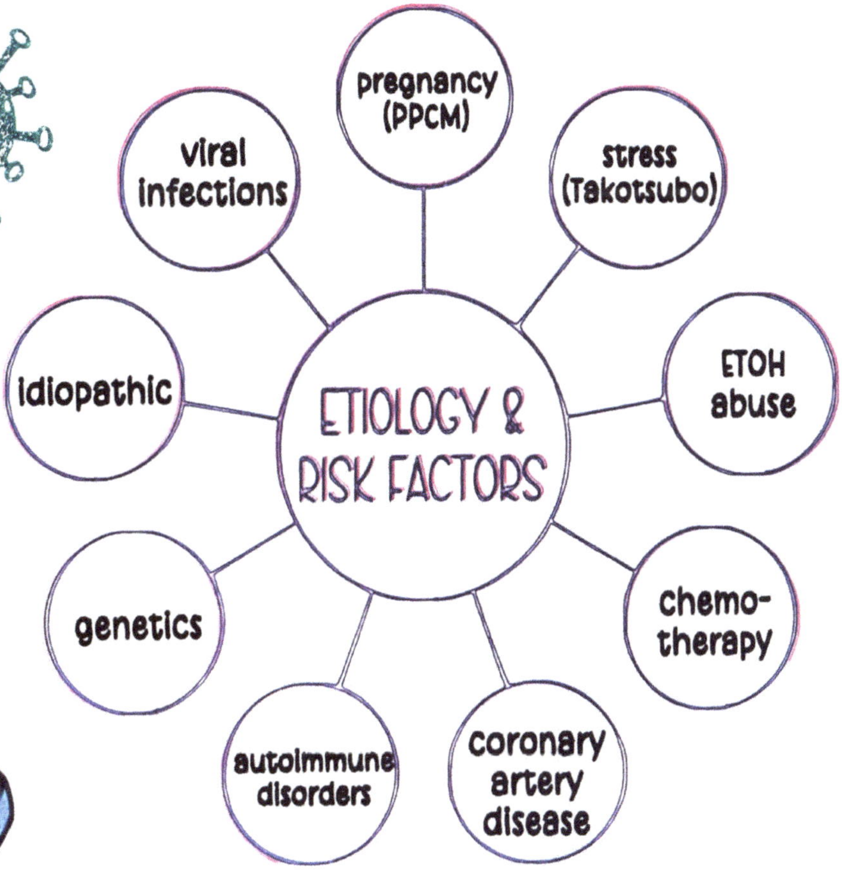

DIAGNOSIS:

echo ⇨ **cardiac cath** ⇨ **12 lead** ⇨ **CXR**

echo
- ↓ EF (HFrEF)
- systolic dysfunction
- LV dilation
- ↓wall thickness
- ventricular thrombi

cardiac cath
- ↓cardiac output
- LV dilation & dysfunction
- ↑LV & RV filling pressures

12 lead
- T wave changes
- septal Q waves
- bundle branch block (BBB)
- A-Fib or NSVT

CXR
- pulmonary edema
- pleural effusion
- cardiomegaly

The signs & symptoms of DCM are the same as HFrEF (heart failure c̄ a reduced ejection fraction)!

TREATMENT:

- ↓preload ⟶ fluid restriction, diuretics, NTG, & ACE-I/ARBs
- ↓afterload ⟶ ACE-I/ARBs & hydralazine + isosorbide dinitrate
- ↑contractility ⟶ + inotropes (Digoxin, dobutamine, milrinone), cardiac resynchronization therapy (CRT), & mechanical support devices (IABP, Impella, LVAD, BIVAD, & ECMO)
- ↓ ♥ remodeling ⟶ ACE-I/ARBs, spironolactone (↓the sympathetic response), & beta blockers
- anticoagulation ⟶ DOACs (Pradaxa, Xarelto, Eliquis)

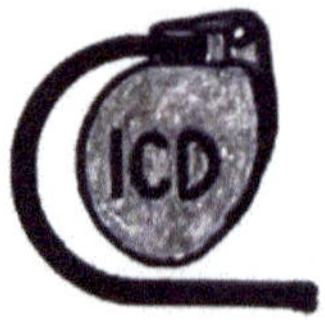

- SCD prevention ⟶ implantable cardiac defibrillator (ICD)
- surgery ⟶ cardiac transplant ♥

BRASH Syndrome

A vicious cycle of severe bradycardia, worsening renal function, & end-organ hypoperfusion that is triggered by AV-nodal blocker(s) and hyperkalemia.

Bradycardia

Renal failure

Av nodal blockade
(beta-blocker or calcium channel blocker)

Shock

Hyperkalemia

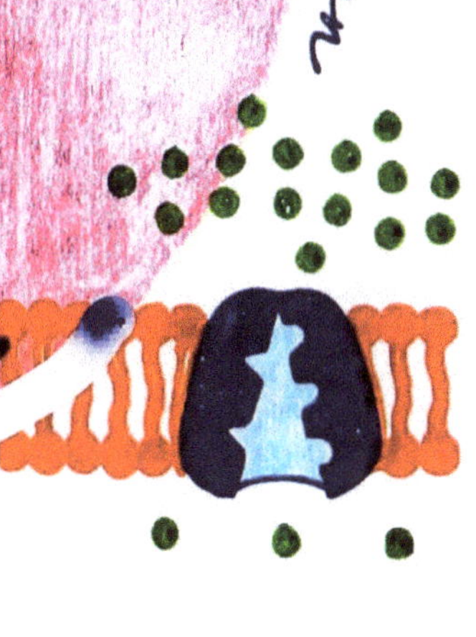

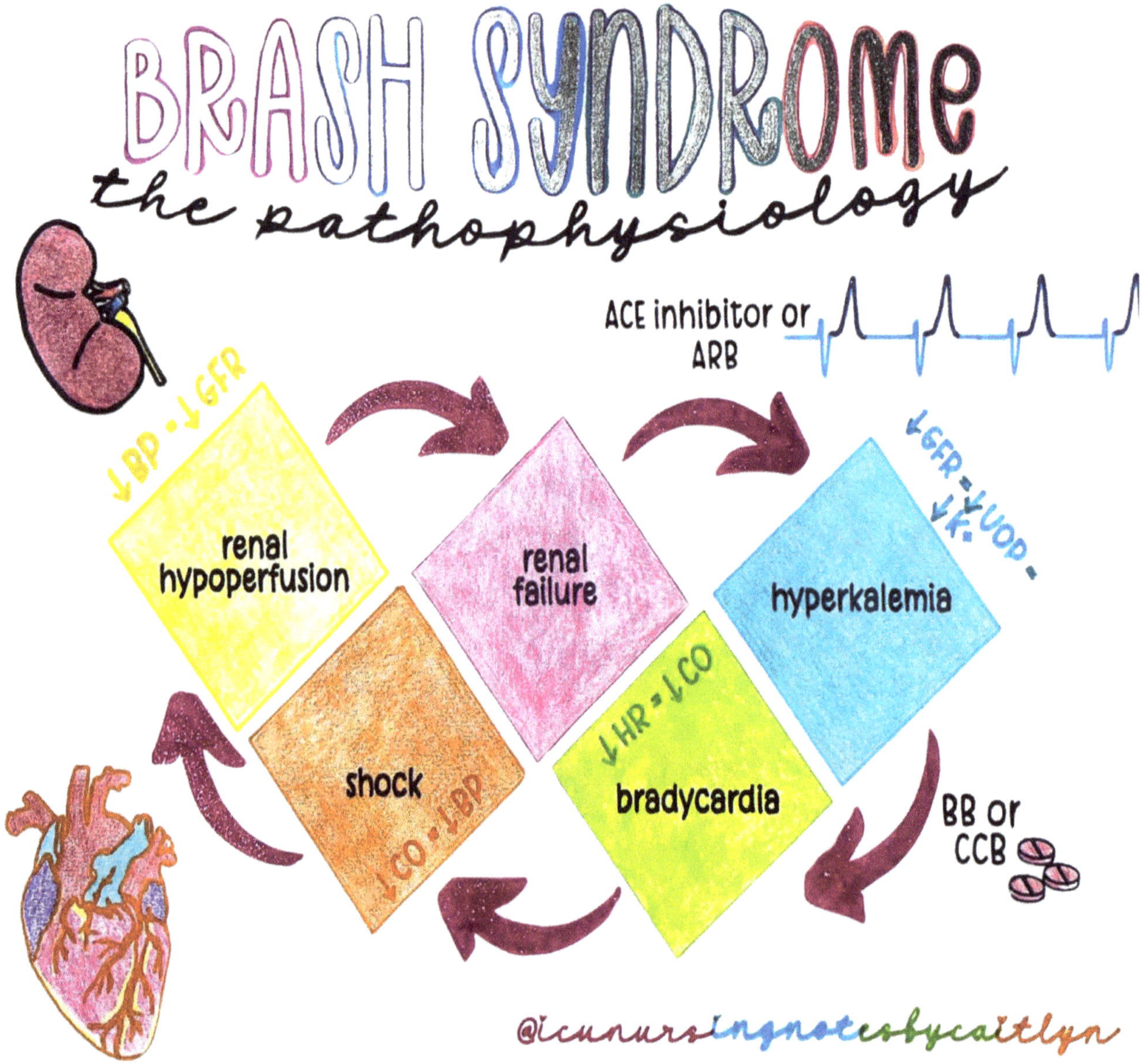
BRASH SYNDROME
the pathophysiology
ACE inhibitor or ARB
↓BP = ↓GFR
renal hypoperfusion
renal failure
↓GFR = ↓UOP = ↑K+
hyperkalemia
shock
↓CO = ↓BP
↓HR = ↓CO
bradycardia
BB or CCB
@icunursingnotesbycaitlyn

Diabetic Ketoacidosis

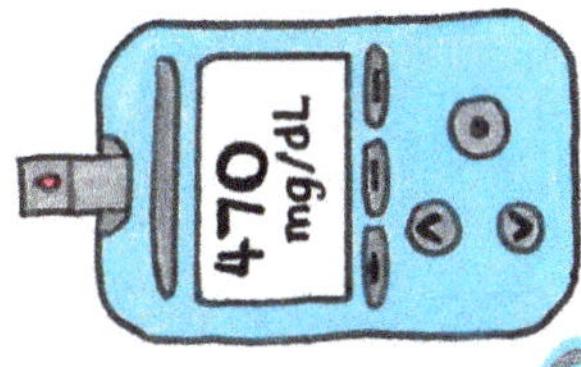

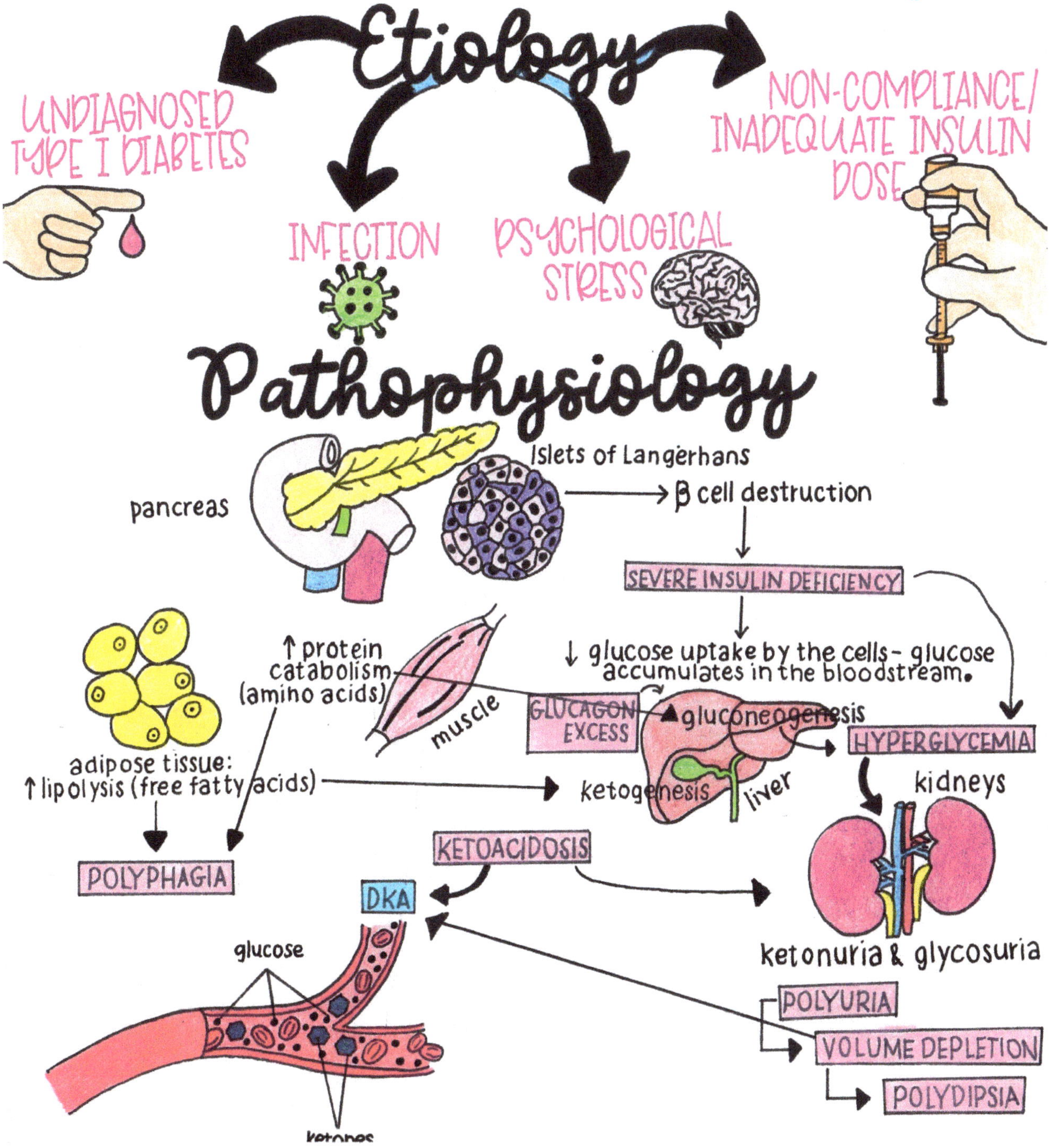

S/S of DKA

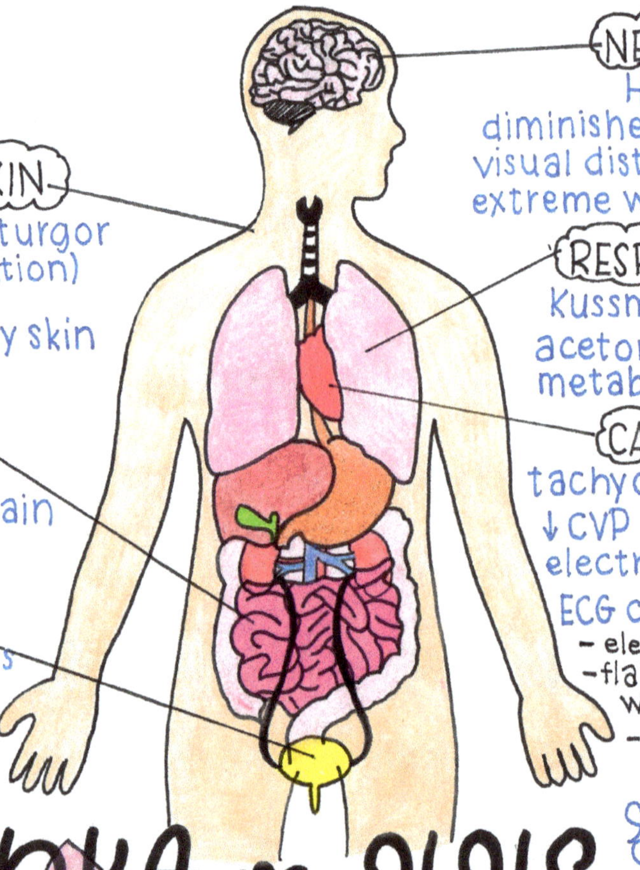

DKA vs. HHS

Hyperglycemic Hyperosmolar Syndrome

DKA

- Usually occurs with Type 1 DM.
- sudden onset
- glucose level is typically 300-800 mg/dL
- Presence of ketones
- metabolic acidosis
- presence of an anion gap (>15)
- relative hypovolemia

HHS

- Usually occurs with Type II DM
- gradual onset
- extreme hyperglycemia (> 600, but can be > 1000)
- Absence of ketones (the body has enough endogenous insulin to prevent ketosis).
- normal blood pH/mild acidosis
- ∅ anion gap
- profound hypovolemia

Medical Management

* Find and treat the underlying cause
* IV fluid resuscitation
* Continuous IV insulin infusion

} reverses metabolic acidosis

* Replace electrolytes

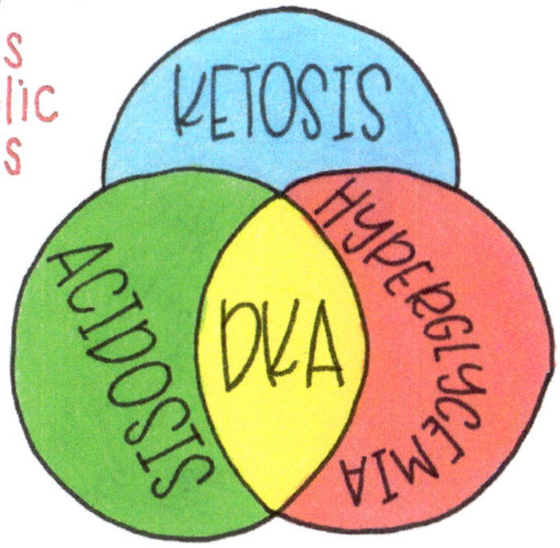

Always know what your patient's K+ level is before you administer IV insulin!!! Treat hypokalemia first.

Insulin drives K+ into the cells, so the serum K+ level can drop quickly → ↑ risk for ♥ arrhythmias.

Nursing Care

- Top 3 priorities: administering IV fluids (liters), monitoring BG closely during insulin infusion (typically hourly) & managing fluid/electrolytes.
- Monitor VS & LOC.
- Monitor ECG for arrhythmias/ectopy.
- Monitor glucose levels hourly, electrolytes (including anion gap), ketones, volume status & the patient's symptoms.
- Follow hospital policy for the frequency of blood glucose checks & insulin gtt titrations; typically q hour (BG) & BMP q 2-4 hrs (varies).
- Assess IV sites frequently for infiltration (especially with peripheral KCl).
- Strict I&O; monitor for S/S of fluid overload; transduce CVP, if available.
- Ensure the patient is NPO until the DKA has been resolved.
- Treat hypokalemia before administering insulin.
- 2-RN verification for insulin administration.
- Remember that human regular insulin is the only type of insulin that can be administered intravenously.
- When transitioning from the insulin gtt to subcutaneous insulin, it's important to continue the IV infusion for 1-2 hours after the subcutaneous dose of basal insulin has been given. This helps to avoid rebound ketoacidosis.

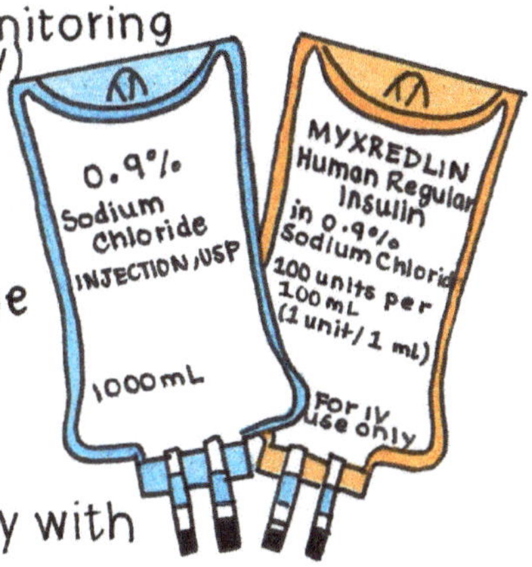

COMPENSATION IN SHOCK

@icunursingnotesbycaitlyn

initial insult that triggers shock

↓tissue perfusion & ↓oxygenation

activation of compensatory mechanisms

↑catecholamine release & ↑cortisol to provide more glucose for energy metabolism

<u>sympathetic activation:</u> ↑HR, ↑BP, ↑contractility & ↑cardiac output

<u>RASS activation:</u> ↑reabsorption of sodium & H2O leads to ↑preload & decreased urine output

As the body's compensatory mechanisms work to ↑cardiac output & SVR, the BP improves.

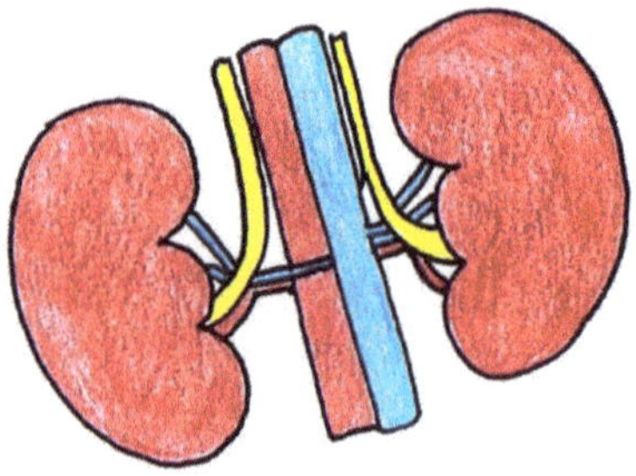

restoration of tissue perfusion & oxygenation

HYPOVOLEMIC SHOCK

ETIOLOGY

what causes it?

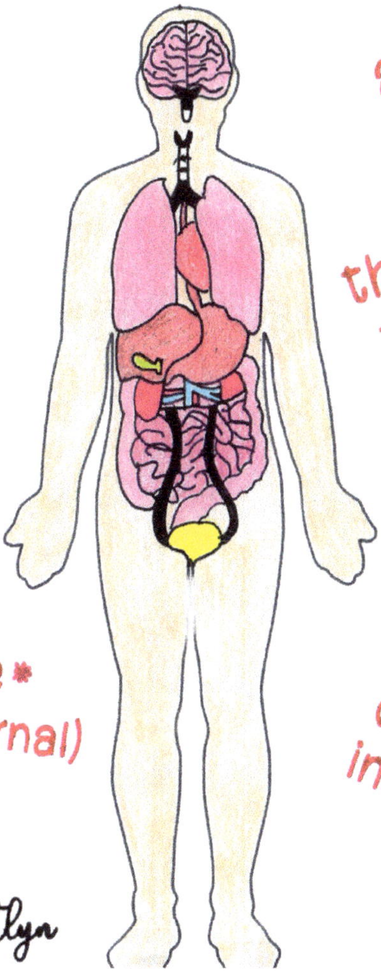

trauma*

burns

osmotic diuresis (DKA)

AVM

PPH

hemorrhage* (internal or external)

GIB

adrenal crisis

third spacing
- acute pancreatitis
- liver failure
- bowel obstruction
- burns
- sepsis

fluid & electrolyte loss

diabetes insipidus (DI)

@icunursingnotesbycaitlyn

PATHOPHYSIOLOGY

Internal or external fluid/blood loss

↓

↓intravascular volume

↓

↓preload (filling pressure)

↓

↓stroke volume (SV)

↑in HR (bracketing ↓preload through ↓stroke volume)

↓

↓cardiac output (CO)

↓

↓mean arterial pressure (MAP)

↓

↓tissue perfusion

↓

↓oxygen & nutrient delivery to cells

↓

multiple-organ-dysfunction syndrome (MODS)

Remember that cardiac output depends on the end-diastolic ventricular pressure, so expect a decrease in cardiac output.

@icunursingnotesbycaitlyn

CVP/RAP, PCWP, CO/CI, & SvO2 will be low; SVR is the only hemodynamic parameter that will be high (because of compensatory vasoconstriction).

SIGNS & SYMPTOMS

- pale, cool & clammy skin
- hypotension c̄ a narrow pulse pressure
- bleeding (hemorrhagic shock)
- tachycardia
- weak, thready pulse
- tachypnea
- restlessness, AMS
- oliguria
- ↑ SVR & ↓ CO/CI
- ↓ CVP, ↓ PCWP, ↓ Svo2
- hemoconcentration
- metabolic acidosis
- elevated lactate

Tachycardia & restlessness are often the first warning signs of impending hypovolemic shock, so it's important to be alert for subtle changes in your nursing assessment (in light of the bigger clinical picture).

TREATMENT

Fix the underlying cause!

IV fluid resuscitation (LR or NS)
Massive transfusion protocol (MTP)
Albumin for third-spacing
Vasopressors to support blood pressure

Think of hypovolemic shock as having no gas in the "vascular tank," so fill it up with fluids!

NURSING CARE

-Continually assess the patient for subtle changes in vital signs, mental status, & end-organ function.
-Prevention is important; know which patients are at risk for developing hypovolemic shock (see page #1). Early recognition is key!
-Monitor & trend hemodynamics to assess the severity of shock & to assess how well the patient is responding to fluid resuscitation.
-Anticipate intubation, central line, Swan-Ganz Catheter, & arterial line placement.
-If the patient doesn't have a Swan-Ganz Catheter or FloTrac but has a central line, then transduce the central venous pressure (CVP) using the distal port.
-Monitor blood pressure & consider the use of vasopressors (first-line: Levophed), especially if the patient isn't fluid responsive.
-Use a pressure bag or a rapid infuser for fluid resuscitation in a hemodynamically unstable patient.
-Frequent neuro assessments & LOC - a decrease in LOC is a sign of advancing shock & airway protection should be your priority!
-Monitor for signs of fluid volume overload.
-Strict I & O and daily weights.
-Frequent cardiac/pulmonary/neurovascular assessments, including pulses.
-Ensure that the IV fluids are running through patent large-bore IV catheters (if not a central line).
-Elevate the patient's legs to help with venous return to the heart (central circulation).
-Monitor core body temperature; consider using a fluid warmer.
-Follow the hospital's massive transfusion protocol (MTP) for hemorrhagic shock.
-Monitor & trend labs (i.e. CBC, electrolytes, ABGs, lactate, etc).
-Continue addressing the underlying cause & treat it!

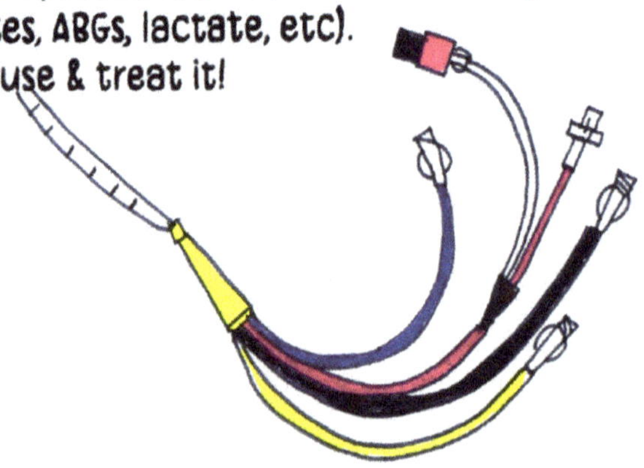

BLOOD TRANSFUSION

BLOOD TYPE COMPATIBILITY

BLOOD TYPE	CAN GIVE TO	CAN RECEIVE FROM
A+	A+, AB+	A+, A-, O+, O-
O+	O+, A+, B+, AB+	O+, O-
B+	B+, AB+	B+, B-, O+, O-
AB+	AB+	EVERYONE
A-	A+, A-, AB+, AB-	A-, O-
O-	EVERYONE	O-
B-	B+, B-, AB+, AB-	B-, O-
AB-	AB+, AB-	AB-, A-, B-, O-

SAFETY CHECKS

2 RN bedside check:

- Valid signed consent form
- Patient's name, DOB, & MRN
- Type of blood product ordered
- ABO/Rh factor
- Unit number
- Expiration date of the blood

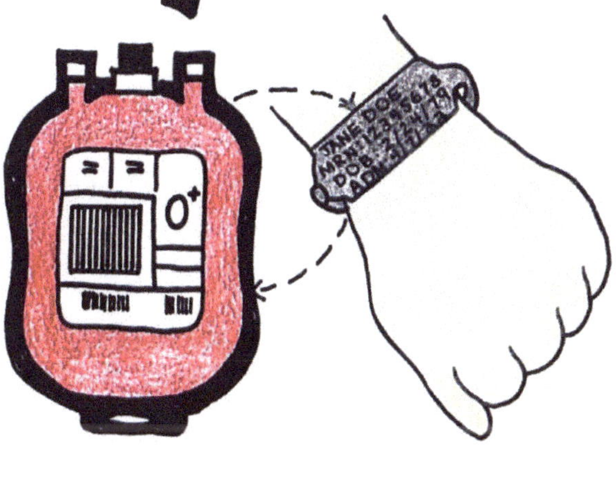

@icunursingnotesbycaitlyn

BLOOD PRODUCTS

Packed Red Blood Cells (PRBCs)

* Prepared from whole blood by removing most of the plasma.
* Indicated for low hemoglobin (usually <7 g/dL), acute sickle cell crisis & blood loss.
* Must be administered within 4 hours.
* Requires ABO & Rh matching before administering.

Platelets

* Used to treat thrombocytopenia, critical bleeding requiring mass transfusion, & conditions involving platelet dysfunction.
* Contraindicated in TTP and HIT.
* Give as quickly as possible

Fresh Frozen Plasma (FFP)

* Replaces clotting factors
* Contains no platelets
* Rh factor & ABO compatibility are required.
* Administer as quickly as possible
* Monitor for hypocalcemia

Cryoprecipitate

* Prepared by thawing FFP & collecting the precipitate; it contains high levels of factor VIII & fibrinogen.
* Used to treat clotting disorders
  - Hemophilia A
  - Von Willebrand disease
* Can also be used to help correct hypofibrinogenemia due to DIC.

ADMINISTERING BLOOD

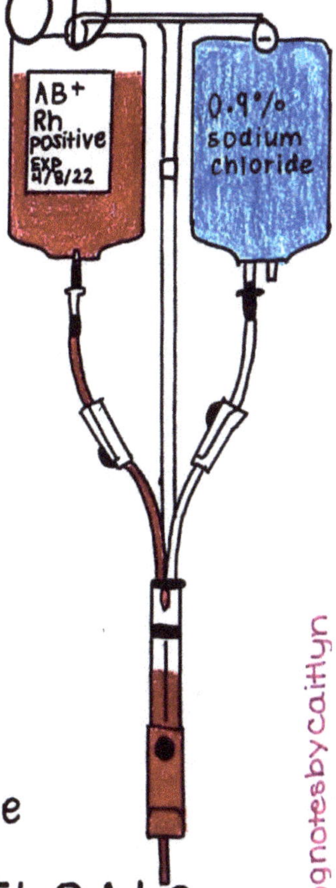

1) Safety checks & 2 RN verification.
2) Obtain pre-transfusion vital signs & a baseline assessment.
3) Ensure patency of the IV line.
4) Hang the NS flush bag & ensure both roller clamps are closed.
5) Spike the NS bag & prime the filter & IV tubing.
6) Close the NS roller clamp & spike the blood bag.
7) Open the blood roller clamp & prime the filter & IV tubing c̄ blood.
8) Load the blood tubing in the IV pump & set the pump to deliver the blood at the desired rate.
9) Flush the IV line, connect the IV tubing to the patient's IV, & begin the infusion.

NURSING CONSIDERATIONS

- Always perform safety checks c̄ another RN.
- Verify that a valid informed consent form has been signed.
- Do not allow blood to hang for > 4 hours
- Start the infusion within 30 minutes of receiving the blood from the blood bank.
- Obtain vital signs before initiating the transfusion, 15 minutes after the transfusion has started, and then q 30 min thereafter.
- A transfusion reaction is most likely to occur within the first 15 minutes of the infusion, so have a strong baseline assessment to assess for any changes.
- Premedicate c̄ an antihistamine (Benadryl) & Tylenol as ordered.
- If you're infusing FFP, keep an eye on your patient's calcium level.
- Administer blood through a 20G or larger (ideally!) IV catheter.
- When administering multiple units of blood under pressure (i.e. trauma), use a blood warmer to prevent hypothermia.
- Monitor for S/S of a transfusion reaction (see pg 4).
- Consider your patient's cardiopulmonary status, age & EF when determining the rate of infusion (higher risk for circulatory overload).

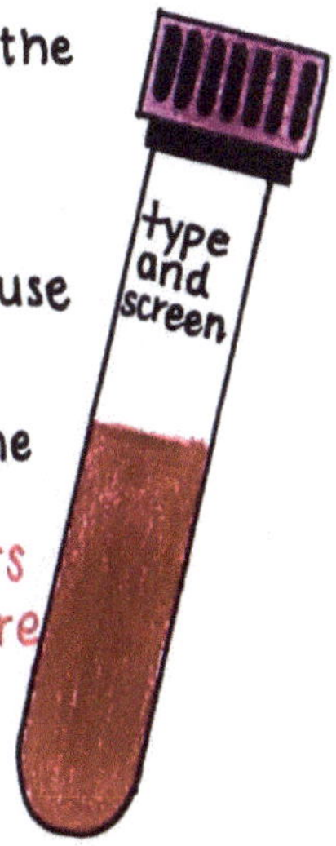

A type & screen is generally only valid for 72 hours (3 days), so consider drawing a new sample before it expires (if you anticipate the need for additional blood transfusions). Make sure there is an order!

TRANSFUSION REACTIONS

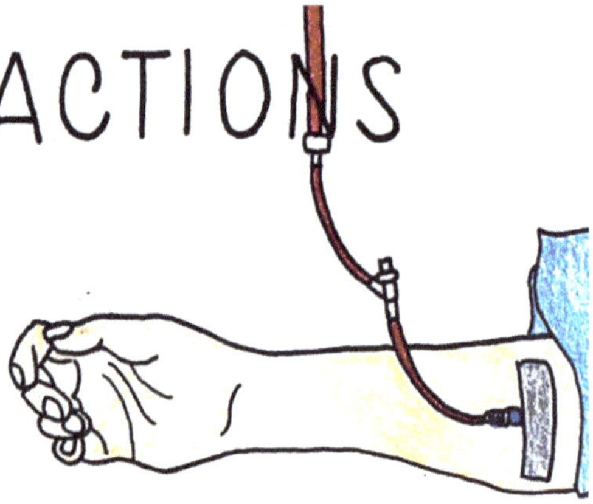

Acute Hemolytic:

- Caused by incompatibility c̄ donor blood.
- S/S: N/V, lower back pain, chest tightness, hypotension & tachycardia, ↓ UOP, hematuria & DIC.
- Tx: airway management, hypotension → vasopressors, diuretics, & management of DIC.

Allergic:

- Caused by a sensitivity reaction to a plasma protein within the blood being transfused.
- S/S (mild): facial flushing, hives/rash
  - → Tx: antihistamines
- S/S (severe): wheezing, ↓ BP, & anaphylaxis.
  - → Tx: epinephrine, airway management, corticosteroids, & vasopressors.

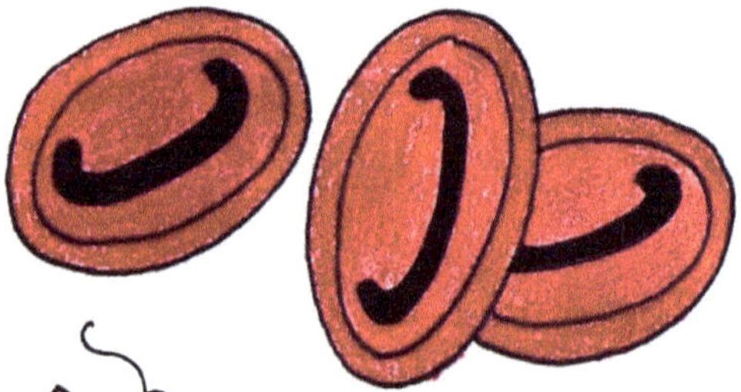

RBCs

Febrile:

- Caused by antibodies to donor leukocytes that remain in the unit of blood.
- S/S: fever, chills, malaise, tachycardia.
- Prevention: pre-medicate with an antipyretic & antihistamine.
- most common transfusion reaction

With all Reactions:

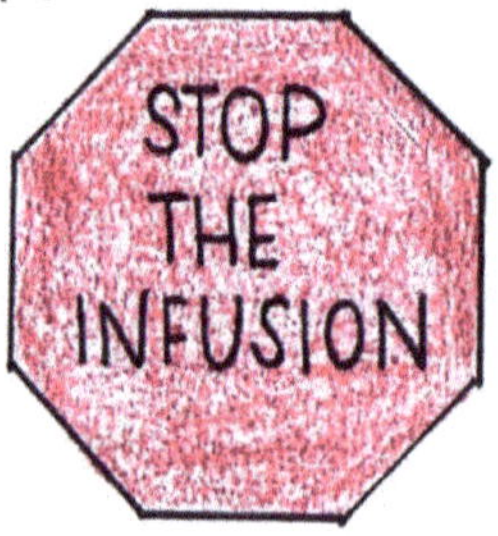

And

Maintain Line c̄ NS

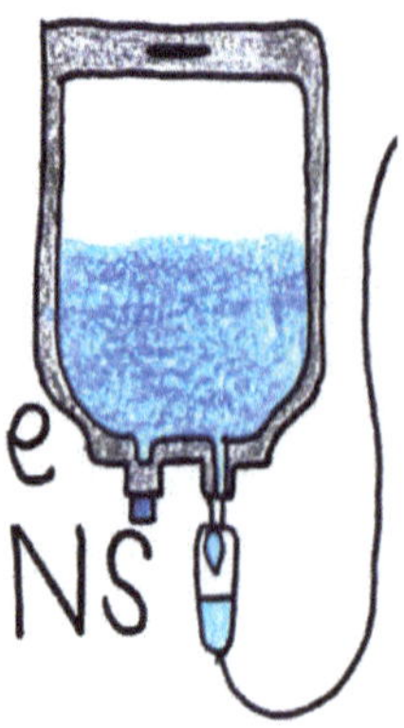

@icunursingnotesbycaitlyn

The Rapid Infuser

Uses

Critically ill patients needing rapid fluid resuscitation (IV fluids and/or blood products).

- Major hemorrhage (i.e. trauma, post-operative, GI bleed, PPH or placental abruption, etc).
- Septic shock
- Hypovolemic shock
- Burns

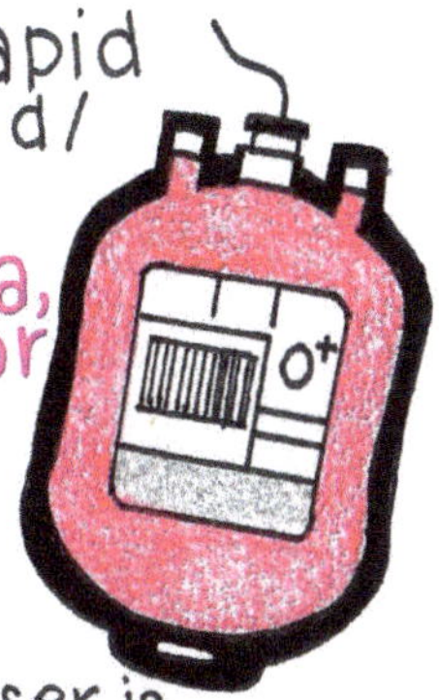

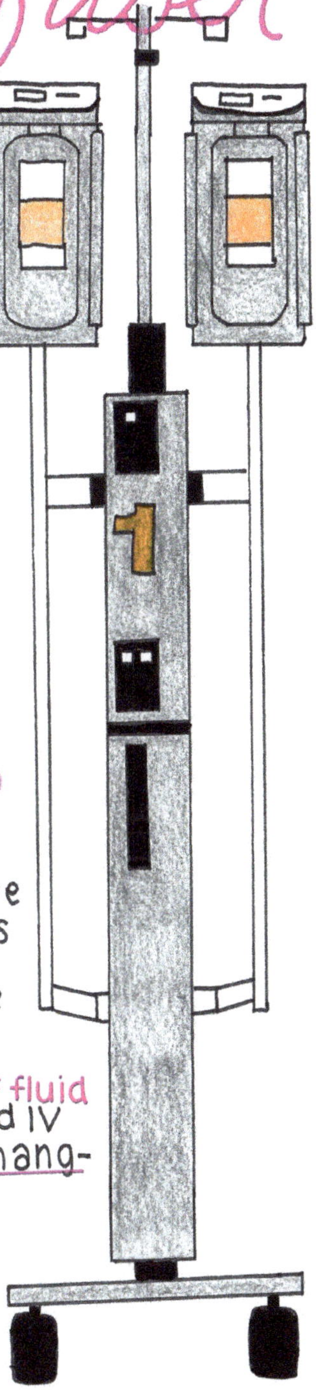

The level I rapid infuser is usually run by a certified IV nurse.

How it Works

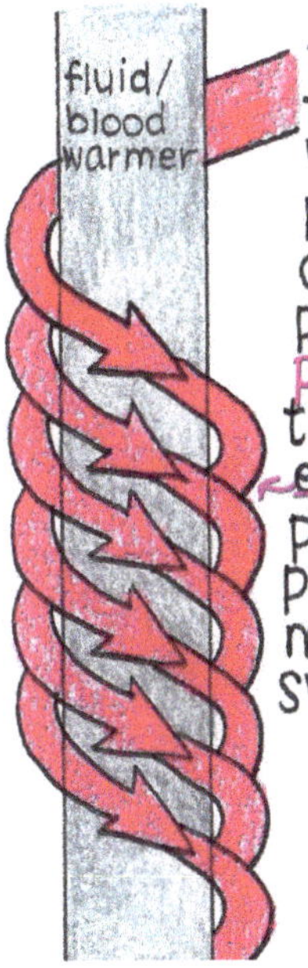

The rapid infuser is used for the massive transfusion of blood products or fluids for resuscitation. The rapid infuser warms IV fluids & blood products & the pressure chambers apply pressure and deliver the prescribed fluids or blood products at a rapid rate (over a liter of fluid per minute!). The device uses specialized IV tubing c̄ a gas vent-filter & a heat exchanger that is designed to expand under pressure. Pressure is maintained by the pressure chambers at a constant 300 mmHg & is turned on/off via a simple switch at the top of each pressure chamber.

The rapid infuser cannot be used to warm platelets, cryo, or granulocytes.

The Rapid Infuser
Nursing Considerations

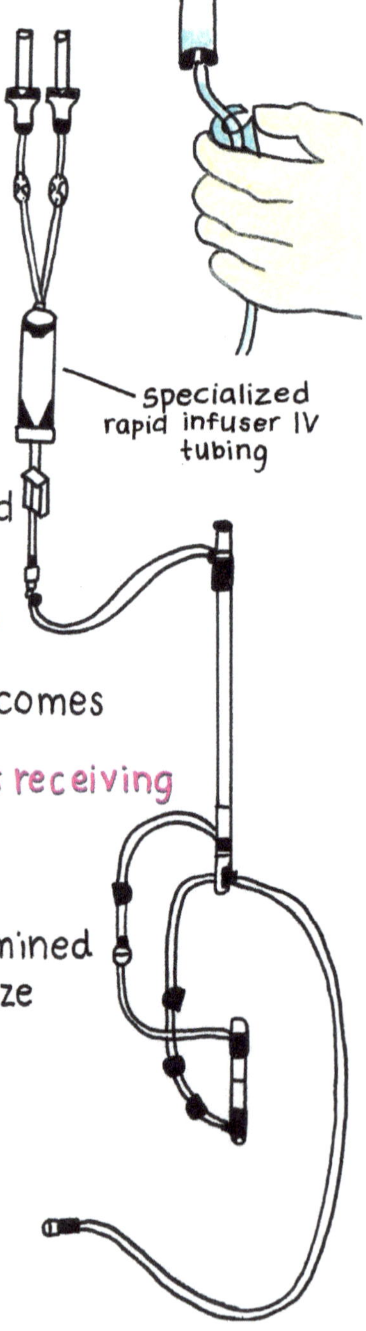

- Monitor core body temperature (risk for hypothermia), and use a Bair Hugger.
- Assess the patient's IV sites frequently (↑ risk of infiltration).
- Monitor urine output & hemodynamic status
- Place a BP cuff on the patient's opposite arm & recycle q 5 min until an art line is placed.
- When spiking a new bag, ensure that all of the air is removed before hanging it in the pressure chamber (just like you would when setting up an arterial line).
- Ensure that all connections are tight & secure.
- Have the next bag of IVF ready to infuse to avoid any delays in infusion.
- Use a marker to keep track of how many bags have been used (timesaver on backtracking & on documentation).
- Replace the filter q 3 hours or when the filter becomes clogged, and the infusion rate slows.
- Monitor the patient's labs & electrolytes (patients receiving large volume fluid resuscitation are at risk for hypokalemia, hypomagnesemia, hypocalcemia, & hypophosphatemia).

Remember that the infusion rate is determined by the size of the IV catheter & not the size of the vein!

Fluids that are inadequately warmed will contribute to hypothermia; fluids that are overly warmed will contribute to hemolysis of the RBCs.

BLOOD LACTATE

PHYSIOLOGY

Lactate (lactic acid) is a byproduct of anaerobic metabolism. Under normal physiologic conditions, the body's tissues use aerobic metabolism to breakdown glucose for energy. If the tissues are deprived of oxygen, though, they revert to using anaerobic metabolism with lactic acid production (byproduct). Lactate levels may be elevated in a critically ill patient for one of two reasons: impaired oxygen delivery (type A lactic acidosis) or impaired oxygen utilization by the cells (type B lactic acidosis). In the ICU, lactate levels are useful for monitoring tissue perfusion status in critically ill patients (particularly those with sepsis & septic shock).

A normal blood lactate level is 0.5 - 1.0 mmol/L!

A lactate level will be more useful when correlated with an ABG or central venous blood gas!

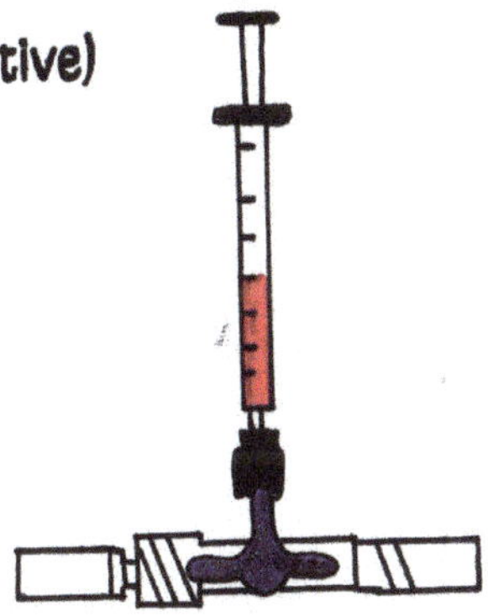

ETIOLOGY

- shock states (septic, cardiogenic, hypovolemic, & obstructive)
- cardiac arrest
- trauma
- rhabdomyolysis
- seizures
- regional ischemia (i.e. mesenteric, etc).
- DKA
- thiamine deficiency
- liver dysfunction (decreased lactate clearance)
- medications (i.e. epinephrine, metformin, etc).

TREATMENT

Depends on the underlying cause: if hypoperfusion or hypoxemia is the culprit, then the treatment is focused on improving tissue perfusion, although sodium bicarbonate is usually used to initially treat lactic acidosis & acidemia.

- shock: IVF, vasopressors, & inotropes.
- regional ischemia: surgery to restore circulation/ remove damaged tissue.
- D/C causative drugs.

An elevated lactate does not necessarily mean "sepsis," & an elevated lactate does not necessarily mean "give more fluid"

HEMODYNAMICS IN SHOCK

	CVP	SVR	PCWP	CO/CI	SVO2
cardiogenic	↑	↑	↑	↓	↓
septic	↓	↓	↓	↑	↑
neurogenic	↓	↓	↓	↑	↓
hypovolemic	↓	↑	↓	↓	↓
obstructive	↑	↑	↑↓	↓	↓

ACUTE RESPIRATORY DISTRESS SYNDROME

PATHOPHYSIOLOGY

SIRS → **lung injury**

damage to the alveolar & pulmonary capillary endothelium → release of proteins, cytokines, & neutrophils into the alveolar space

↑ alveolar-capillary membrane permeability & pulmonary edema → type II alveolar cell damage causes ↓ surfactant production

atelectasis & hypoxemia occur: pulmonary vasoconstriction

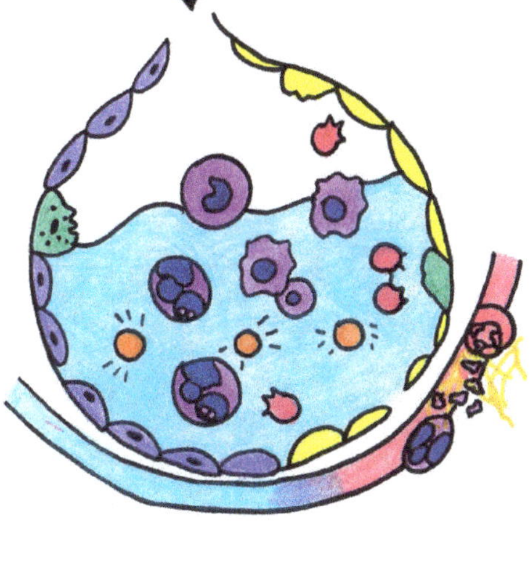

- respiratory acidosis
- refractory hypoxemia
- PHTN
- irreversible lung damage
- cardiac failure
- MODS

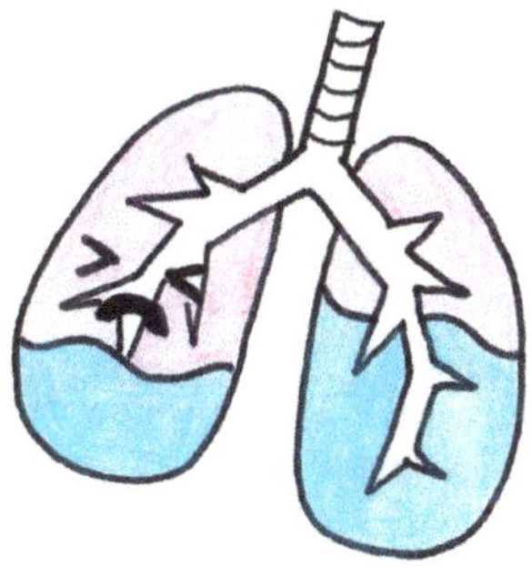

ETIOLOGY

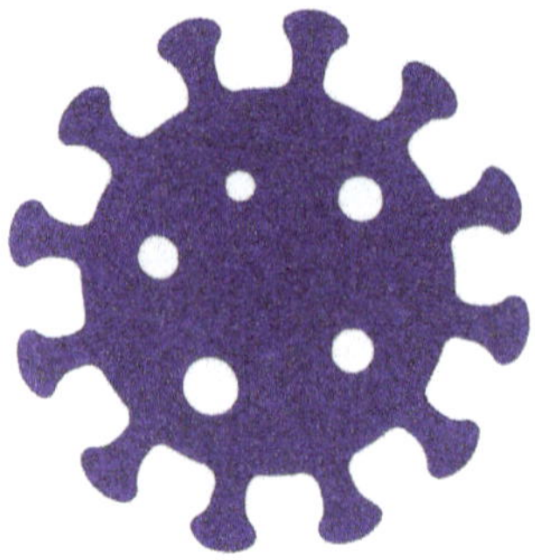

- septic shock
- trauma
- DIC
- acute pancreatits
- multiple blood transfusions (TRALI)
- near-drowning
- PNA/aspiration
- inhalation injury
- CPB

SIGNS & SYMPTOMS

- refractory hypoxemia, cyanosis
- dyspnea, tachypnea & tachycardia
- noncardiogenic pulmonary edema
- diffuse crackles
- oliguria
- bilateral pulmonary infiltrates on CXR
- worsening P/F ratio (<200) & increased A-a gradient
- PAWP <18 mmHg
- AMS (elevated PaCO2, low PaO2)

TREATMENT

- treat the underlying cause (i.e. abx for
- sepsis)
- mechanical ventilation (LTVV & ↑ PEEP)
- VV-ECMO
- prone positioning
- + inotropes, vasopressors & diuretics
- inhaled pulmonary vasodilators
- fluid management (neutral/net negative)
- supportive care to ↓ O2 consumption (temperature control with antipyretics, deep sedation, NMB with paralytics)

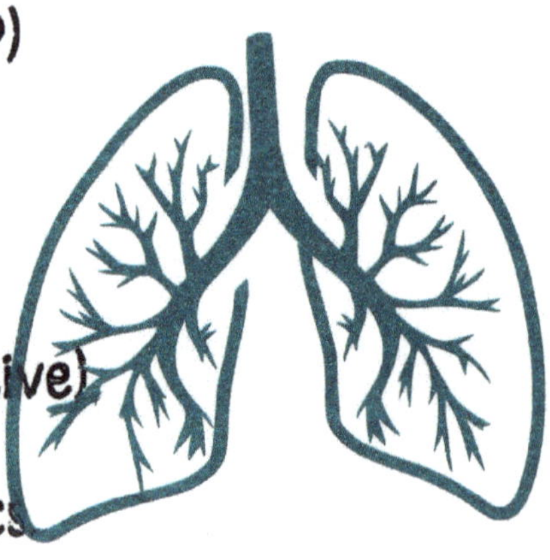

- Monitor serial ABGs & trend lactate levels.
- When increasing PEEP, monitor for hypotension (decreased venous return).
- Monitor hemodynamics & trends in pulmonary artery pressure (PAP) & wedge pressure (PCWP), if a Swan-Ganz catheter is in place (increasing pressures indicate further deterioration & worsening pulmonary edema).
- Proning is important & evidence-based! Prone for at least 16 hours.
- Anticipate the need for VV-ECMO, if refractory hypoxemia persists.
- Pain & anxiety management.
- Allow permissive hypercapnia in these patients.
- Address pain, fever, restlessness/agitation, & ventilator dyssynchrony - all of which increase oxygen consumption.
- Achieve appropriate sedation level to facilitate patient-ventilator synchrony.
- Train-of-four (TOF) monitoring for paralytics: ensure that these patients are deeply sedated to RASS -5 & do not decrease sedative/analgesic gtts while paralyzed.
- Implement preventative measures for ventilator-associated pneumonia (VAP).
- Strict I&O, daily weights & conservative fluid management.
- PI, PUD & VTE prophylaxis.
- Reduce the risk of secondary infections (i.e. CLABSI, VAP, UTI).
- Address goals of care.

NURSING CARE

AUTO-POSITIVE END EXPIRATORY PRESSURE (AUTO-PEEP)

A complication of mechanical ventilation that typically affects patients c̄ obstructive airway disease!

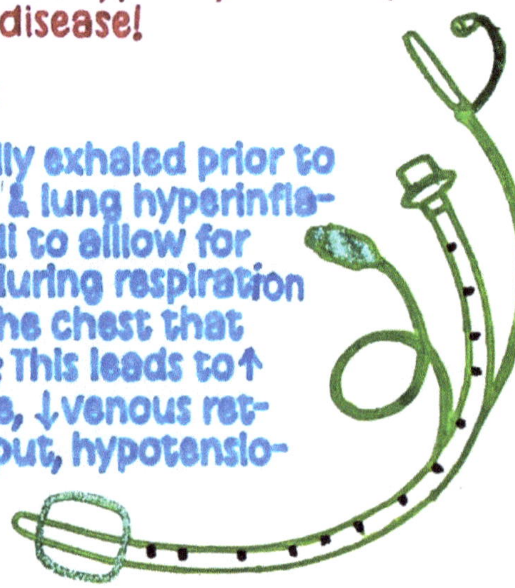

PATHOPHYSIOLOGY:

Auto-PEEP occurs when a breath can't be fully exhaled prior to the next inhalation, resulting in "air trapping" & lung hyperinflation. Air needs to move in & out of the alveoli to allow for gas exchange. Trapped air within the lungs during respiration creates additional positive pressure within the chest that exceeds the PEEP value set by the ventilator. This leads to ↑ intrathoracic pressure, ↑ peak airway pressure, ↓ venous return, ↓ preload, ↓ afterload (SVR), ↓ cardiac output, hypotension, barotrauma, ventilator dyssynchrony, & hypoxemia!

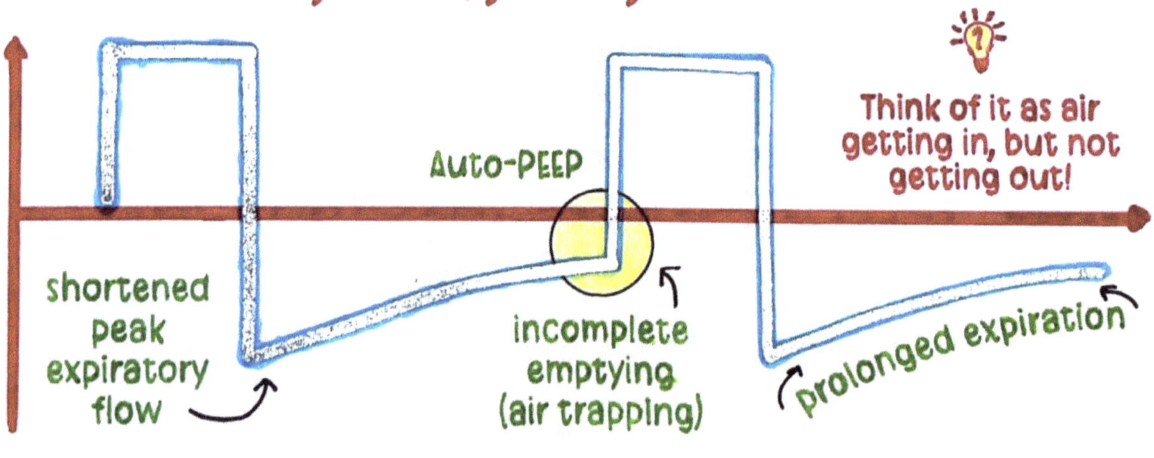

HOW TO CORRECT AUTO-PEEP?

- Treat the underlying cause
- ↓ the inspiratory time &/or ↑ the expiratory time
- ↓ the tidal volume (TV)
- ↓ the respiratory rate

PULMONARY EMBOLISM

RISK FACTORS

- venous stasis (post-op, prolonged immobility, A-fib, CHF, etc).
- hypercoagulability (cancer, oral contraceptive use, hormone replacement therapy, blood dyscrasias, pregnancy/post-partum).
- endothelial damage (history of VTE, trauma, IVDA, surgery, chemotherapy, diabetes, sepsis)

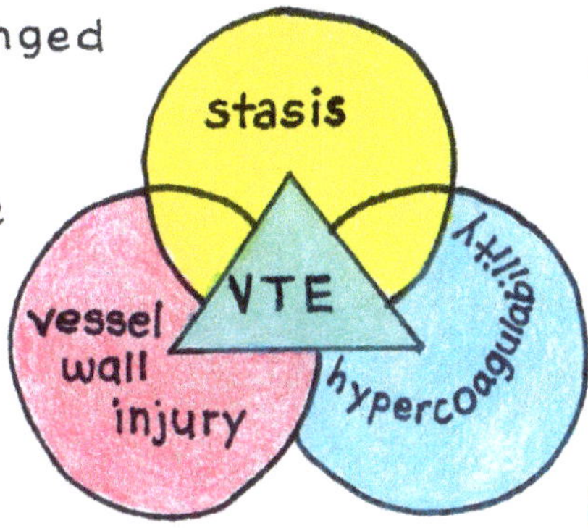

PATHOPHYS

A pulmonary embolism (PE) occurs when an embolus (thrombotic or nonthrombotic) lodges in the pulmonary arterial system and disrupts blood flow to the lungs. A blood clot typically forms in a vein of the lower extremities and breaks free from the vessel wall and travels to the lungs via the bloodstream. Obstruction of the pulmonary arterial system has both pulmonary and hemodynamic consequences. Pulmonary effects: ↑ alveolar dead space, bronchoconstriction, and compensatory shunting that leads to hypoxemia. Hemodynamic effects: ↑ PVR and ↑ right ventricular workload.

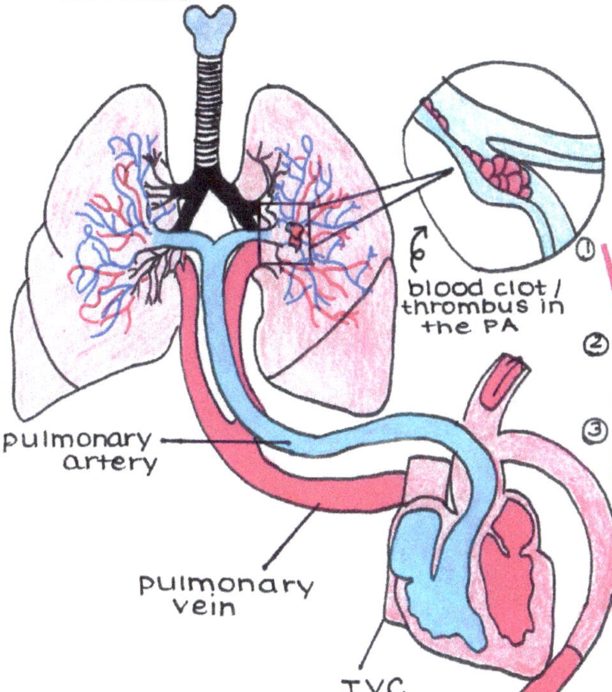

VIRCHow's Triad:

1. **VI**: vessel injury
2. **R**: reduced blood flow
3. **CH**: hypercoagulability

DX

- ★ pulmonary angiogram
- ★ V/Q scan
- ★ U/S – DVT extremities
- ★ ABG – ↓ PaO_2
- ★ CT scan

S/S

- tachycardia, tachypnea
- dyspnea
- chest pain
- crackles
- diaphoresis, anxiety
- sudden right-sided ♥ failure
- increased pulmonary artery pressures (PAP)

TREATMENT

- respiratory support (O_2)
- suspected PE: anticoagulants (LMWH or fondaparinux), direct thrombin inhibitor or factor Xa inhibitor, warfarin (Coumadin)
- acute PE c̄ hemodynamic instability: thrombolytics (alteplase/tPA)
- catheter-assisted thrombolysis (EKOS)
- pulmonary embolectomy
- vena cava filter

Remember that the alveoli are *ventilated*, but there is *lack of perfusion* (V/Q mismatch)!

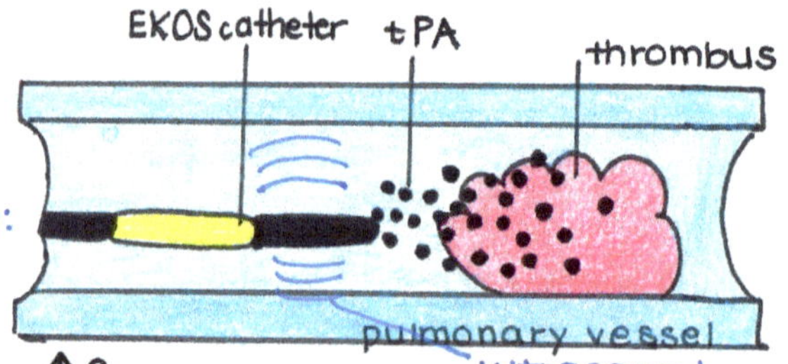

catheter-assisted thrombolysis

NURSING CARE

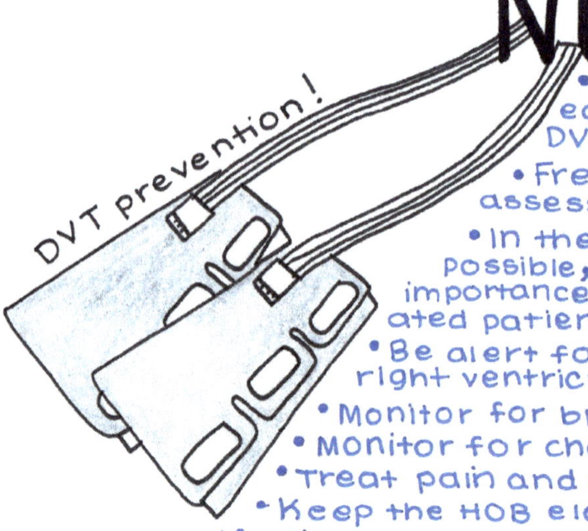

- Prevention is key* (encourage early ambulation, if possible, implement DVT prophylaxis interventions, etc).
- Frequent cardiac and pulmonary assessments.
- In the ICU, ambulation is not always possible, but don't underestimate the importance of passive ROM exercises for intubated patients!
- Be alert for signs of cardiogenic shock and right ventricular failure.
- Monitor for bleeding (H and H, urine, gums, etc)
- Monitor for changes in the ABGs.
- Treat pain and anxiety.
- Keep the HOB elevated to facilitate lung expansion.
- If using an EKOS catheter, verify that the coolant and thrombolytic infusion rates are accurate.

CHEST TUBES

@icunursingnotesbycaitlyn

INDICATIONS

- pneumothorax (closed and open).
- empyema
- hemothorax + hemopneumothorax
- pleural effusions
- open chest wound
- post- CT surgery (mediastinal chest tube)

Chest tube insertion sites vary based on the type of drainage to be removed (air: 2nd ICS at the MCL, fluid: 5th or 6th ICS, midaxillary line, etc).

PHYSIOLOGY

The pleural space is normally lubricated by a small amount of pleural fluid that allows the pleurae to move s̄ friction during respiration. When an excess of fluid and/or air enters the pleural space, it alters intrapleural pressure and causes partial or total lung collapse.

A chest tube, connected to a negative pressure closed drainage system, allows air and/or fluid to drain from the pleural space but not re-enter the pleural space (one-way valve).

A chest tube will re-establish normal lung mechanics and facilitate lung re-expansion by restoring negative pressure within the pleural space.

THE THREE CHAMBERS

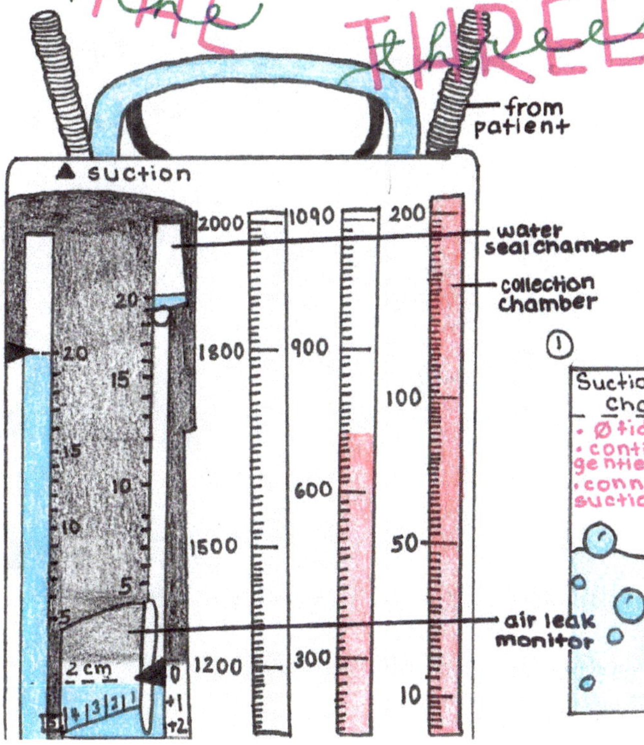

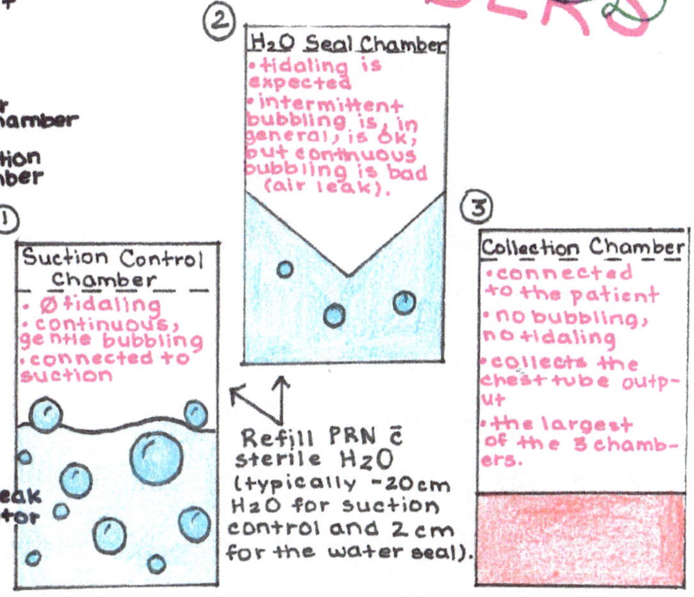

NURSING CARE

♡@icunursingnotesbycaitlyn

- Focused pulmonary assessment: RR, WOB, oxygenation, lung sounds, incision site, subcutaneous emphysema, amount/consistency of drainage, etc.
- Chest tubes are painful! Address pain.
- Monitor water levels in the water-seal and suction control chambers; it will evaporate over time, so add sterile H_2O PRN to maintain the prescribed levels.
- Check for tidaling (fluctuations in the water-seal chamber c̄ respiratory effort)
  → troubleshoot in the absence of tidaling: kinks in the tubing, tube compression, problem c̄ the wall suction regulator, etc.

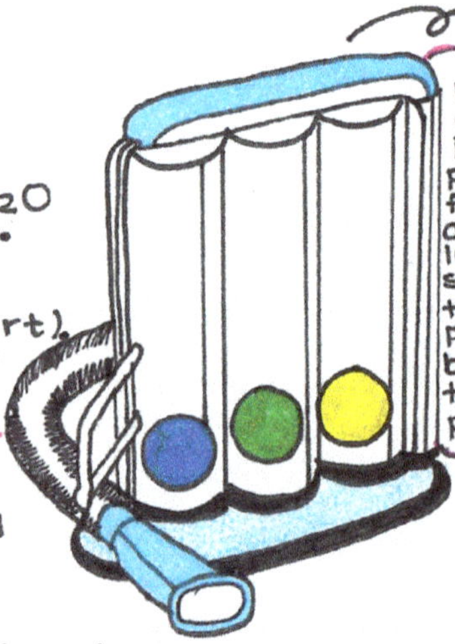

Deep breathing/coughing is important for promoting fluid drainage and for facilitating lung re-expansion, so be sure to teach your patient this, but don't forget to address pain first!!

💡 Don't expect tidaling c̄ complete lung re-expansion or c̄ mediastinal chest tubes.

- Suspect a possible air leak if there is continuous bubbling in the water-seal chamber; check by briefly clamping the tubing at different intervals until the source of the air leak is found.
- Keep at the bedside: Kelly clamps, container of sterile H_2O (dislodgement → creates a temporary water seal), occlusive sterile dressing/tape, another chest tube drainage system).

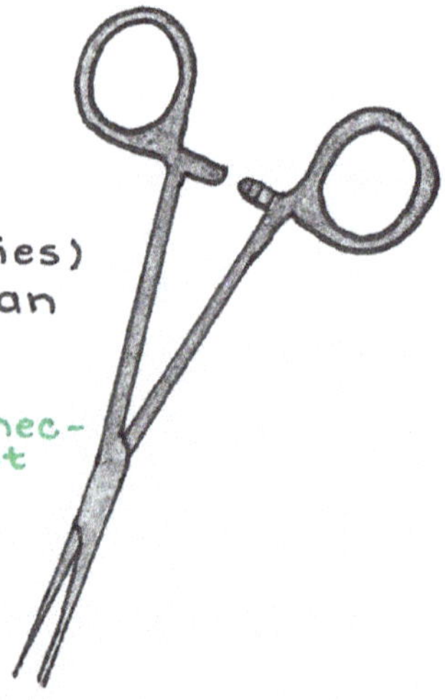

- Change the dressing PRN / per facility protocol (varies)
- Avoid clamping the tube (exceptions: checking for an air leak or changing the system).
- Replace the system when it's full.
  → tip: set it up using sterile technique before disconnecting the old one to minimize the time that the chest tube is clamped!
- Assess the color/amount/consistency of drainage, mark it on the drainage unit, and document it as output in I's and O's.
- Always make sure that the drainage system remains below the level of the chest.

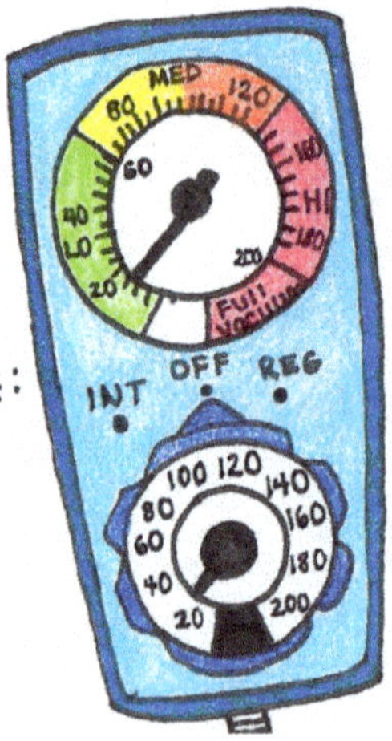

Connect the suction tubing to the drainage system and the suction/vacuum regulator on the wall.

STOP & Do Your Chest Tube Assessment:

→ **S**ite
→ **T**ubing
→ **O**utput
→ **P**atency

The Cardiac Conduction System

@icunursingnotesbycaitlyn

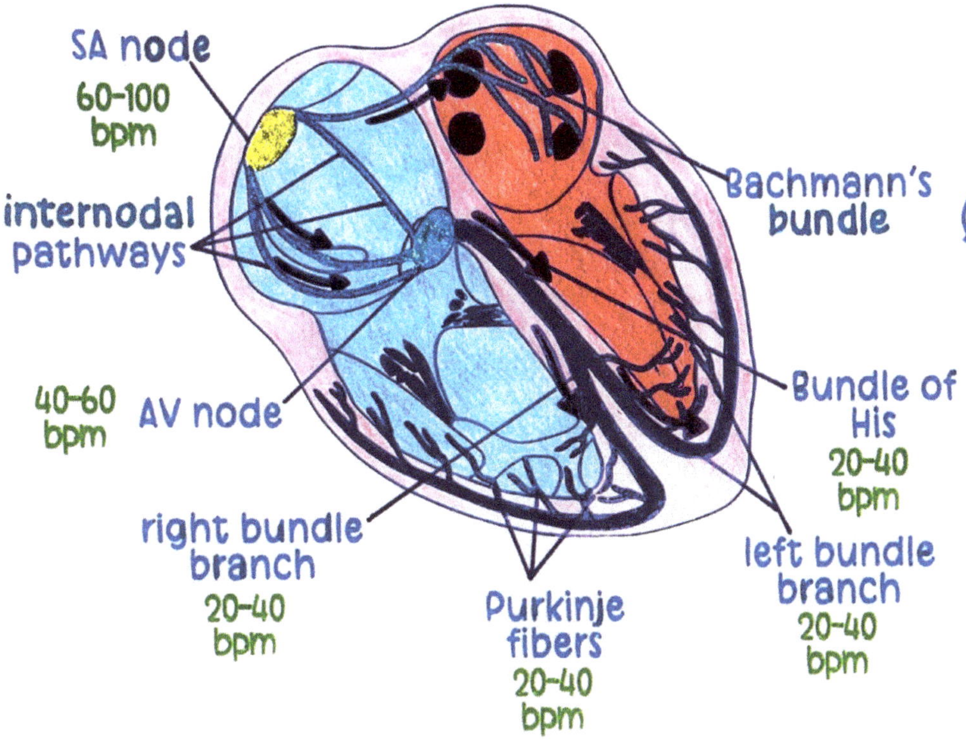

SA node → internodal pathways → AV node → Bundle of His → bundle branches → Purkinje fibers

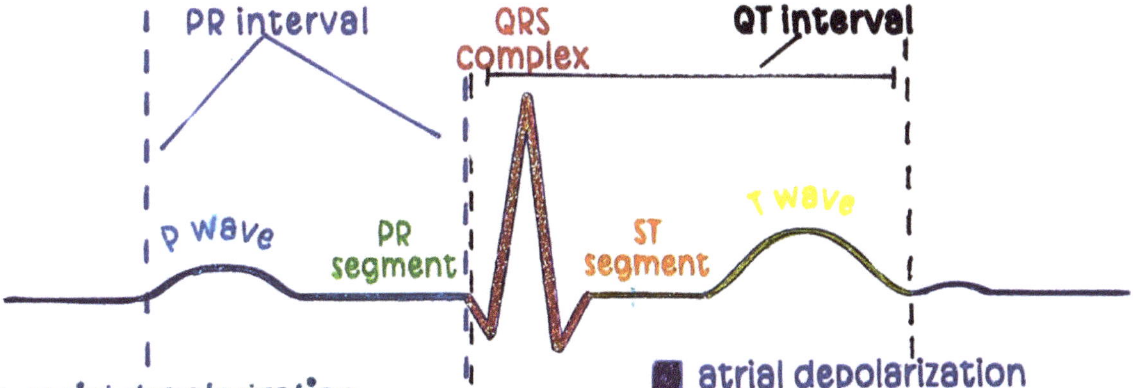

- atrial depolarization
- ventricular depolarization
- ventricular repolarization
- atrial depolarization & AV nodal delay
- isoelectric period of depolarized ventricles
- length of ventricular depolarization& repolarization

The Coronary Sinus

Located on the posterior aspect of the left atrium, the CS is the largest coronary vein that drains deoxygenated blood from the coronary circulation into the right atrium during atrial systole

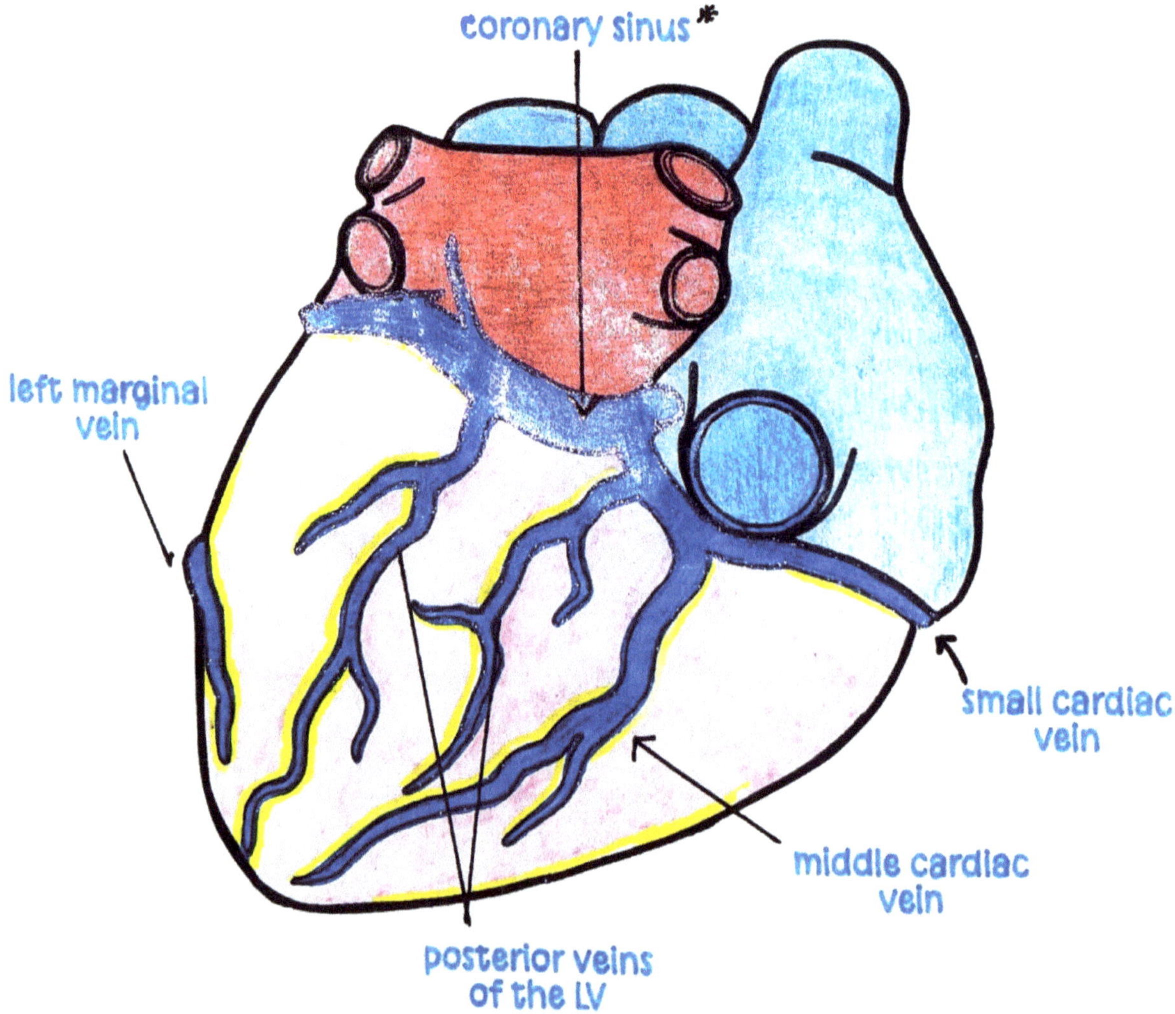

Sauza, P. (2020). Coronary sinus

The CS is used for left ventricular lead placement c̄ biventricular pacemakers (cardiac resynchronization therapy), & cannulation of the CS is useful for mapping left-sided accessory pathways or for evaluating left-sided tachyarrhythmias (i.e. A-Fib) for radiofrequency (RF) ablation!

VENTRICULAR TACHYCARDIA

@cunursingnotesbycaitlyn

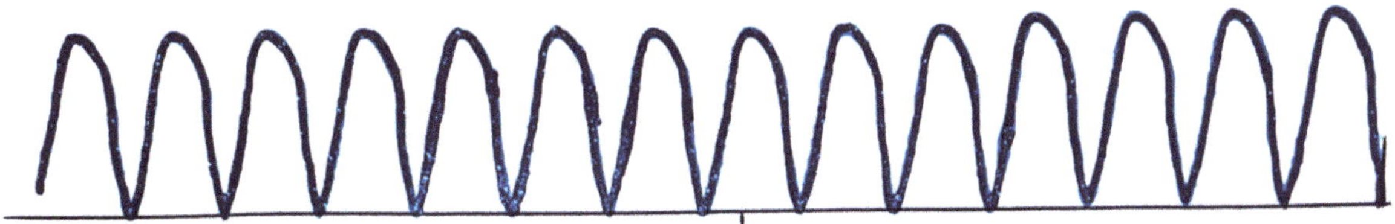

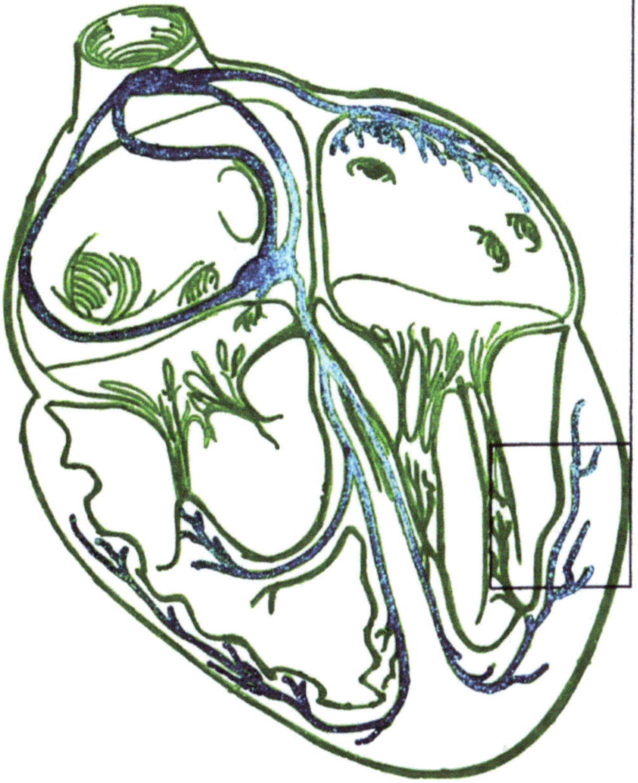

A dysrhythmia originating from an ectopic pacemaker in the ventricles (rather than the SA node) at a rate between 100 and 250 bpm. VT may be non-sustained (≤30 seconds) or sustained (≥ 30 seconds).

Sustained VT causes a ↓ in cardiac output because of ↓ventricular diastolic filling times & the loss of atrial kick (secondary to the rapid ventricular rate); this can cause severe hypotension & ↓myocardial perfusion; VT can deteriorate into ventricular fibrillation.

monomorphic VT

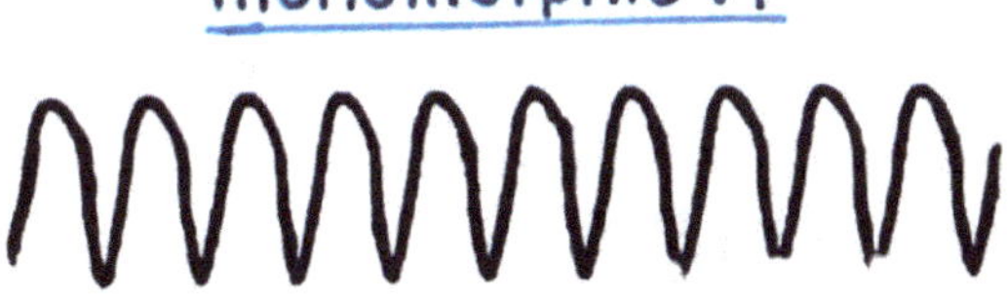

the QRS looks the same from beat-to-beat

polymorphic VT

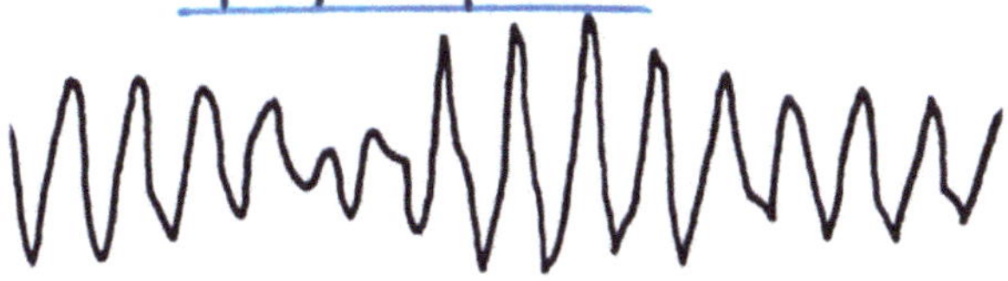

the QRS complexes vary randomly in shape

VENTRICULAR TACHYCARDIA PART II

Risk Factors:

- myocardial ischemia
- coronary artery disease
- cardiomyopathy
- valvular heart disease
- HFrEF
- drug toxicity
- QT prolongation
- drug toxicity
- congenital ♥ disorders
- acid-base imbalance
- electrolyte imbalance(s)

Acute VT Treatment:

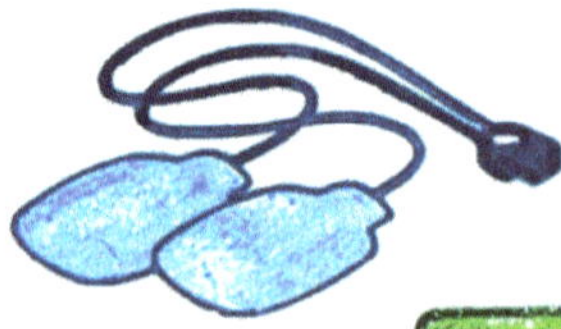

- **stable VT**: IV antiarrhythmic (amio, lido, procainamide)
- **unstable VT**: cardioversion, IV amiodarone, & BP support
- **pulseless VT**: CPR & early defibrillation, epi
- **torsades**: IV $MgSO_4$, cardioversion or CPR + defibrillation, possible overdrive pacing/Isuprel infusion

Nursing Considerations:

- First step: always check for a pulse!
- Put defib pads on your patient (if they aren't on already)!
- Remember your ABCs (airway, breathing & circulation).
- Be familiar with & follow your ACLS algorithms.
- Remember that VT can progress to V-Fib → be prepared for this.
- Recognize & understand the different types of VT (monomorphic vs. polymorphic), because the treatment will vary.
- Don't give IV amiodarone (or most antiarrhythmics) to a patient in torsades, because it will further prolong the QT interval & worsen the patient's condition.

@cunursingnotesbycaitlyn

VT STORM

A state of cardiac electrical instability characterized by ≥ 3 episodes of sustained ventricular tachycardia (VT) requiring cardioversion (VT c̄ a pulse), defibrillation (pulseless VT), or ICD shocks within a 24-hour period.

PATHOPHYSIOLOGY:

The pathophysiology of VT storm isn't entirely understood, but it's thought to be caused by a catecholamine surge/adrenergic storm 2/2 an underlying disease process & a trigger that sends the heart into overdrive. Most patients who present c̄ VT storm have underlying structural heart disease.

a trigger

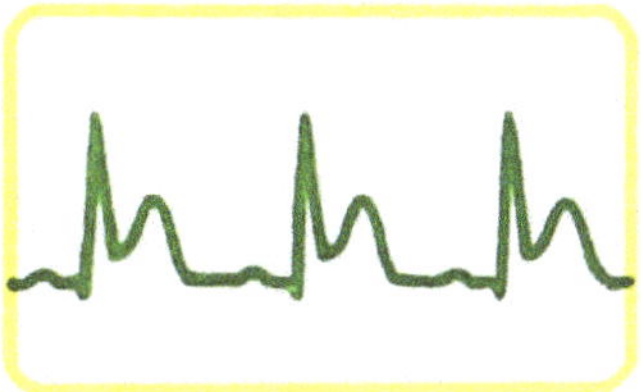

- myocardial ischemia
- electrolyte imbalances
- thyrotoxicosis
- heart failure
- infection
- hypoxia
- drugs

underlying ♥ disease

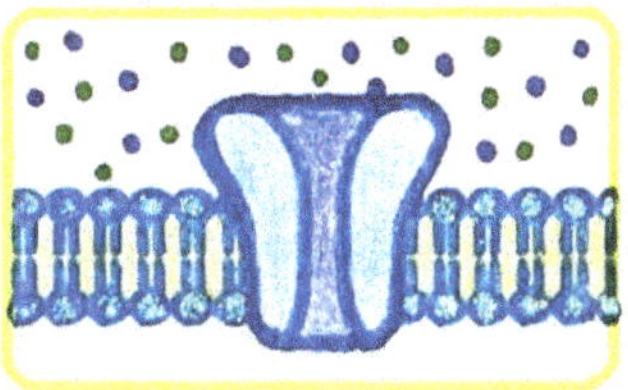

- ischemic heart disease
- channelopathies
  - Brugada Syndrome
  - CPVT, LQTS, & SQTS
- cardiomyopathies
- cardiac sarcoidosis
- LV dysfunction

sympathetic surge

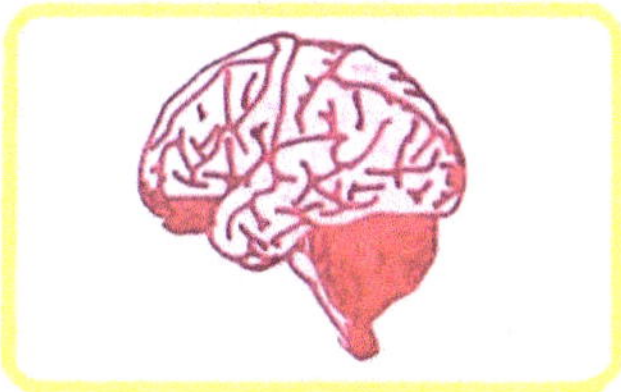

- underlying disease process
- recurrent shocks
- pain/stress

MANAGEMENT

- Antiarrhythmics (amiodarone, lidocaine, procainamide)
- ↓ the sympathetic response via a beta blockade (esmolol or propranolol), sedation/analgesia, & stellate ganglion block (last-ditch effort for mitigating a sympathetic storm).
- Defibrillation (pulseless VT) or cardioversion (VT c̄ a pulse).
- Identify & treat underlying reversible causes. Device interrogation & possible reprogramming for patients c̄ ICDs.
- Mechanical circulatory support for hemodynamic instability (IABP, Impella, or ECMO).
- Catheter ablation.

@icunursingnotesbycaitlyn

Catecholaminergic Polymorphic VT

A genetic cardiac ion channelopathy, which presents c̄ polymorphic or bidirectional ventricular tachycardia induced by physical or emotional stress, in the presence of a structurally normal heart & c̄ a typically normal resting ECG.

UNDERSTANDING THE PATHO: IT'S ALL ABOUT CALCIUM

Most cases of CPVT (60%) result from a mutation in the RyR2 gene that encodes a protein called the cardiac ryanodine receptor (RyR2) - a calcium ion ($Ca2^{+}$) channel that regulates intracellular $Ca2^{+}$ release from the sarcoplasmic reticulum (SR) in cardiac muscle cells.

When it comes to myocardial contractility, calcium is the most important ion!

@icunursingnotesbycaitlyn

CPVT is the result of too much intracellular calcium. A genetic defect in the $Ca2^{+}$ channels of the sarcoplasmic reticulum (RyR2) in cardiac muscle cells causes $Ca2^{+}$ to "leak" intracellularly during diastole (ventricular relaxation) in response to adrenergic/sympathetic stimulation (i.e. physical exercise, emotional stress, etc). This disrupts normal $Ca2^{+}$ homeostasis, resulting in intracellular calcium overload & electrical instability that can precipitate delayed afterdepolarizations (DADs) & triggered activity - both of which can induce VT/VF.

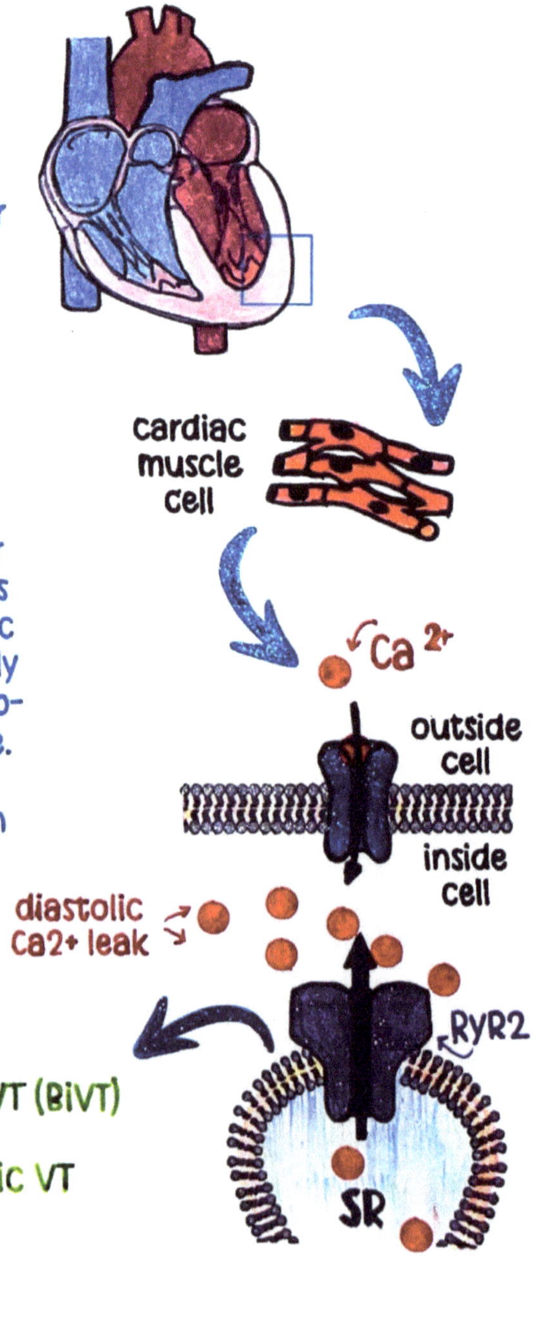

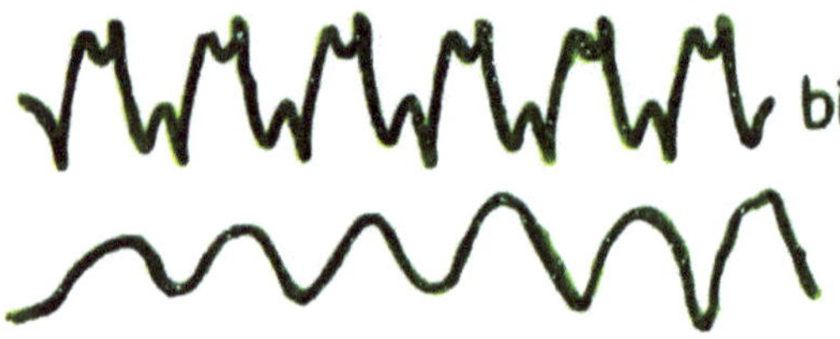

bidirectional VT (BiVT)

polymorphic VT

CPVT

Catecholaminergic **P**olymorphic **V**entricular **T**achycardia

MANAGEMENT

LIFESTYLE CHANGES

avoid...

competitive sports

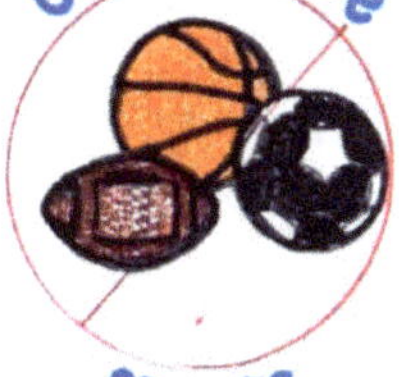

stimulants

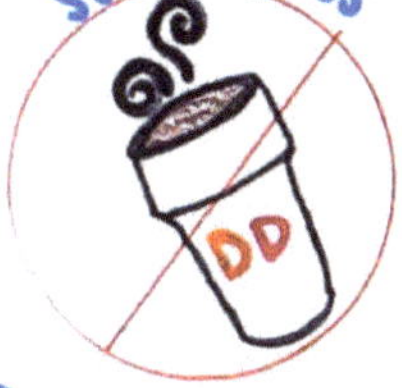

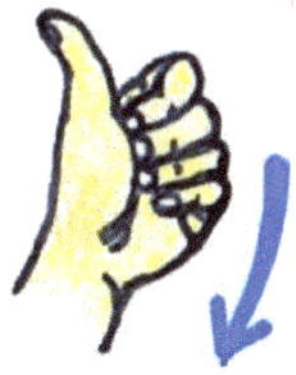

low-intensity exercise

\+

NON-SELECTIVE BETA BLOCKER

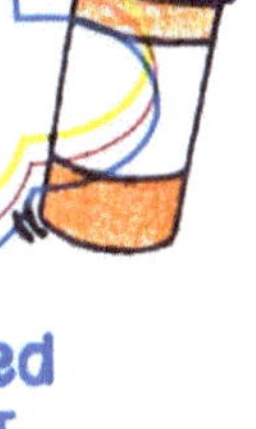

Nadolol is the preferred beta blocker for CPVT.

Flecainide (antiarrhythmic) can be used as an adjunct to nadolol for recurrent VT.

LEFT CARDIAC SYMPATHETIC DENERVATION (LCSD)

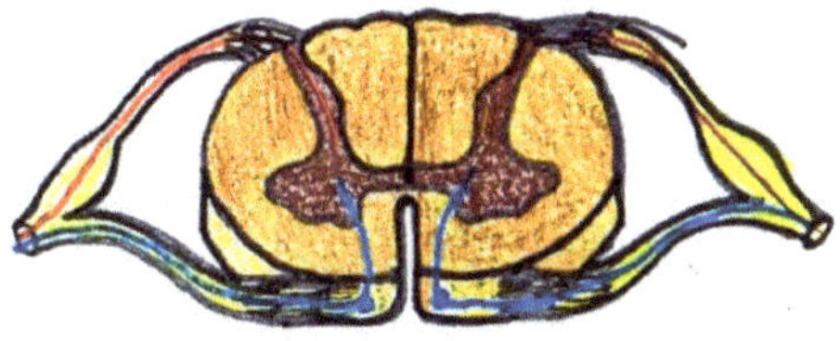

A surgical procedure for refractory CPVT that prevents norepinephrine release in the heart, ↑ the threshold for ventricular fibrillation (VF).

ICD (& beta blockers)

This is the last resort for refractory CPVT. These patients are sensitive to catecholamines, so an ICD shock will ↑ their sympathetic drive, precipitating an electrical/VT storm!

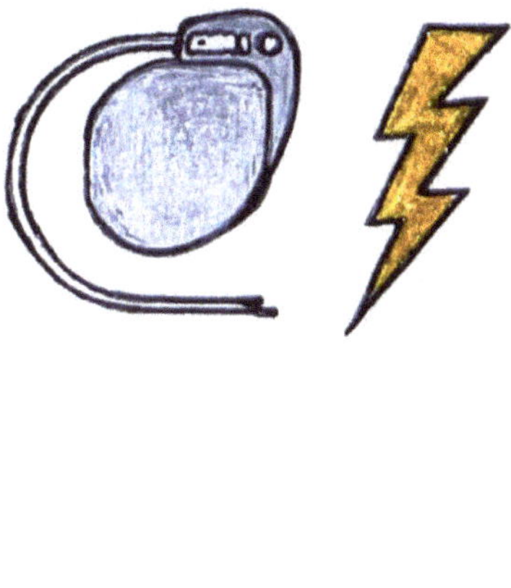

Brugada Syndrome

An autosomal-dominant genetic disorder that affects the cardiac muscle cells' ability to conduct an action potential & causes sudden cardiac death (SCD) in patients c̄ structurally normal hearts.

@icunursingnotesbycaitlyn

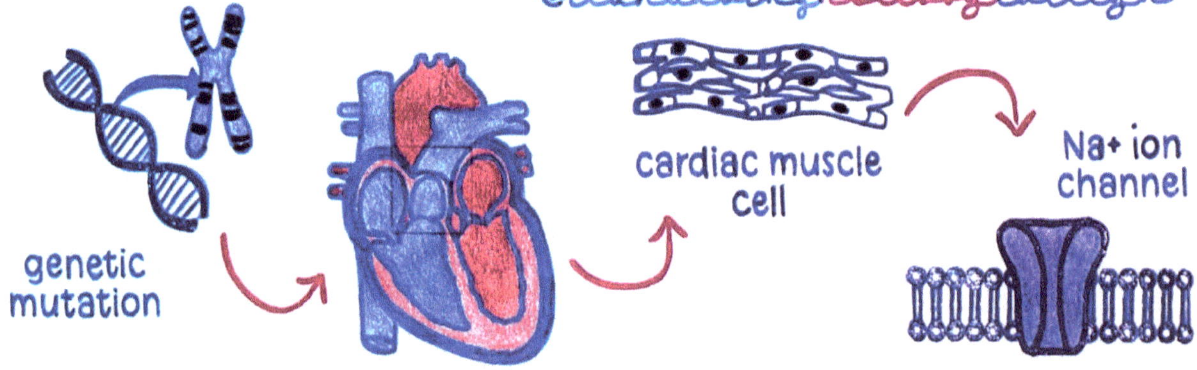

Brugada Syndrome is caused by a mutation in the SCN5A gene that codes for sodium ion channels in the cell membranes of cardiac muscle cells. Loss of functional sodium ion channels impairs the heart's ability to conduct an action potential, causing some regions of the heart to repolarize abnormally. These regions become vulnerable to a reentrant loop that can induce ventricular tachycardia (VT) or ventricular fibrillation (VF).

ECG Findings

ST-elevation in V1, V2, & V3 (right precordial leads)

pseudo-right bundle branch block (RBBB)

Type I

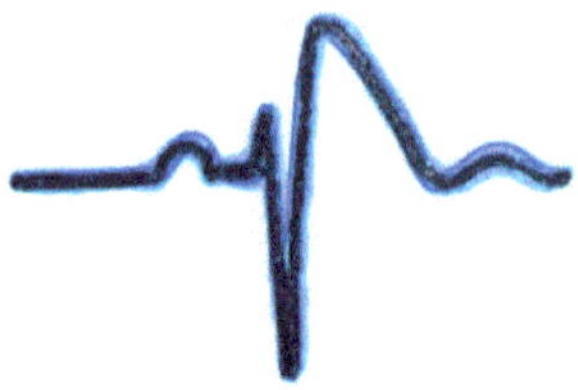

ST-elevation & inverted T wave (most common)

Type II

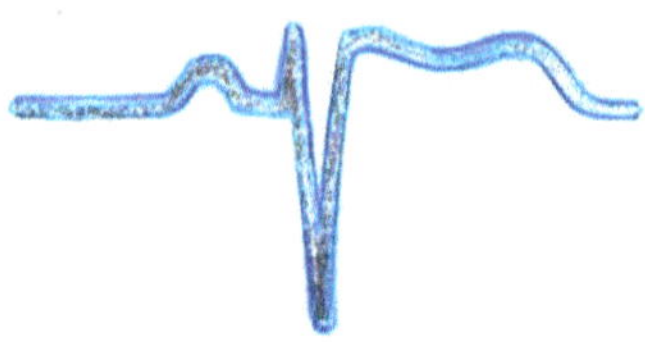

"saddleback" ST-elevation

Type III

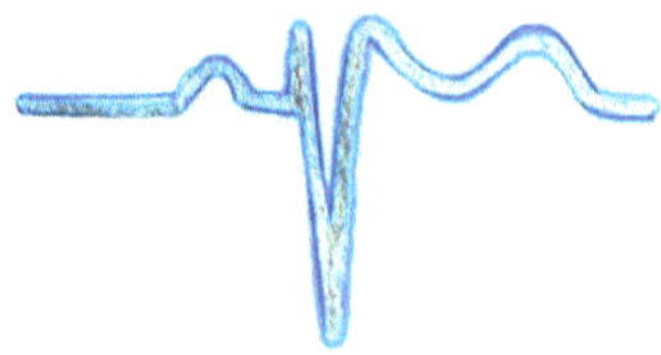

Type I or II morphology c̄ <2 mm of ST-elevation

Atrioventricular Reentrant Tachycardia

A type of supraventricular tachycardia (SVT) associated c̄ Wolff-Parkinson-White (WPW) syndrome.

@lcunursingnotesbycaitlyn

AVRT

orthodromic

impulse travels down the AV node & up the accessory pathway

antidromic

impulse travels down the accessory pathway & up the AV node

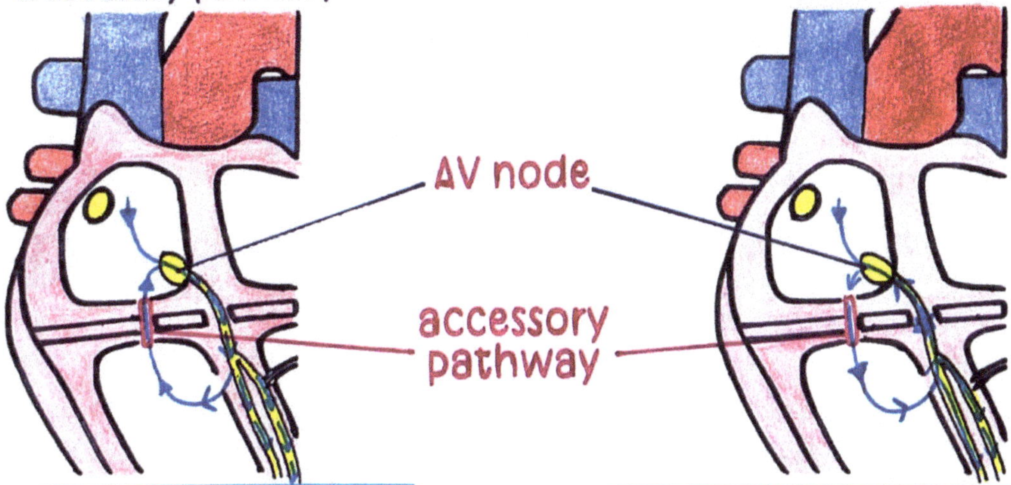

orthodromic

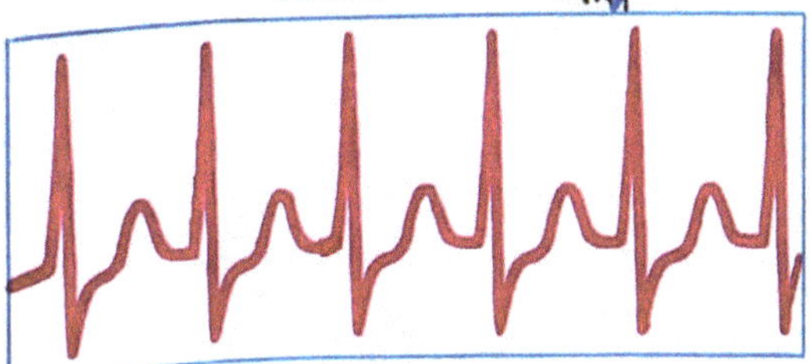

- most common WPW AVRT (90-95%)
- narrow-complex
- classic "SVT" appearance

antidromic

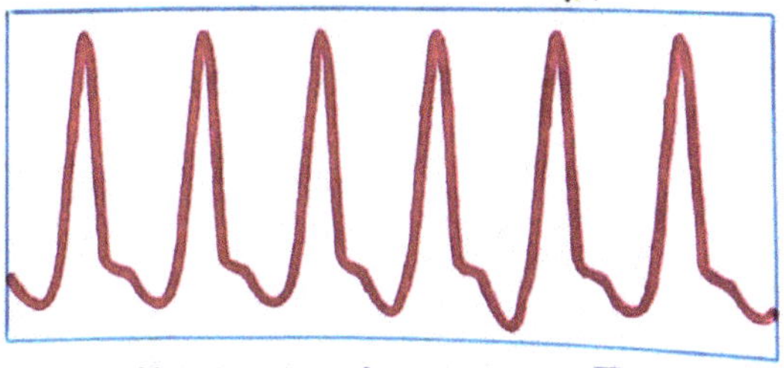

- usually seen in A-Fib c̄ WPW
- less common
- wide-complex
- looks like V-Tach!

WPW PATTERN

The constellation of ECG abnormalities related to the presence of an atrioventricular (AV) accessory pathway.

W P W

- **W**ave (delta)
- **PR** interval is short
- **W**ide QRS complex

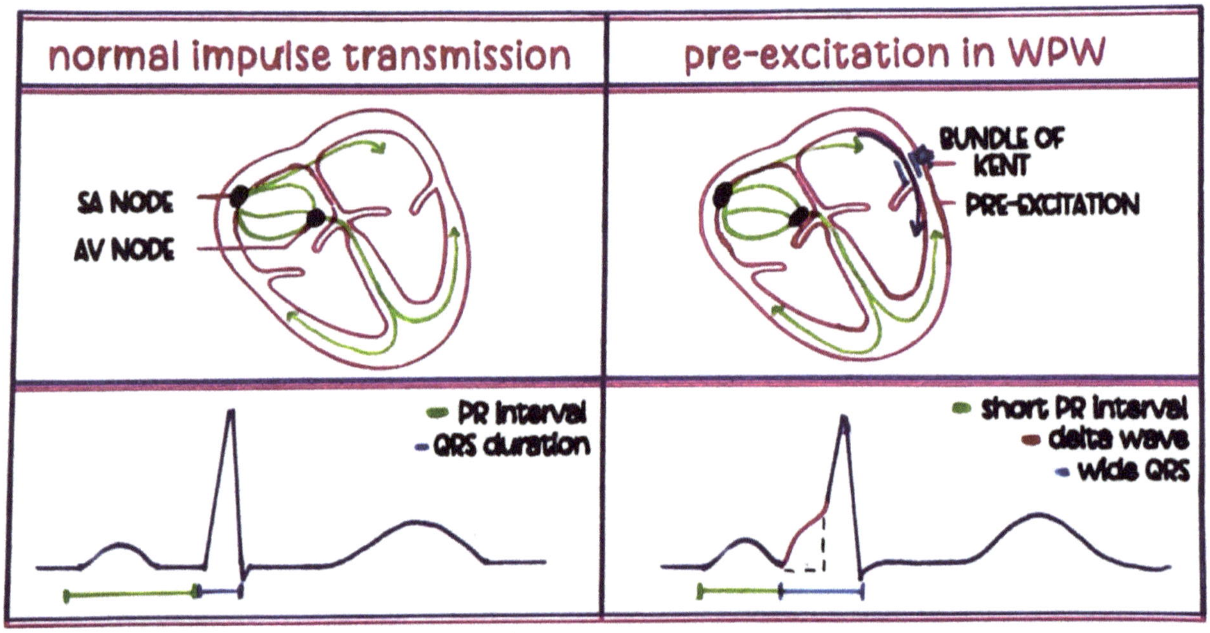

delta wave — premature ventricular depolarization

short PR interval — loss of normal AV node delay

wide QRS — fusion of accessory pathway conduction c̄ normal AV nodal conduction

R-ON-T PHENOMENON

Ventricular depolarization (R wave) coincides c̄ the vulnerable period of repolarization (T wave) of the preceding beat, possibly precipitating ventricular tachycardia or fibrillation (VT/VF).

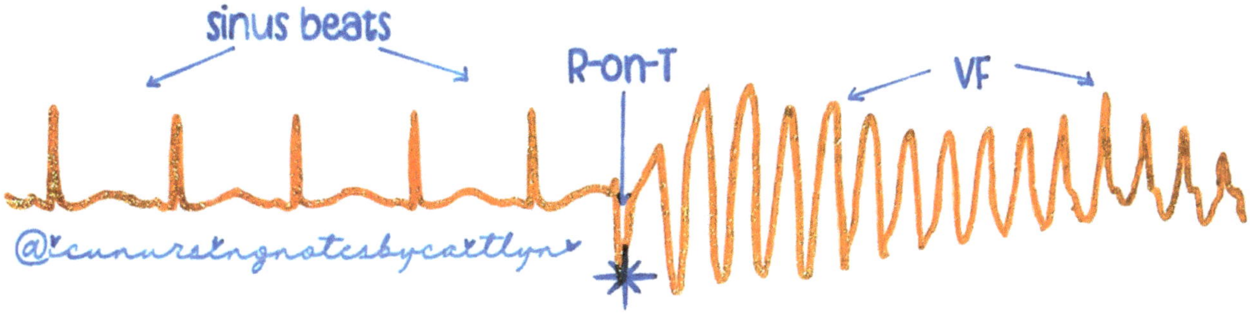

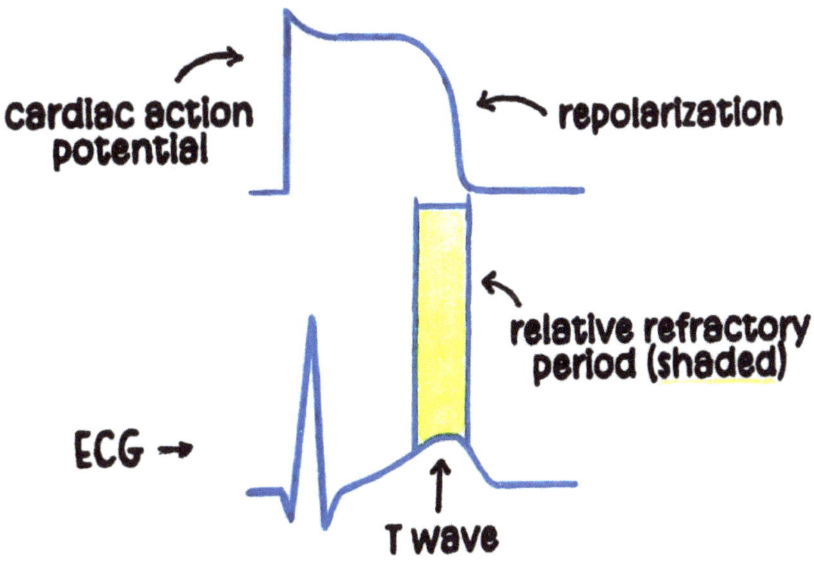

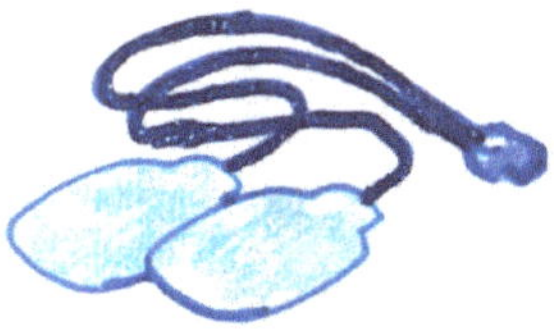

The relative refractory period coincides c̄ the T wave on an ECG!

PHYSIOLOGY

The last half of the T wave coincides c̄ the relative refractory period (RRP) of the cardiac cycle, & it represents ventricular repolarization. If a premature ventricular contraction (PVC) or a pacing stimulus (in the setting of under-sensing) is strong enough to depolarize the cardiac cells when only part of the myocardium is repolarized, it can induce VT or VF, as individual segments of the heart muscle depolarize independently of one another.

Commotio Cordis

@icunursingnotesbycaitlyn

A phenomenon in which ventricular fibrillation/cardiac arrest is induced following blunt force trauma to the chest during the heart's repolarization period (T wave).

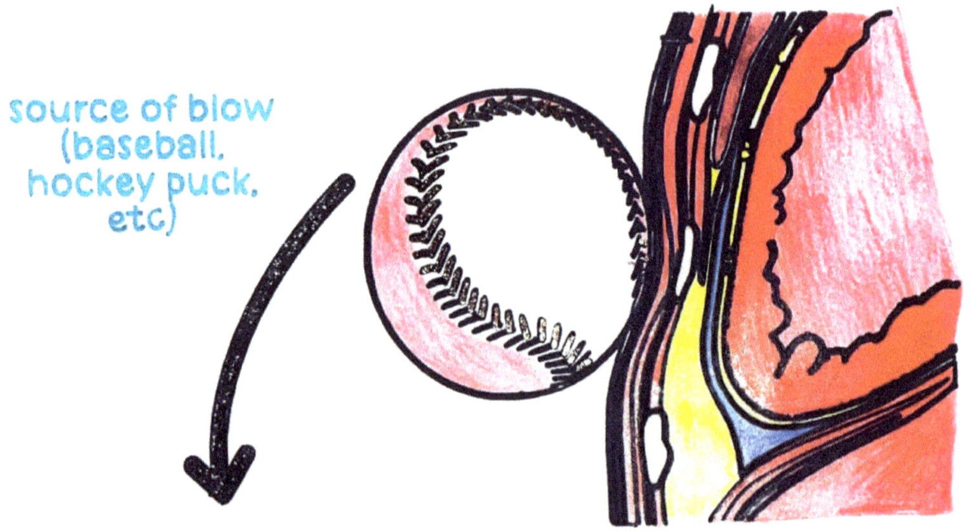

Commotio cordis is Latin for "agitation of the heart."

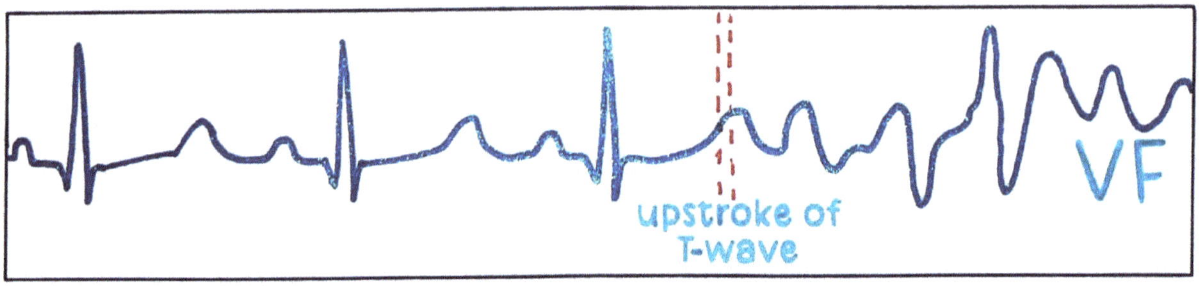

PATHOPHYSIOLOGY

The cardiac cycle starts c̄ atrial depolarization (P-wave) & ends c̄ ventricular repolarization (T-wave). The force to the chest, in & of itself, does NOT cause sudden cardiac arrest; commotio cordis is related to the time of impact during the cardiac cycle; the timing of the impact must be perfectly synchronized with the upstroke of the T-wave (ventricular repolarization) - the most vulnerable part of the cardiac cycle. Commotio cordis is most common in young athletes (Stevenson & Jalife, 2021).

Holiday Heart Syndrome

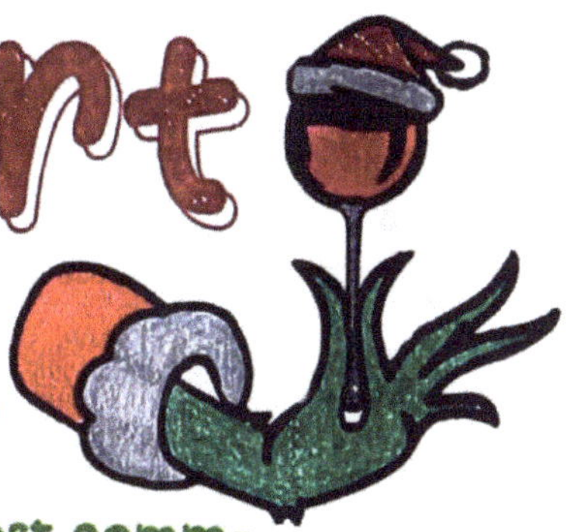

Transient alcohol-induced atrial arrhythmias (most commonly A-Fib) associated c̄ binge drinking during the holiday season in people who don't have underlying heart disease.

PATHOPHYSIOLOGY

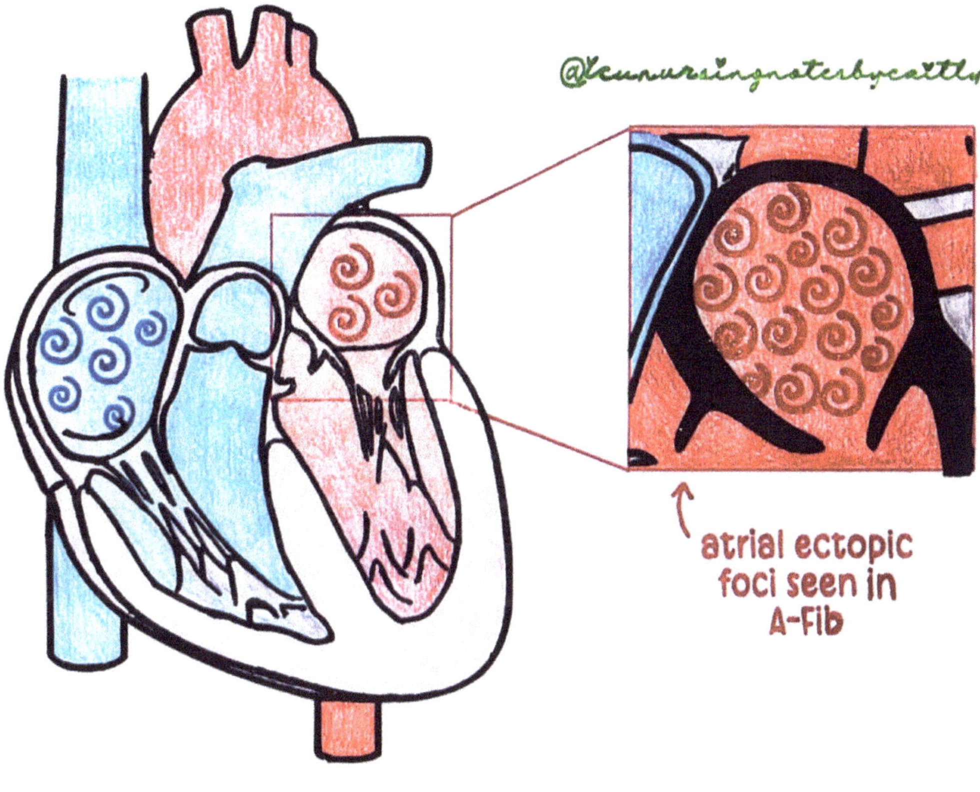

Although the pathophysiology of alcohol-induced arrhythmias isn't fully understood, excessive ETOH intake produces various electrophysiologic, cellular, & autonomic effects that may precipitate A-Fib. Several mechanisms have been proposed to explain holiday heart syndrome: cardiac conduction interference facilitating re-entry, shortening of the atrial refractory period, ↑ sympathetic & parasympathetic activity, & an ↑ in plasma-free fatty acids and catecholamines (norepi & epi).

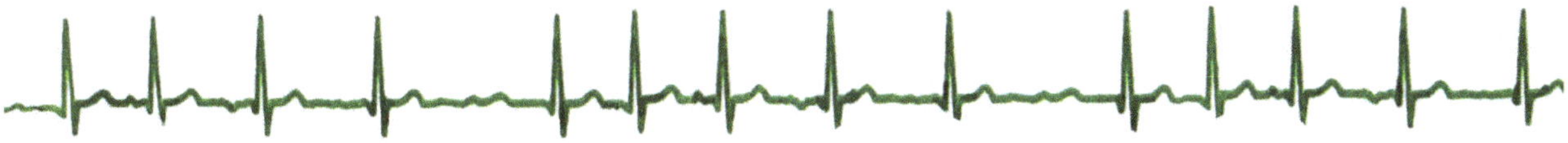

Leadless Pacemakers

INDICATIONS

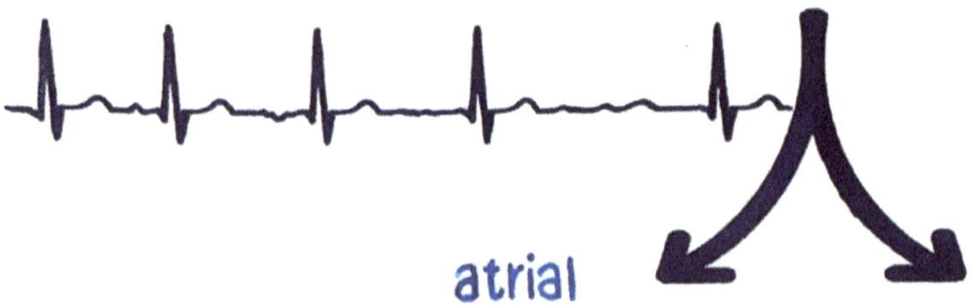

atrial fibrillation

AV block

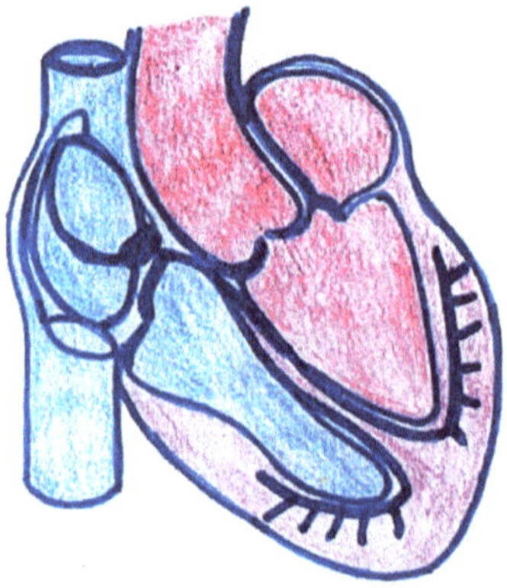

WHEN SHOULD A LEADLESS PACER BE CONSIDERED?

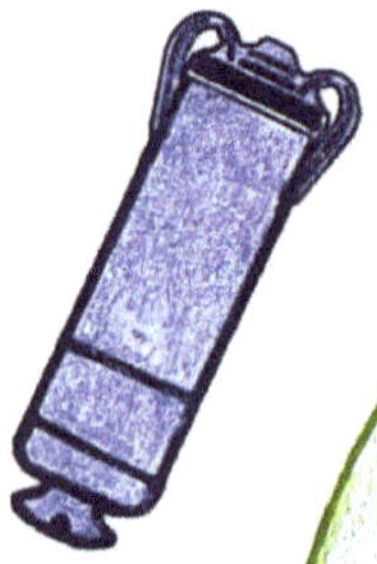

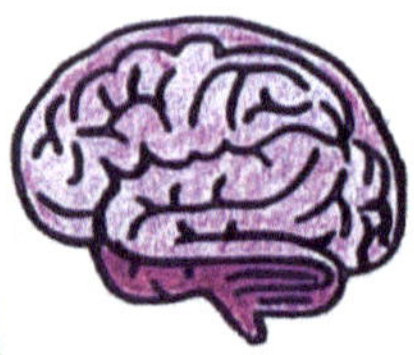

- ESRD on HD
- cognitive impairment/ inability to comply c̄ activity restrictions
- high infection risk
- limited venous access

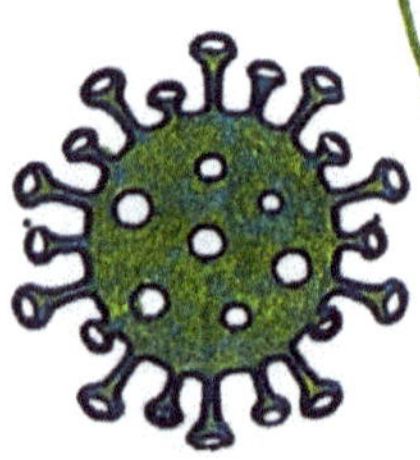

@icunursingnotesbycaitlyn

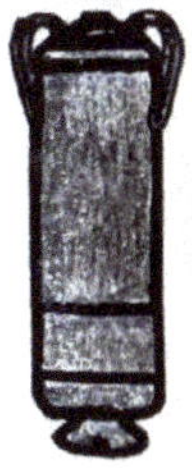

The Micra™: THE LEADLESS PACEMAKER

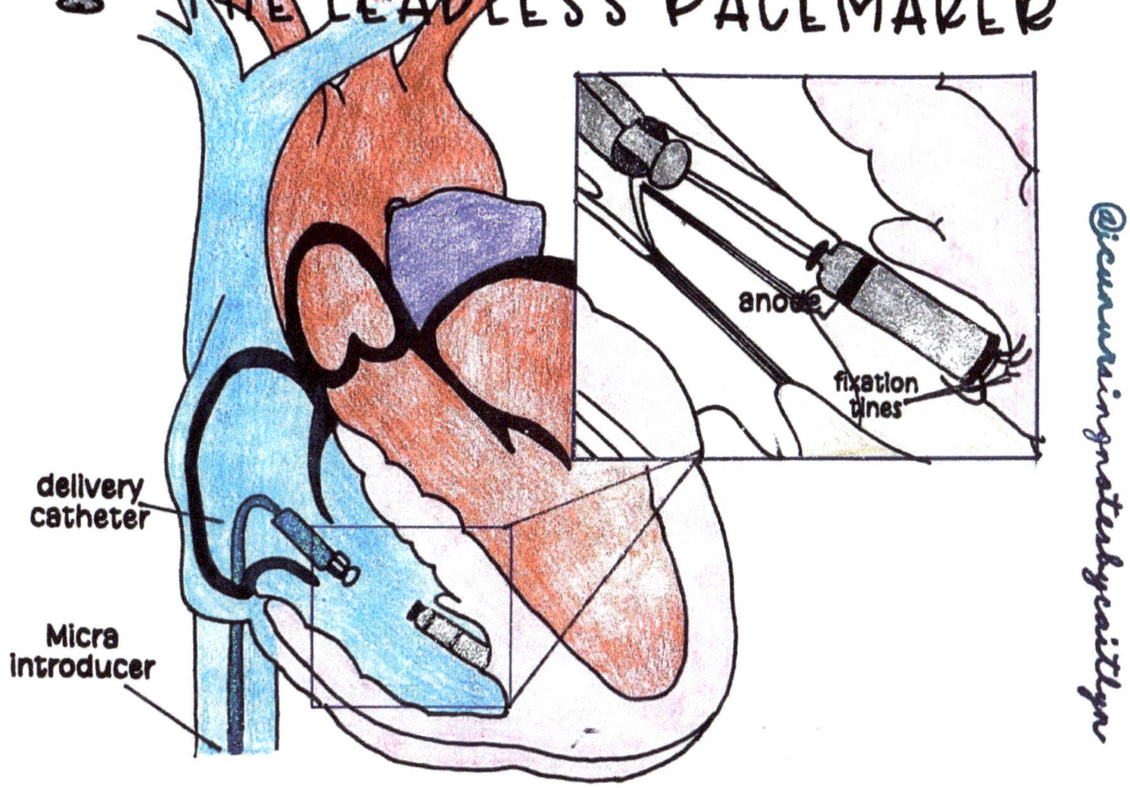

The Micra™ is a single-chamber, & leadless pacemaker that is delivered percutaneously via the femoral vein through a catheter delivery system. It's implanted directly inside the right ventricle where it affixes to the myocardium via fixation tines. It delivers electrical impulses that pace the heart through an electrode located at the end of the device, eliminating the need for a device pocket/chest incision & a transvenous pacing lead.

The Micra is the world's smallest pacemaker, and it's about the size of a vitamin capsule (Medtronic)!

Nursing Care of a Patient c̄ a Leadless Pacemaker

- Get a post-procedure 12-lead ECG.
- Assess the venous access site frequently for bleeding & for development of a hematoma.
- Maintain bedrest for 4-6 hours (follow your hospital's policy). Keep the HOB <30 (Reverse Trendelenburg may be more comfortable for your patient than lying completely flat).
- Closely monitor for S/S of right ventricular perforation & development of a pericardial effusion and possible tamponade – anticipate the need for an echo, pericardiocentesis, & emergency surgery (depending on severity).

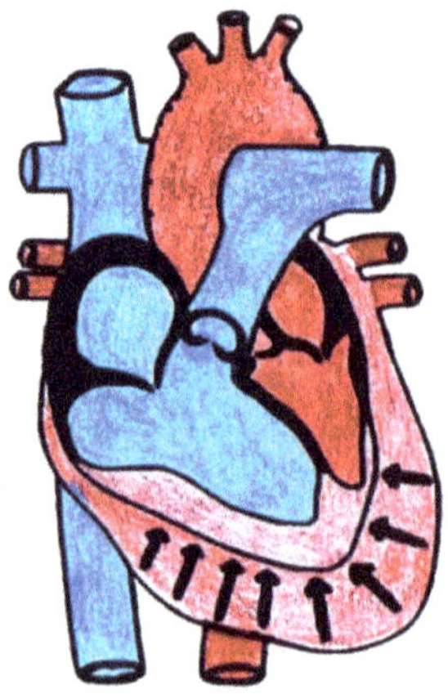

Signs & symptoms of cardiac perforation: c/p, hemodynamic instability, dyspnea, & abdominal pain.

- Monitor for vital sign changes, c/p or palpitations, diminished pulses, & color/temperature of the affected extremity.
- Monitor the patient's ECG for failure to pace or capture, oversensing & undersensing.

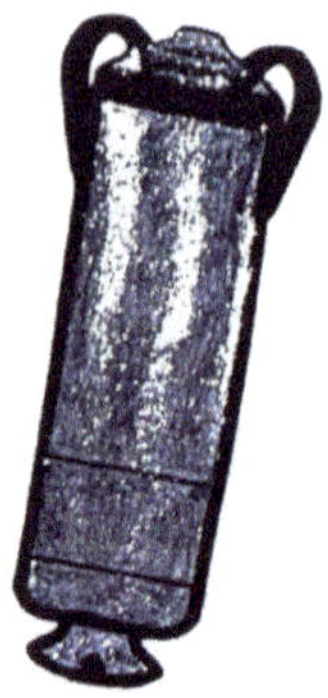

- Although it's rare, device migration is a possible complication that can occur after insertion of a leadless pacemaker, so keep this in mind.
- Unlike traditional pacemakers, leadless pacemakers do not require any activity restrictions (other than avoiding strenuous exercise for 1 week post-procedure).
- Leadless pacemakers are MRI-compatible, so it's ok for your patient to have a MRI, if needed.
- The position of a leadless pacemaker is confirmed under fluoro, so a post-procedure CXR is typically not required.

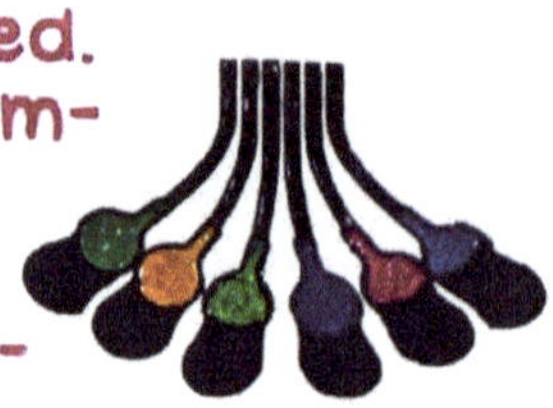

- Ensure that your patient has his/her pacemaker ID card & instructions before discharge!

@icunursingnotesbycaitlyn

BUNDLE BRANCH BLOCKS

An electrical impulse is blocked from passing through the right or left bundle branch, so the right & the left ventricles do not depolarize ("contract") simultaneously. The ventricle affected by the blocked bundle depolarizes slower than the unaffected ventricle, which results in the hallmark widened QRS

Use leads V1 and V6 to determine whether a block is in the right bundle or the left bundle!

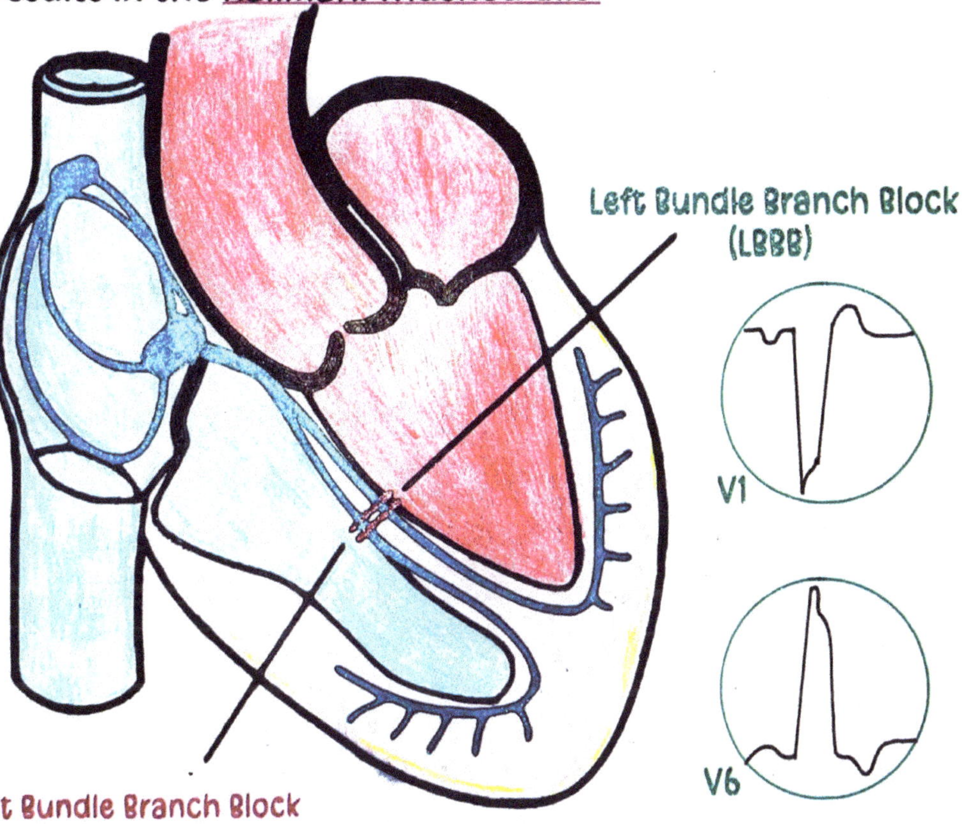

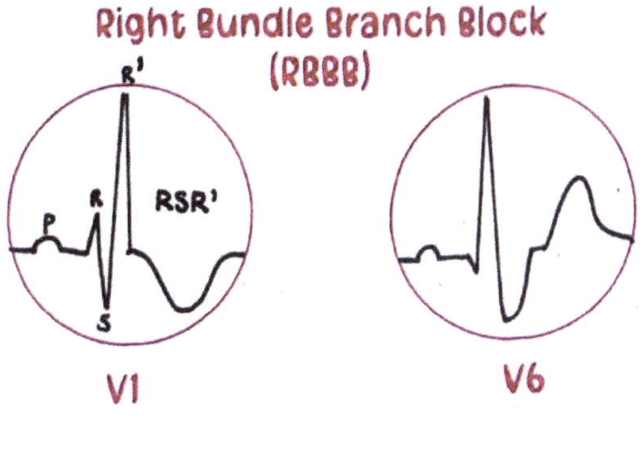

Normal cardiac conduction:
SA node
↓
AV node
↓
Bundle of His
↓
left/right bundle branches
↓
Purkinje fibers

@icunursingnotesbycaitlyn

PVC PATTERNS MADE EASY!

@icunursingnotesbycaitlyn

VENTRICULAR BIGEMINY

ventricular bigeminy

every other beat is a PVC

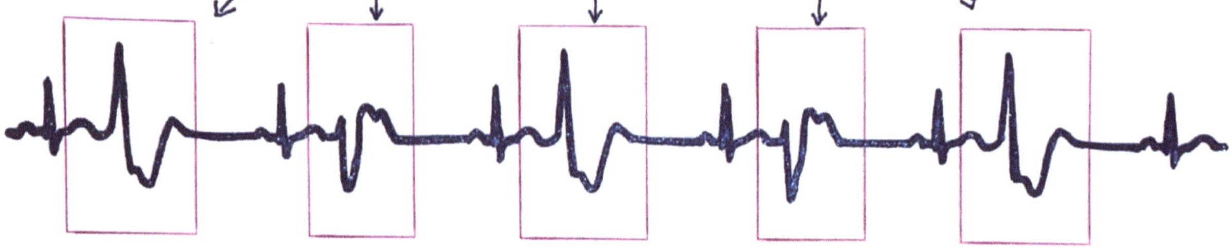

VENTRICULAR TRIGEMINY

ventricular trigeminy

every third beat is a PVC

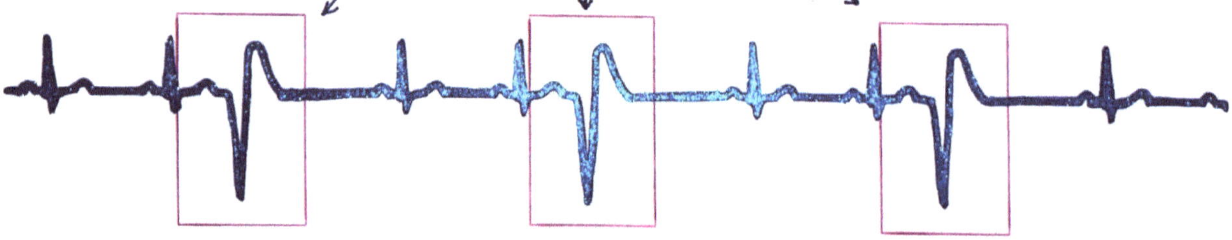

VENTRICULAR QUADGEMINY

ventricular quadgeminy

every fourth beat is a PVC

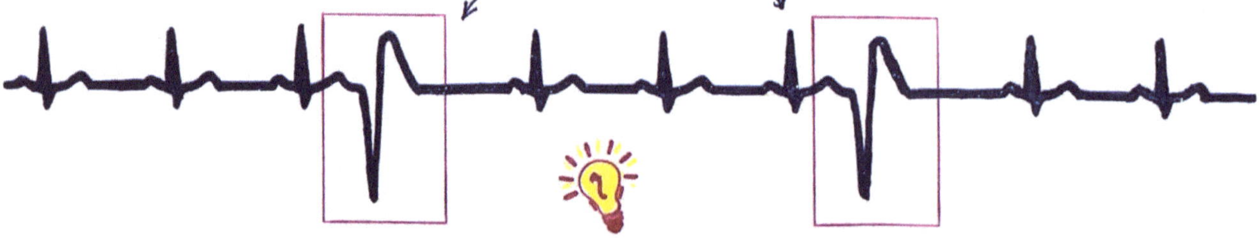

These aren't rhythms: they're patterns. There will be an underlying rhythm (i.e. NSR, sinus brady, etc). We describe the underlying rhythm first followed by the PVC pattern present (i.e. sinus rhythm c̄ ventricular bigeminy)!

VENTRICULAR FIBRILLATION

Rapid firing of multiple ventricular ectopic foci causes the ventricles to quiver (rather than cohesively contract): lack of coordinated ventricular contraction leads to a sudden loss of cardiac output and, ultimately, cardiac arrest.

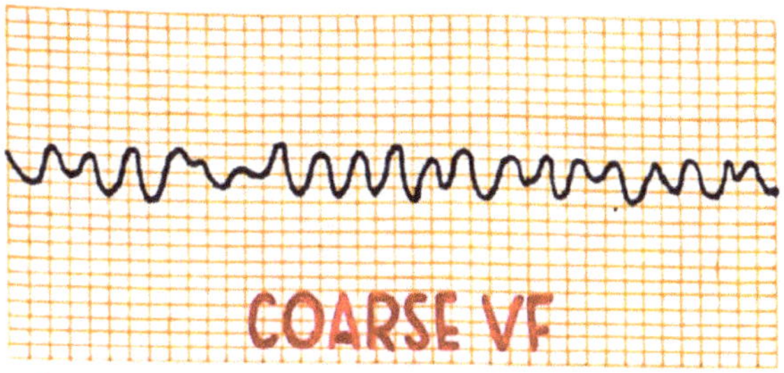

COARSE VF

indicates recent onset VF that is more responsive to defibrillation than fine VF!

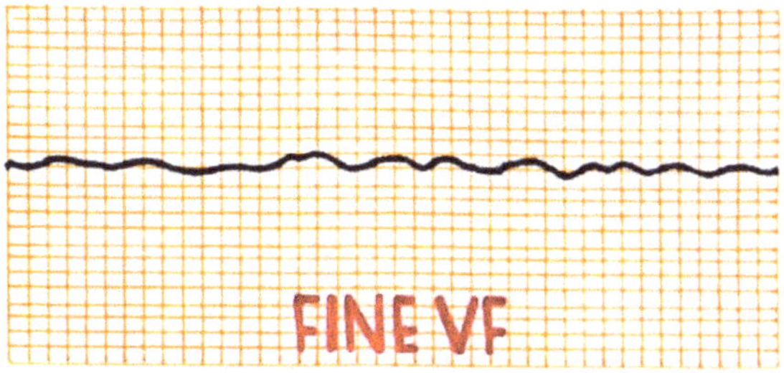

FINE VF

less likely to respond to defibrillation (more hypoxic & acidodic).

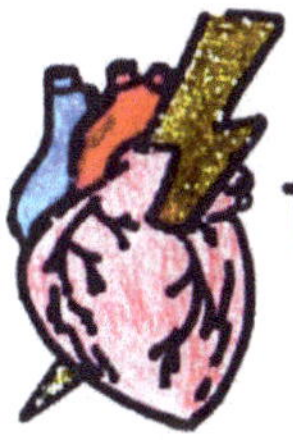

@icunursingnotesbycaitlyn

There is no cardiac output or pulse c̄ VF: always remember to DEFIB FOR V-FIB!

CAUSES

- acute MI
- untreated V-tach
- R-on-T phenomenon
- cardiomyopathy
- coronary artery disease
- long QT syndrome (LQTS)
- Brugada syndrome
- acid base & electrolyte imbalances

TREATMENT

- early defibrillation & CPR
- 1 mg IV/IO epinephrine q 3-5 min
- 300 mg IV/IO amiodarone (preferable to lidocaine)

you can give an additional 150 mg IV/IO amio bolus for refractory VF!

Antiarrhythmics (amio/lido) are generally used if defibrillation is unsuccessful.

TORSADES DE POINTES

"twisting of the points"

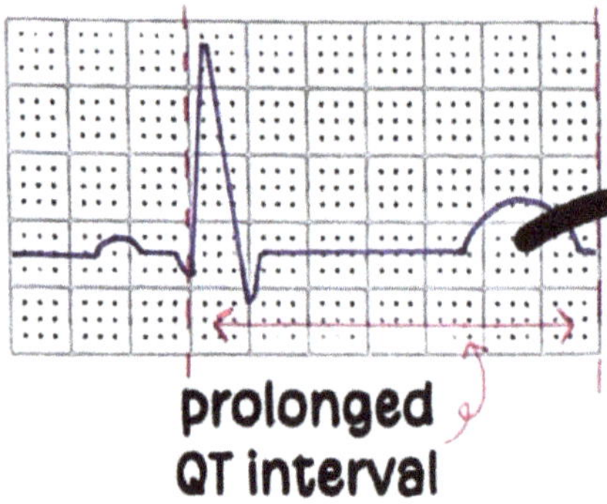

Torsades has the potential to resolve spontaneously or deteriorate into V-fib/VF!

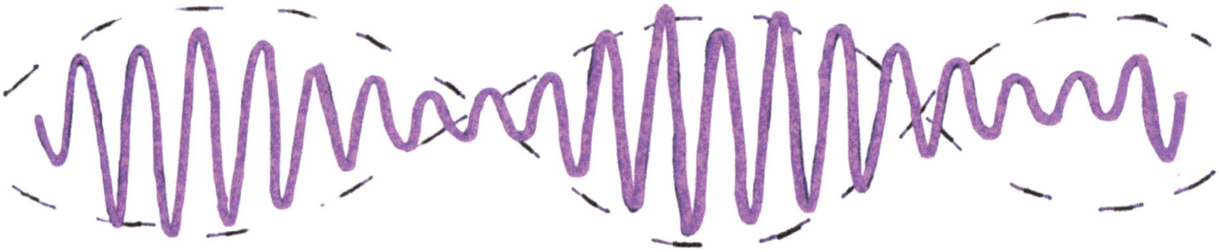

A type of polymorphic VT characterized by a long QTc & wide QRS complexes that "twist" around the isoelectric line!

ETIOLOGY

electrolyte imbalances

hypokalemia
hypomagnesemia
hypocalcemia

drug-induced prolonged QT interval

antiarrhythmics
antibiotics
antipsychotics
Zofran
methadone

other causes

congenital
myocardial ischemia
bradycardia R/T sick sinus syndrome (SSS) or ♥ block

@♡icunursingnotesbycaitlyn

TORSADES DE POINTES

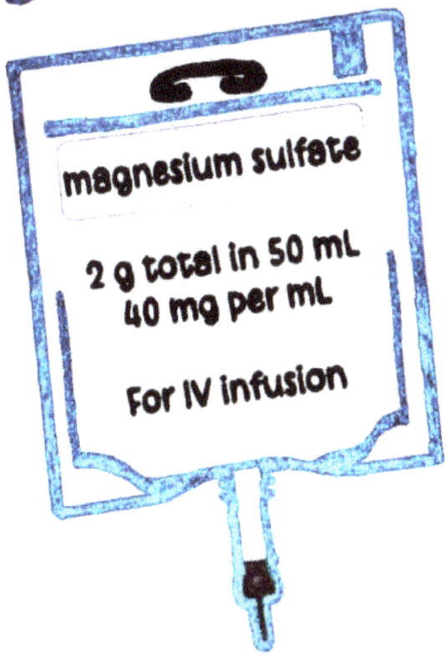

Treatment :

- electrolyte repletion
- IV magnesium
- IV Isuprel (if unresponsive to IV MgSO4)
- overdrive pacing
- defibrillation + CPR (if pulseless)
- cardioversion (unstable c̄ a pulse)

You wouldn't want to give amiodarone in the setting of torsades because it will actually further prolong the QT interval!

Nursing Care!

- First, check a pulse. No pulse? ⟶ Start CPR! Pulse? ⟶ Give 1-2 grams of IV MgSO4.
- If the patient has a long QTc, grab a bag of mag & IV tubing for the bedside (don't spike the bag, but have it there just in case you need it!).
- Know which medications to avoid if a patient already has a prolonged QT interval (Zofran, Benadryl, antipsychotics, most antiarrhythmics, antibiotics, etc).
- For a patient who continues to have intermittent runs of torsades, despite treatment c̄ IV MgSO4, ↑ the HR c̄ IV Isuprel may also help. Why? It ↑ the HR & shortens the QT interval, ↓ the risk of the "R-on-T phenomenon" that can lead to TdP.
- Correct any electrolyte abnormalities, especially in your high-risk patients.
- Remember that TdP can sometimes resolve spontaneously, but it can also progress to V-Fib.

@♡icunursingnotesbycaitlyn

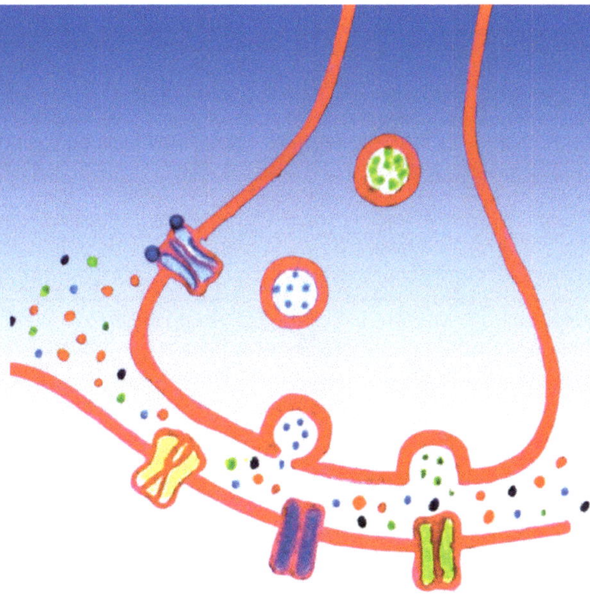

PHARMACOLOGY

pharmacology

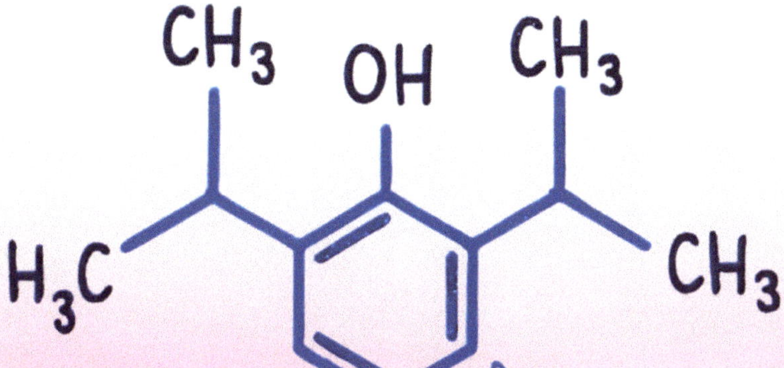

propofol

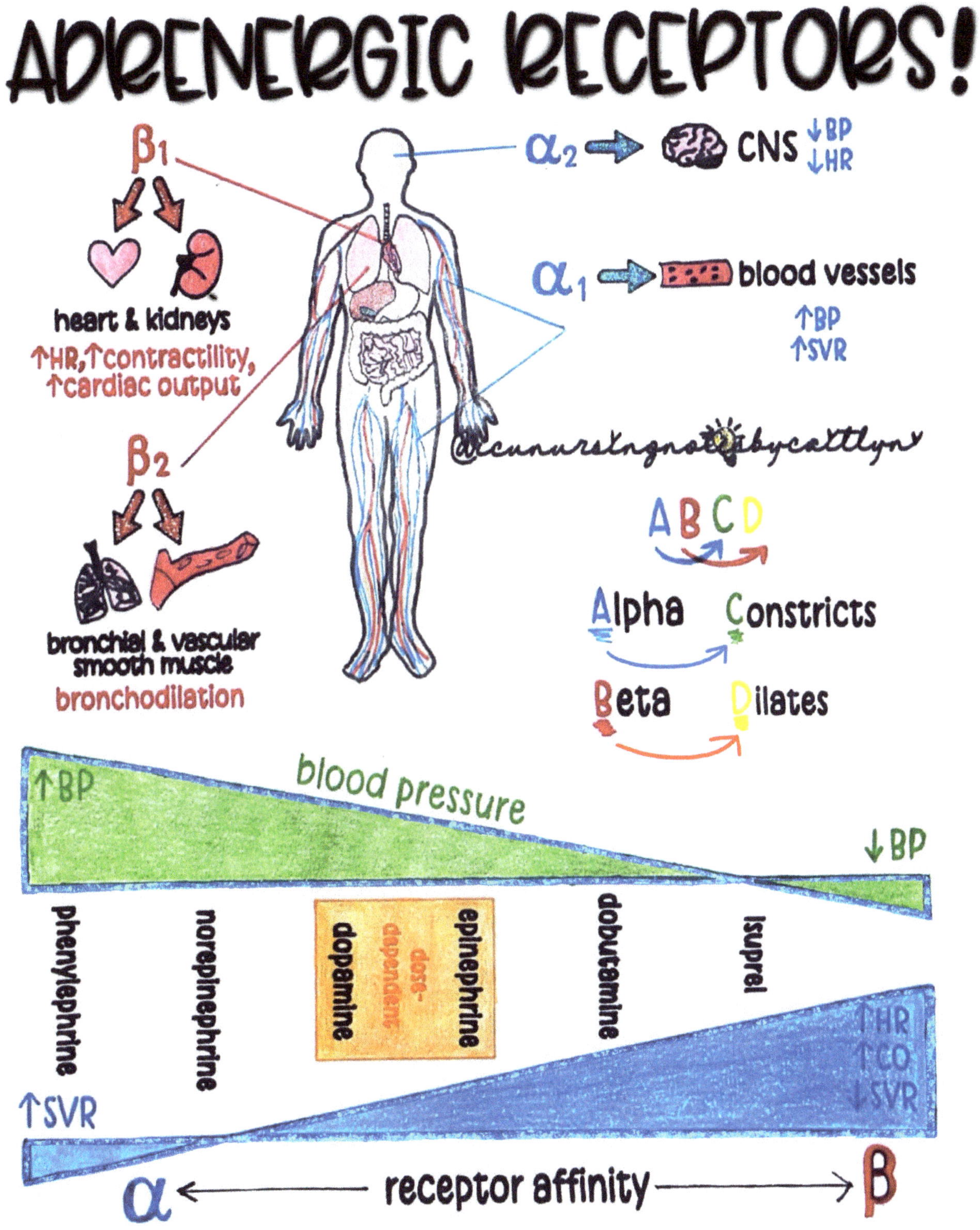

Drawing inspired by the work of Rishi Kumar, MD.

Common ICU Drips

Vasopressors

Gtt	Use	Starting Dose*	Titration*	Max Dose*	Notes
Levophed	↑ BP	5 mcg/min	2 mcg/min q 2 min	40 mcg/min	alpha effects > beta effects
vasopressin	↑ BP	0.04 units/min	non-titratable	N/A	used in combo c̄ other pressors enhances Levo
Neo	↑ BP	20 mcg/min	10 mcg/min q 2 min	400 mcg/min	↑ SVR
epi	↑ BP	1 mcg/min	2 mcg/min q 2 min	40 mcg/min	Higher doses are not better, monitor for ↑ HR.
dopamine	↑ BP	5 mcg/kg/min	2 mcg/kg/min q 5 min	20 mcg/kg/min	monitor for ↑ HR, & arrhythmias

Vasodilators

Gtt	Use	Starting Dose*	Titration*	Max Dose*	Notes
nicardipine	↓ BP	5 mg/hr	2.5 mg/hr q 5 min	15 mg/hr	monitor HR/BP
esmolol	↓ BP	load 0.5 mg/kg over 1 min, then 50 mcg/kg/min	50 mcg/kg/min q 15 min	300 mcg/kg/min	decreases BP, HR, AV conduction
Nipride	↓ BP	0.25 mcg/kg/min	0.5 mcg/kg/min q 5 min	10 mcg/kg/min	watch for cyanide toxicity!

Miscellaneous Gtts

Gtt	Use	Starting Dose*	Titration*	Max Dose*	Notes
propofol	sedation	10 mcg/kg/min	10 mcg/kg/min q 5 min	100 mcg/kg/min	change IV tubing q 12 hrs, monitor triglycerides, ↓ BP
Precedex	sedation	0.2 mcg/kg/hr	0.1 mcg/kg/min q 30 min	1.4 mcg/kg/min	watch for ↓ BP & bradycardia, can be used in non-intubated pts
diltiazem	↓ HR, conversion to NSR	5 mg/hr	5 mg/hr q 15 min	15 mg/hr	know what the HR goal is
amio	VT/VF	loading dose, then infusion @ 1 mg/min x 6 hrs, then 0.5 mg/min x 18 hrs	1 mg/min x 6 hrs, then 0.5 mg/min x 18 hrs	N/A	use filtered IV tubing, onset takes hours, typically starts c̄ a bolus

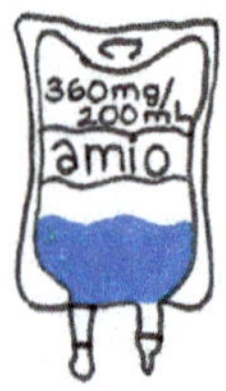

* May vary by facility, but a general guideline

@icunursingnotesbycaitlyn

ADENOSINE

@icunursingnotesbycaitlyn

indications:

stable supraventricular tachycardia (SVT)

- AVNRT
- AVRT

side effects:

- dyspnea
- hypotension
- facial flushing
- chest pain
- lightheadedness

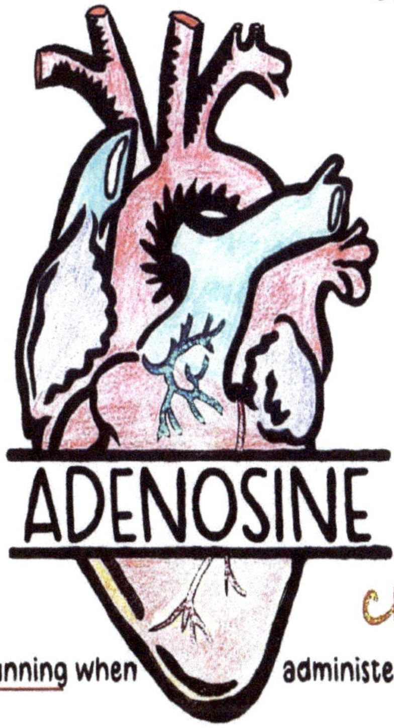

pharmacology:

Adenosine is an antiarrhythmic that slows impulse conduction through the heart's AV node & causes transient AV block; this terminates any reentrant circuit involving the AV node (AVNRT & AVRT)!

nursing considerations:

- Always have a 12-lead ECG running when administering adenosine & have defib pads on the patient.
- Continuous cardiac monitoring & vital signs.
- Have the code cart & a defibrillator at the bedside; ensure it's ready to be used, if needed.
- Warn the patient ā you give it!
- Know adenosine's contraindications (i.e. 2nd or 3rd degree AV block, bundle branch block, sick sinus syndrome, A-Fib/atrial flutter, VT & asthma, etc).
- Expect a brief period of asystole while the rhythm abates.
- Administer adenosine via rapid IV push through the IV port closest to the patient (very short half-life) & follow c̄ a 20 cc flush.
- Use a three-way stopcock (adenosine & NS flush) to ensure that the adenosine gets to the heart quickly.
- Remember to hold pressure on the flush syringe while you push the adenosine (or the adenosine can back up into the flush syringe).

Amiodarone

a class III antiarrhythmic (K+ channel blocker) used for the acute & prophylactic treatment of ventricular tachycardia (VT) & ventricular fibrillation (VF)

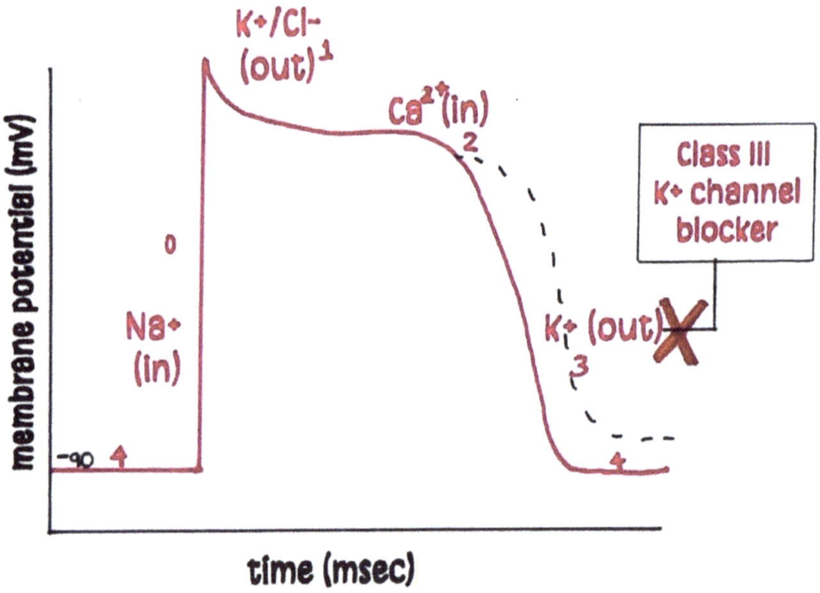

- ↑refractory period of the AV node/slows conduction
- ↑action potential duration
- Prolongs PR & QTc intervals
- vasodilatory effects

SIDE EFFECTS

- hypotension
- bradycardia
- arrhythmias (AV block)
- N/V, H/A
- skin discoloration
- pulmonary toxicity
- hepatotoxicity
- thyroid dysfunction
- photosensitivity
- visual changes

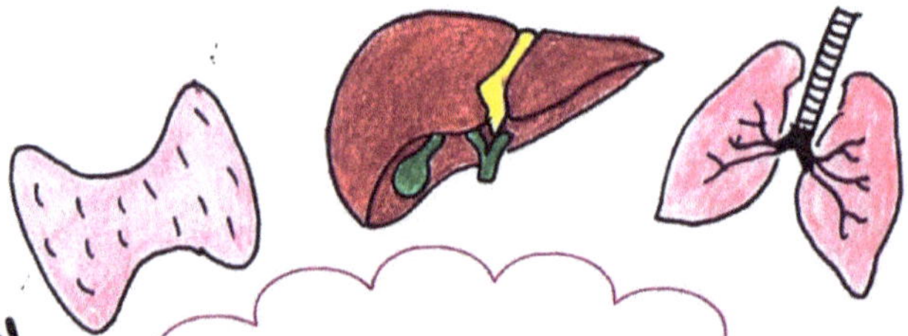

Use the mnemonic "PFTs, LFTs, & TFTs," to help you remember amiodarone's effects on the lungs, liver & thyroid c̄ long-term use!

Nursing Considerations

-Monitor for hypotension & bradycardia c̄ IV administration, especially when administering a bolus. Be prepared to potentially pace a patient, if needed, & have atropine readily available when initiating a gtt.

-Always administer IV amio through an in-line filter and, ideally, through a central line. If administering peripherally, frequently monitor the IV site for phlebitis.

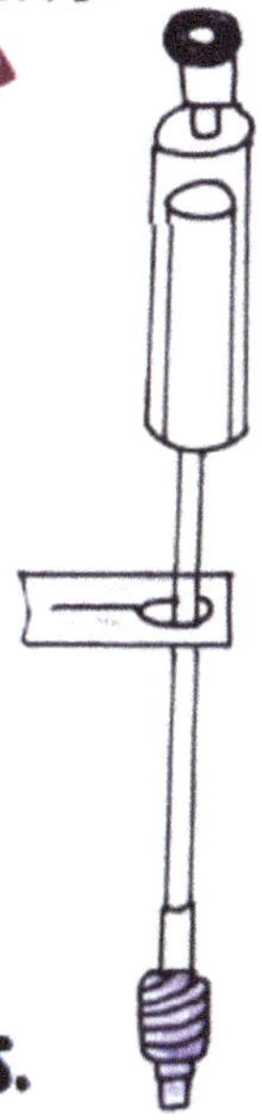

-Monitor labs & look for uptrends in LFTs. Replete electrolytes PRN.

- Monitor for ventricular dysrhythmias & AV heart block.

-Amiodarone will prolong the QTc, so be cautious of administering other QTc-prolonging medications.

-IV amio is typically ordered as a bolus followed by a maintenance infusion (1 mg/min x 6 hours, then 0.5 mg/min x 18 hours). Ensure that you know the plan for when the drip is complete (i.e. D/C entirely, continue the infusion, or transition to PO).

-Amio has a very long half-life (average is 58 days)! This ↑ the risk for toxicity.

-Amio has a lot of drug-drug interactions → key ones to know: ↑ levels of digoxin, warfarin, phenytoin, carvedilol, & cyclosporine.

-If your patient is on warfarin, anticipate the need to make dose adjustments for a therapeutic INR.

@icunursingnotesbycaitlyn

Know Your Antidotes!

opioids	naloxone (Narcan)
benzos	flumazenil (Romazicon)
heparin	protamine sulfate
warfarin	Vitamin K
digoxin	Digibind
beta blockers	glucagon
calcium channel blockers	calcium chloride
Tylenol	acetylcysteine
MgSO4	calcium gluconate
K+	IV insulin + dextrose
paralytics	acetylcholinesterase inhibitors

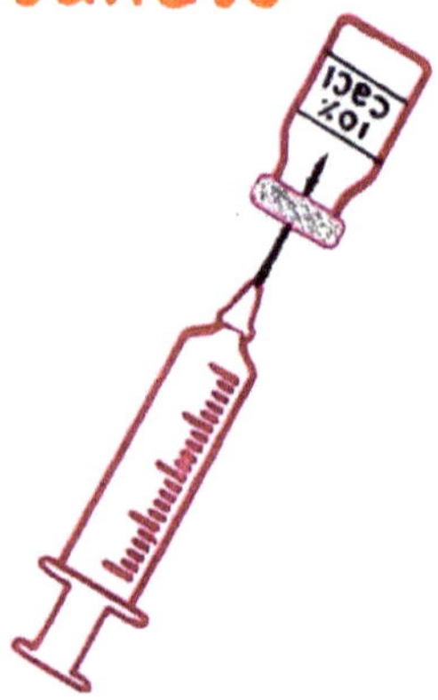

IV uses

- symptomatic bradycardia
- some heart blocks that occur at the nodal level (it will not work for blocks below the AV node)

pharmacology

Atropine ↑s heart rate & ↑s impulse conduction through the AV node by blocking the effects of the vagus nerve on the SA & AV nodes of the heart. When a bradycardic patient is given atropine, it works against the vagus nerve to ↑HR (think of it as removing the parasympathetic "brake" on the heart)!!

@icunursingnotesbycaitlyn

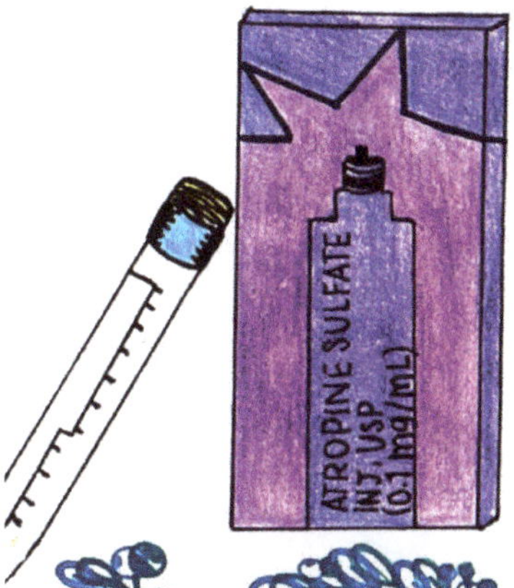

atropine

nursing considerations!

- Typical dosing is 1 mg IV q 3-5 min (max dose is 3 mg) per ACLS guidelines.
- Doses <0.5 mg &/or pushing atropine too slowly can cause rebound bradycardia.
- Know atropine's side effects: tachycardia & ↑MVO2 (myocardial oxygen demand), arrhythmias, dry mouth, urinary retention, ↓K+, & H/A.
- Make sure that there are pacer/defib pads on the patient!
- If atropine fails to ↑HR, be prepared to transcutaneously pace the patient & to possibly start a dopamine/epi gtt, and anticipate TVP placement.
- Atropine will not work for a patient c̄ Mobitz Type II or complete (3rd degree) heart block. It's also ineffective in patients c̄ heart transplants, because they lack vagal nerve innervation.
- Atropine ↑ myocardial oxygen consumption (MvO2) & can worsen ischemia in a patient c̄ coronary artery disease (CAD).
- In the cath lab, if intervening in the RCA, have atropine available & have pacer/defib pads on the patient (remember that the RCA supplies the SA node)!

drug class & use

An IV <u>direct thrombin inhibitor</u> used as an alternative to heparin for acute coronary syndrome (ACS), PCI, mechanical circulatory support, & cardiopulmonary bypass <u>when heparin is contraindicated</u> (i.e. heparin-induced thrombocytopenia/HIT).

how it works

Bivalirudin works by selectively binding to circulating & clot-bound thrombin (thrombin that is trapped in established clots). <u>Without thrombin, fibrinogen can't convert to fibrin, producing an anticoagulant effect.</u>

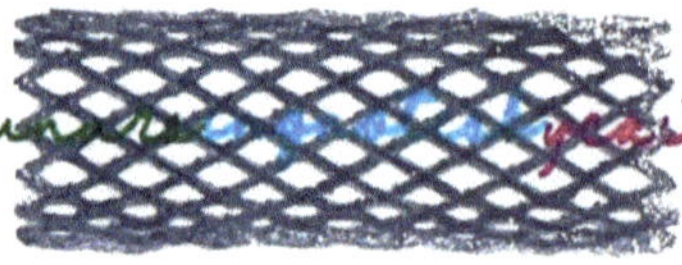

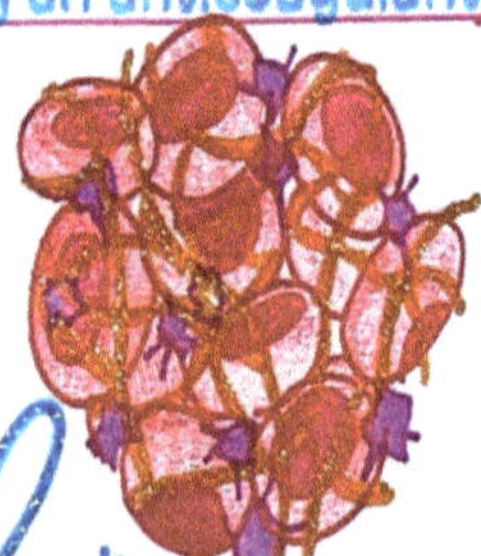

bivalirudin (Angiomax)

nursing considerations

- <u>Know your patient's renal function</u> - the infusion rate should be ↓ for patients c̄ renal insufficiency.
- The usual dose is 0.75 mg/kg IV bolus followed by a continuous IV infusion of 1.75 mg/kg/hr for up to 4 hours s/p PCI. After 4 hours, a low-rate infusion (0.2 mg/kg/hr) may or may not be continued for up to 20 hours.
- Monitor for bleeding, hypotension, & signs of acute stent thrombosis (AST) in patients c̄ STEMI undergoing PCI c̄ Angiomax (<u>higher incidence of AST in patients treated c̄ Angiomax compared to those treated c̄ heparin</u>)!
- Unlike heparin, there is no antidote for Angiomax, but it does have a shorter half-life (wears off more quickly) & a lower bleeding risk!
- Check an activated clotting time (ACT) 5 minutes after administering the initial bolus dose; if it isn't therapeutic (<250 sec), then an additional bolus can be given (0.3 mg/kg).
- Angiomax <u>does NOT dissolve existing clots</u>; it prevents further clot formation.

Check an ACT!

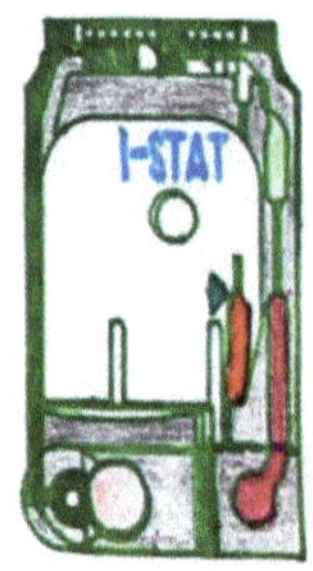

CANGRELOR

Why It's Used

It's a fast-acting IV P2Y12 inhibitor used to ↓ the risk of periprocedural MI, repeat coronary revascularization, & stent thrombosis in patients undergoing percutaneous coronary intervention (PCI) who haven't been pre-treated c̄ a PO P2Y12 inhibitor (i.e. ticagrelor, clopidogrel, or prasugrel) & who aren't being given a GP IIb/IIIa inhibitor (i.e. eptifibatide or tirofiban).

How it Works

Activated platelets release adenosine diphosphate (ADP) that binds to P2Y12 receptors on platelets, triggering a cascade of events that lead to platelet aggregation. Cangrelor binds reversibly to these receptors, preventing signaling & activation of platelets by ADP.

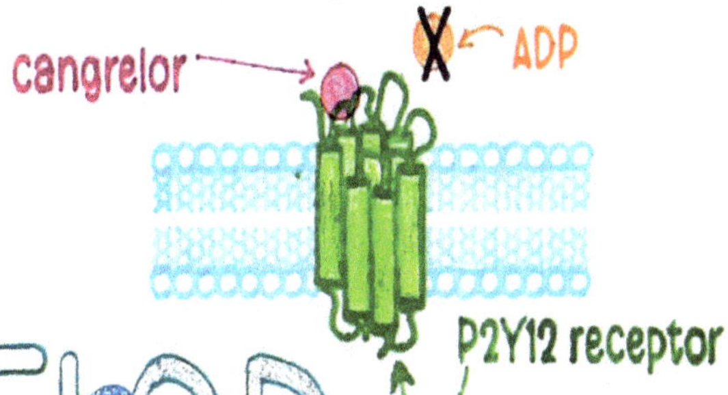

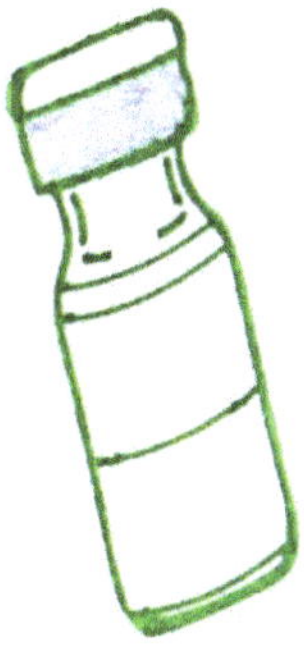

Nursing Considerations

- Cangrelor is ideal for patients who are unable to take a PO P2Y12 inhibitor (i.e. intubated patients, N/V, shock states, etc) & in patients requiring surgery (5-7 day drug washout period for PO antiplatelets).
- It has a quick on-off capability; it starts working within 2 minutes following IV administration, & platelet function returns to the patient's baseline within 1 hour of D/C'ing the infusion.
- Monitor for bleeding; Cangrelor has a higher bleeding risk than the other drugs in this class.
- Transient dyspnea can occur in some patients.
- It's given as a weight-based IV bolus (30 mcg/kg) prior to PCI followed by an IV infusion (4 mcg/kg/min) for at least 2 hours or for the duration of the PCI (whichever is longer).
- Reconstitute a 50 mg cangrelor vial c̄ 5 cc of sterile water & add to a 250 cc bag of NS or D5W to yield a final concentration of 200 mcg/mL. Once mixed, it's stable for 12 hours. Remove the initial bolus dose from the diluted bag (200 mcg/mL), NEVER from the reconstituted vial!
- Administer through a dedicated IV line.
- Cangrelor doesn't replace the oral P2Y12 inhibitors! A loading dose of a P2Y12 inhibitor is given to maintain platelet inhibition. A ticagrelor loading dose can be given at any time during the cangrelor infusion or immediately after D/C'ing it, but clopidogrel & prasugrel can only be given after the infusion is D/C'd because they will compete c̄ cangrelor for the receptor site! @icunursingnotesbycaitlyn

Clopidogrel Resistance

Reduced effectiveness of clopidogrel (Plavix) in patients who are poor metabolizers of the drug 2/2 genetic variations in the CYP2C19 enzyme.

DRUG INDICATIONS

- acute coronary syndrome (ACS)
- prevention of stent thrombosis s/p PCI
- peripheral arterial disease (PAD)
- stroke

@icunursingnotesbycaitlyn

PATHOPHYSIOLOGY OF "NON-RESPONDERS"

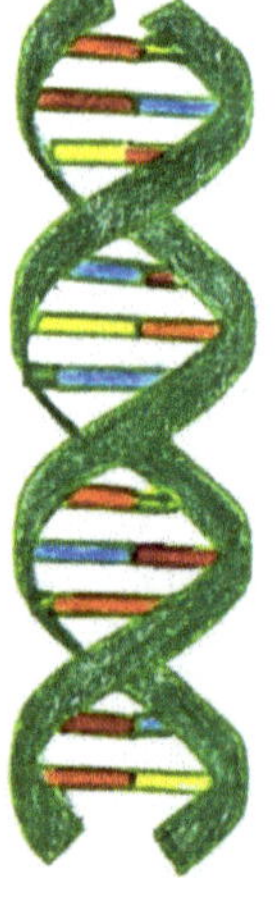

Clopidogrel (Plavix) is a $P2Y_{12}$ inhibitor that exerts its anti-platelet effects by blocking $P2Y_{12}$ ADP receptors on platelets. Because it's a prodrug, it requires a two-step metabolism that involves multiple enzymes, including CYP2C19– the liver enzyme needed to convert clopidogrel to its active form so that it can function in the body!

People c̄ variant forms of the CYP2C19 gene (≈ 30% of the population) cannot metabolize clopidogrel to its active form & will, therefore, not benefit from it. These patients are often referred to as "Plavix non-responders" & are at a ↑ risk for cardiac events & adverse outcomes after PCI or ACS when given clopidogrel as part of DAPT!

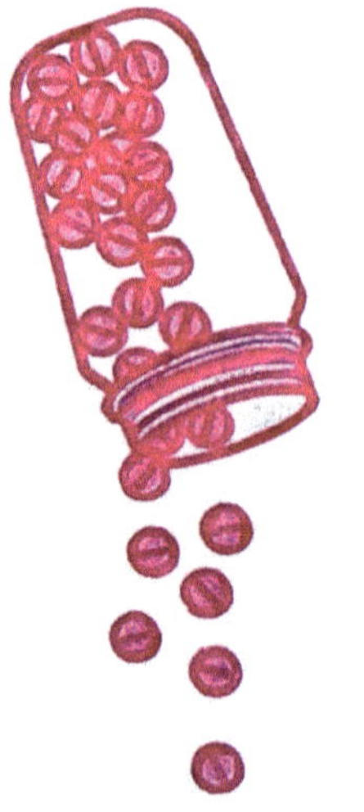

THE ALTERNATIVES:

- ticagrelor (Brilinta)

or

- prasugrel (Effient)

Genetic testing will confirm if a patient is a Plavix non-responder.

DRUG CLASS & INDICATIONS

A selective alpha-2 adrenergic agonist c̄ sedative, anxiolytic, & mild anesthetic properties that is used for:

- sedation of intubated patients
- spontaneous breathing trials (SBT)
- adjunct to general anesthesia
- procedural sedation
- ETOH withdrawal

@icunursingnotesbycaitlyn

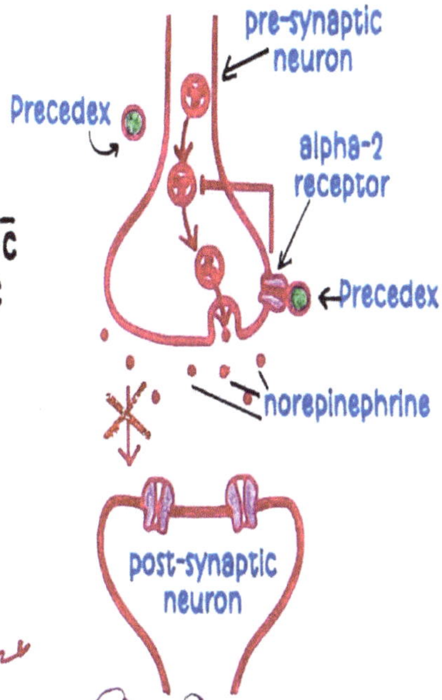

HOW IT WORKS

Dexmedetomidine selectively binds to presynaptic alpha-2 receptors (mostly in the locus coeruleus of the brain), inhibiting norepinephrine release & inducing hyperpolarization of neurons; this, in turn, terminates the propagation of pain signals & induces sedation and mild analgesia!

dexmedetomidine

(PRECEDEX)

NURSING CONSIDERATIONS:

- Monitor for bradycardia & hypotension 2/2 ↓ sympathetic nervous system activity.
- It has a rapid onset of action & a short half-life, so consider a loading dose (1 mcg/kg) over 10 min before starting a continous IV infusion (0.2-0.7 mcg/kg/hr). Consider slowing or omitting the loading dose if your patient's BP &/or HR are on the lower end of normal.
- Titrate the gtt according to the ordered RASS goal. Wait at least 30 min between titrations to avoid the risk of hypotension.
- Dexmedetomidine does not cause respiratory depression, so it can be used to bridge patients through the entire extubation process (i.e. unlike propofol, dexmedetomidine doesn't have to be D/C'd prior to extubation). It can also be used safely in non-intubated patients.
- Remember that sedation doesn't replace pain control! If your patient still seems uncomfortable & you continue to ↑ the infusion rate, treat the pain! Consider adding an analgesic.

diltiazem (CARDIZEM)

USES:

- supraventricular tachycardias c̄ RVR (A-Fib/flutter or paroxysmal SVT)
- prevention of radial artery spasm (cardiac cath)
- hypertension
- chronic stable angina

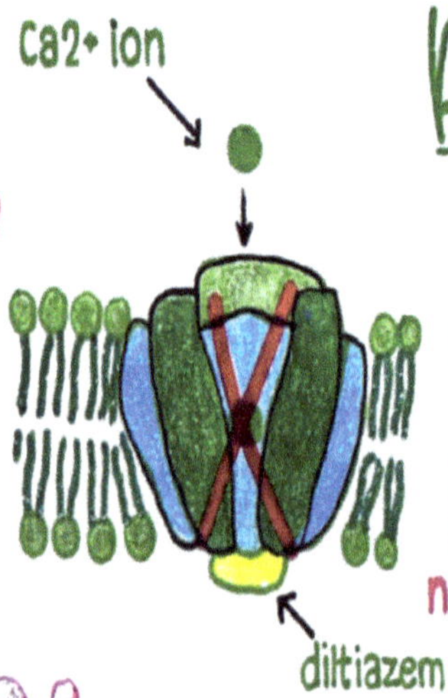

PHARMACOLOGY:

Diltiazem is a class IV antiarrhythmic/calcium channel blocker that ↓s cardiac contractility, ↓s the heart rate & ↓s blood pressure by blocking the influx of Ca^{2+} ions into myocardial, cardiac nodal, & arterial smooth muscle cells.

NURSING CONSIDERATIONS:

- Don't give IV diltiazem to a patient c̄ a known history of heart failure c̄ a low EF (HFrEF) or LV dysfunction 2/2 its negative inotropic effects. It will exacerbate the patient's heart failure & will likely cause hemodynamic instability in these patients!
- Know its contraindications: sick sinus syndrome or 2nd/3rd degree heart block (without a pacemaker), Wolff-Parkinson-White (WPW), hypotension, ↓ ejection fraction (<40%)/LV dysfunction, cardiogenic shock, acute MI, VT, & beta blockade.
- For ongoing control of the ventricular rate in patients c̄ A-Fib/flutter, a continuous IV infusion of diltiazem is typically initiated at a dose range of 5-15 mg/hr (titrated according to the desired HR). 2 IV boluses of diltiazem are usually given before initiating a gtt.
- Monitor HR, blood pressure & cardiac rhythm; watch for bradycardia, heart block, & hypotension.
- Monitor for S/S of heart failure (strict I&O, daily weight, pulmonary congestion, edema, JVD, etc).
- IV diltiazem and an IV beta blocker shouldn't be given within a few hours of each other.
- Monitor K^+ levels, as hypokalemia ↑s the risk of arrhythmias. @icunursingnotesbycaitlyn

CLASS & USES

A predominant beta-1 adrenergic agonist & inodilator
(+ inotrope & vasodilator)
used for:

- acute decompensated ♥ failure
- cardiogenic shock
- dobutamine stress echo
- cardiac surgery

HOW IT WORKS

β_1 >>> β_2 > α_1

β_1:
↑contractility
↓ESV = ↑SV = ↑CO
↑heart rate

β_2:
vasodilation
↓SVR (afterload)

α_1:
vasoconstriction
(minimal)

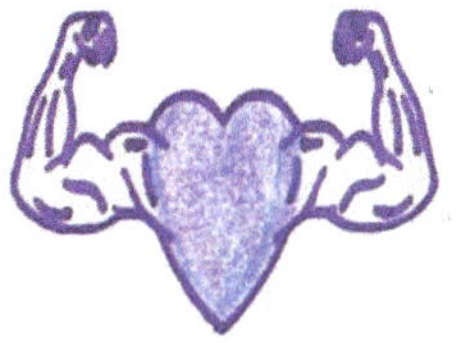

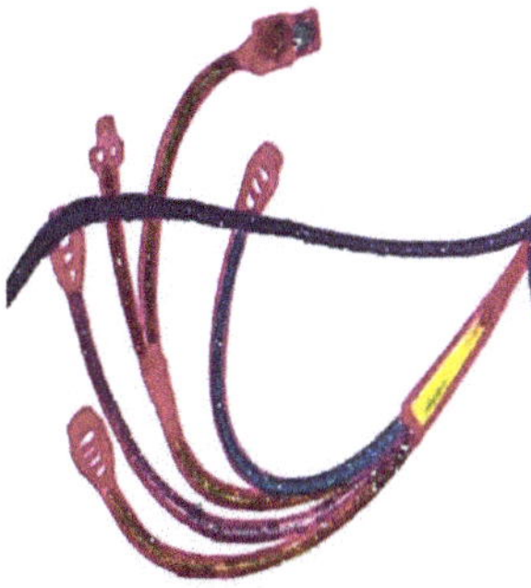

dobutamine

♥ NURSING CONSIDERATIONS ♥

@icunursingnotesbycaitlyn

- Dobutamine can worsen hypotension in the setting of inadequate preload, so optimize fluid volume status first!
- Know the most common side effects: tachycardia (↑chronotropy), ventricular ectopy (PVCs) & arrhythmias, dyspnea, & ↑ or ↓ BP, & hypokalemia.
- Dobutamine can have variable effects on BP: it can ↑ systolic blood pressure because ↑ stroke volume (SV), but it can also ↓ BP in some patients.
- Strict I&O: if it's working, there should be an ↑ urine output (↑cardiac output = ↑UOP)!
- If your patient has A-Fib, giving Digoxin before starting a dobutamine gtt can ↓ the risk of A-Fib c̄ RVR.
- Dobutamine isn't ideal inotrope for patients on chronic beta-blocker therapy (milrinone is preferred in this case).
- If your patient has a Swan-Ganz/PAC, monitor & trend CO/CI, SVR, PAWP, & SvO2. Ideally, you should see an overall ↑ in CO/CI, ↓ SVR, ↓ PAWP, & ↑ SvO2.
- Dobutamine is indicated for short-term inotropic support; after a few days, drug tolerance can develop 2/2 the down-regulation of beta receptors.
- Its short half-life & rapid onset make it easily titratable; titrate according to the ordered hemodynamic parameter(s) (usually CO/CI rather than MAP)!
- Question the use of dobutamine in the setting of acute MI, beta blocker use, hypokalemia, hypovolemia, VT/VF, & A-Fib.

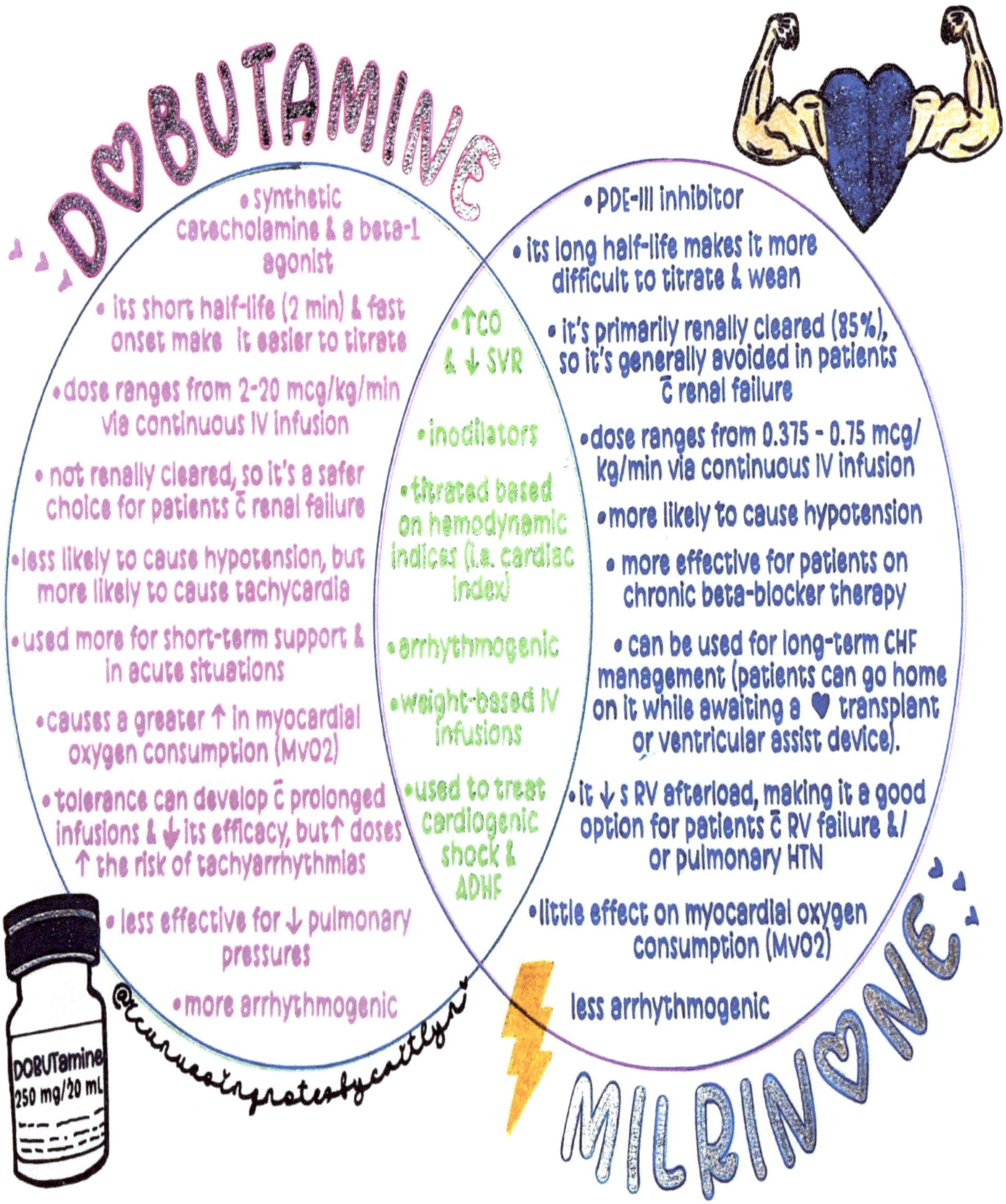
DOBUTAMINE
• synthetic catecholamine & a beta-1 agonist
• its short half-life (2 min) & fast onset make it easier to titrate
• dose ranges from 2-20 mcg/kg/min via continuous IV infusion
• not renally cleared, so it's a safer choice for patients c̄ renal failure
• less likely to cause hypotension, but more likely to cause tachycardia
• used more for short-term support & in acute situations
• causes a greater ↑ in myocardial oxygen consumption (MvO2)
• tolerance can develop c̄ prolonged infusions & ↓ its efficacy, but ↑ doses ↑ the risk of tachyarrhythmias
• less effective for ↓ pulmonary pressures
• more arrhythmogenic
• ↑CO & ↓ SVR
• inodilators
• titrated based on hemodynamic indices (i.e. cardiac index)
• arrhythmogenic
• weight-based IV infusions
• used to treat cardiogenic shock & ADHF
• PDE-III inhibitor
• its long half-life makes it more difficult to titrate & wean
• it's primarily renally cleared (85%), so it's generally avoided in patients c̄ renal failure
• dose ranges from 0.375 - 0.75 mcg/kg/min via continuous IV infusion
• more likely to cause hypotension
• more effective for patients on chronic beta-blocker therapy
• can be used for long-term CHF management (patients can go home on it while awaiting a ♥ transplant or ventricular assist device).
• it ↓ s RV afterload, making it a good option for patients c̄ RV failure &/ or pulmonary HTN
• little effect on myocardial oxygen consumption (MvO2)
less arrhythmogenic
MILRINONE
DOBUTamine
250 mg/20 mL
@icunursingnotesbycaitlyn

DUAL ANTIPLATELET THERAPY (DAPT)

aspirin (indefinitely) 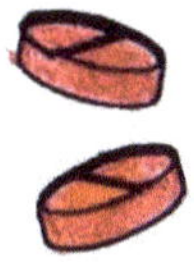

&

P2Y12 inhibitor
ticagrelor (Brilinta)
clopidogrel (Plavix)
prasugrel (Effient)

Who?

Patients c̄ ACS s/p PCI c̄ coronary stenting or CABG.[1]

What?

Patients are prescribed aspirin in combination c̄ a P2Y12 inhibitor (clopidogrel, ticagrelor, or prasugrel).

When?

[3] Optimal DAPT duration post-PCI is 12 months (ASA is taken indefinitely)!

How?

Antiplatelets make platelets less "sticky" & ↓ platelet aggregation to keep the stent(s) from clotting off.

A patient is typically given an initial loading dose of a P2Y12 inhibitor (at the time of PCI) followed by a daily maintenance dose.[2]

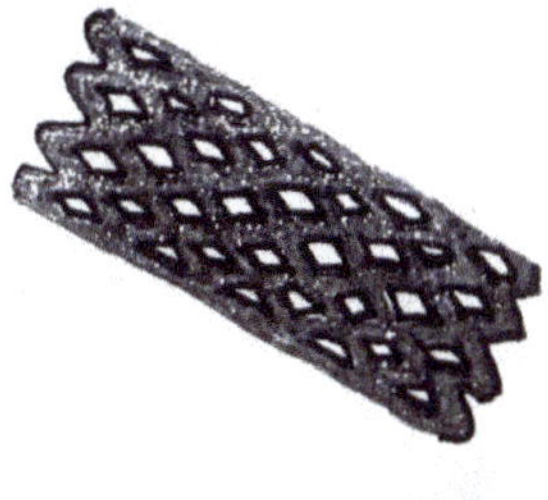

Why?

DAPT has been shown to reduce the risk of stent thrombosis & ischemic events post-PCI & ↓s the risk of vein graft occlusion post-CABG.[4]

@icunursingnotesbycaitlyn

P2Y12 Inhibitors Made Easy!

	clopidogrel (Plavix)	prasugrel (Effient)	ticagrelor (Brilinta)
DOSING	loading dose: 600 mg maintenance: 75 mg daily	loading dose: 60 mg maintenance: 10 mg daily	loading dose: 180 mg maintenance: 90 mg BID
NURSING CONSIDERATIONS	• up to 30% of patients are Plavix "non-responders" (genetic resistance)![5] • its effectiveness is ↓ by amio, calcium channel blockers, NSAIDs & PPIs.[6] • slower onset • monitor for bleeding!	• contraindicated in patients c̄ a history of a TIA/stroke &/or patients ≥ 75 yrs-old.[6] • faster onset & more potent than Plavix but has an ↑ bleeding risk.[6] • works quickly • monitor for bleeding	• not ideal for patients who are likely to be non-compliant! • works quickly but has a shorter half-life.[6] • very expensive – make sure that your patient's insurance covers it! • monitor for bleeding

@icunursingnotesbycaitlyn

@icunursingnotesbycaitlyn

EPINEPHRINE

* greater effect on the ♥
* non-selective: affects all receptors
  - beta effects (↑inotropy & chronotropy) > alpha effects (vasoconstriction)
* ↑SVR, ↑BP, ↑MAP, ↑HR, ↑CO & ↑contractility
* Used for ♥ arrest, anaphylactic shock, & refractory hypotension (not responsive to Levo & vaso)
* can cause hyperglycemia, ↑lactate, & hypokalemia
* routes: IV, SQ, IM, inhalation
* more arrhythmogenic effects

Both

- inopressors
- endogenous catecholamines
- alpha & beta agonists
- easily titratable (short-acting)
- can cause ischemia
- vesicants (central line is ideal)

NOREPI (LEVO)

* greater effect on the blood vessels
* more selective: more of an alpha than beta agonist (less inotropy & chronotropy, more vasoconstriction)
* ↑SVR, ↑BP, ↑MAP: little effect on HR, SV & CO
* first-line pressor for shock states & hypotension
* can cause reflex bradycardia
* IV administration only
  - fewer side effects & less potent than epi (acts on fewer receptors)

EPTIFIBATIDE (INTEGRILIN)

indications

- acute coronary syndrome (ACS)
- percutaneous coronary intervention (PCI)

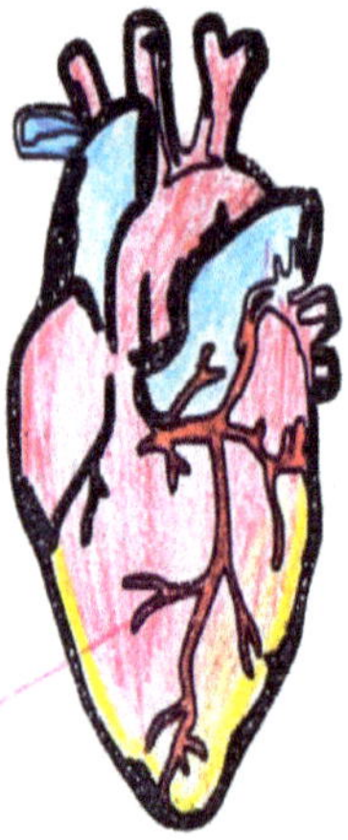

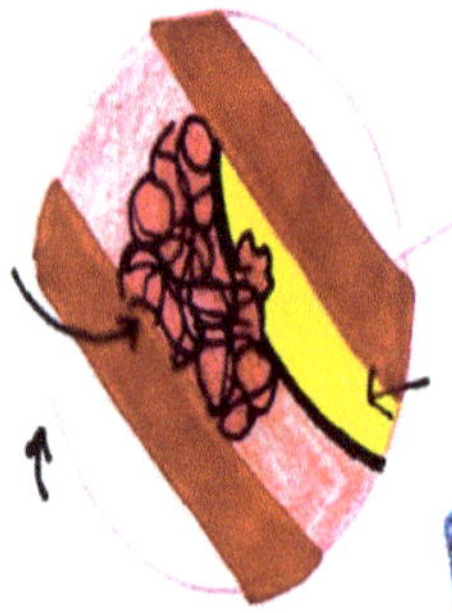

pharmacology

Eptifibatide (Integrilin) is classified as an antiplatelet & a glycoprotein (GP) IIb/IIIa inhibitor that inhibits platelet aggregation (clumping together) by blocking special receptors on platelets; this ↓ the ability of the platelets to form clots within the coronary arteries.

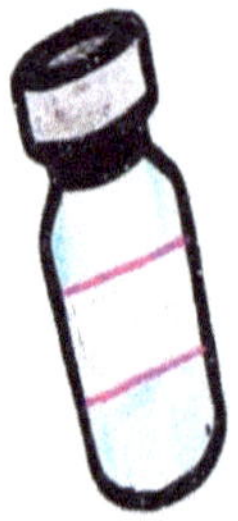

nursing considerations

- It's a high-alert medication!
- The infusion rate is determined by the patient's body weight & renal function.
- Patients c̄ renal insufficiency will need a dose reduction (Integrilin is renally cleared).
- Integrilin is typically only given in an intensive care unit or a cardiac cath lab.
- Monitor for bleeding (vascular access sites, GI/GU, etc) & thrombocytopenia.
- Monitor platelet count, ACT (target ACT is 200 to 300 sec for a PCI), CBC, aPTT, & HgB.
- Typically given as a 180 mcg/kg IV bolus followed by a 2 mcg/kg/min gtt (you can give a second bolus 10 minutes after the first bolus PRN).
- Integrilin is given in conjunction c̄ ASA & heparin.
- Onset is immediate c̄ a half-life ≈ 2.5 hrs.

fentanyl

INDICATIONS:

- induction & maintenance of anesthesia
- procedural sedation
- acute post-operative pain
- pain control in intubated patients

HOW IT WORKS:

Fentanyl is a mu-opioid receptor agonist & opioid analgesic that binds to stereospecific pain receptors in the central nervous system (CNS). It increases pain threshold, alters pain perception, & inhibits ascending pain pathways in the body.

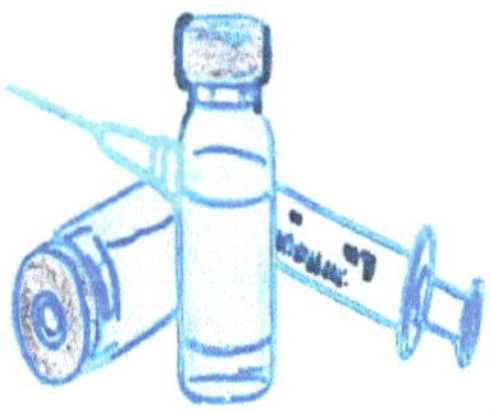

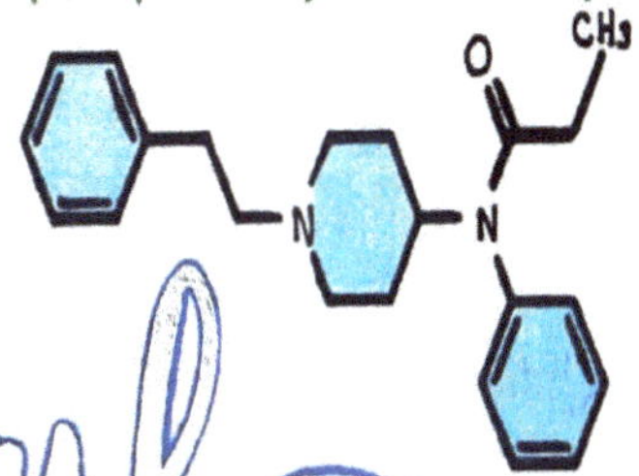

NURSING CONSIDERATIONS:

@icunursingnotesbycaitlyn

- Fentanyl is 100x more potent than morphine! 100 mcg of fentanyl ≈ 10 mg of morphine! Fentanyl is less likely to cause hypotension than morphine 2/2 lack of histamine release.
- Fentanyl can be administered via several routes: IV, transdermal, intranasal, intrathecal, & sublingual; this is because fentanyl is highly lipophilic!
- It has a rapid onset of action, & peak effects are achieved within minutes of IV administration.
- The respiratory depressant effect often lasts longer than the analgesic effect.
- When administered as a continuous IV infusion, it has a high context-sensitive half-time, so, if the gtt has been infusing for > 3-4 hours, anticipate that it's going to take several hours before your patient is ready to extubate after discontinuing the fentanyl infusion!
- Monitor RR (risk of respiratory depression), SpO2, EtCO2, HR, & BP, and always have a code cart, BVM, & suction readily available!
- Patients c̄ COPD are more sensitive to the respiratory depressant effects of fentanyl. Ensure that you assess your patient's respiratory status first!
- Fentanyl is a better choice of analgesic in patients c̄ renal failure &/or hemodynamic instability.
- Naloxone (Narcan) is the reversal agent (antidote) for fentanyl.
- Rapid IV administration of fentanyl at higher doses (i.e. high-dose fentanyl induction) has been associated c̄ bradycardia, hypotension, & rigidity in the chest wall muscles. Since the introduction of more balanced anesthetics & enhanced recovery protocols for cardiac surgery patients, this induction technique isn't used as often.

Lasix

indications:

- CHF
- acute pulmonary edema
- HTN
- FVE R/T heart, kidney, &/or liver failure

@icunursingnotesbycaitlyn

pharmacology:

Lasix is a loop diuretic that acts on the loop of Henle within the nephron of the kidney to ↑ urine output & rid the body of excess fluid (i.e. promote diuresis).

It blocks the reabsorption of Na^+, K^+ & Cl^- and, therefore, water back into the bloodstream (remember: H_2O follows salt); this ↓ the intravascular volume & ↓ preload/LVEDP!

Lasix also causes a transient venodilation that helps relieve dyspnea in the setting of HF & ↓ PAP/PCWP, ↓ BP.

side effects:

- ↓ K^+, Na^+, Cl^-, Ca^{2+}, Mg^{2+}
- hyperglycemia
- hyperuricemia
- muscle cramps
- orthostatic hypotension
- dizziness
- dehydration
- tinnitus (rapid IVP)

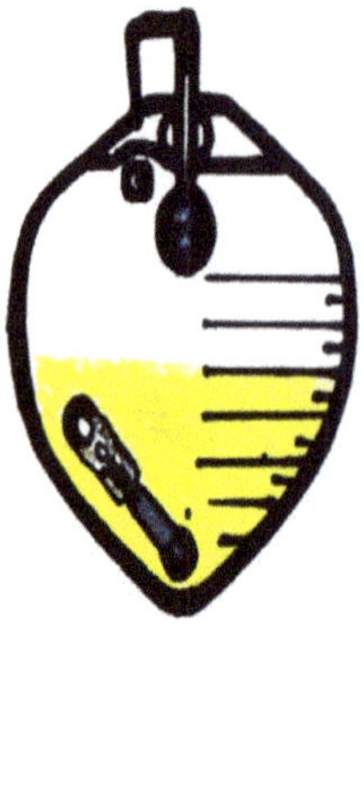

nursing considerations:

-strict I&O (includes IV gtts), daily weights & fluid restriction

-Monitor for hypotension: recycle the BP ā you administer an antihypertensive or nitrate, if the patient is actively diuresing.

-Monitoring electrolytes is important; replete PRN & consider drawing a K^+/Mg^{2+} level for ↑ ectopy & a high UOP.

-Before giving Lasix, ask yourself, "why?" Does your patient still have signs of fluid overload (i.e. crackles, JVD, etc)? What's the patient's diuresis goal?

-If your patient isn't responding to an ↑ in the dose & frequency of intermittent IVPs, consider advocating for more aggressive diuresis (i.e. Bumex/Diuril) or possibly a Lasix gtt.

-Expect to administer a higher than usual Lasix dose to a patient c̄ renal &/or heart failure!

IV heparin

indications

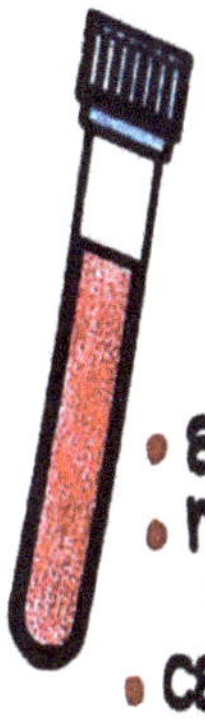

- DVT & PE
- DVT prophylaxis
- atrial fibrillation
- cardiac catheterization
- acute coronary syndrome (ACS)
- mechanical circulatory support devices (IABP, Impella, & ECMO)
- cardiopulmonary bypass (CPB) for open-heart surgery
- hemodialysis & CRRT
- disseminated intravascular coagulation (DIC)
- maintain implanted port patency (heparin flush)

pharmacology

Heparin is an anticoagulant that interferes c̄ normal coagulation by interfering c̄ the clotting cascade & thrombin formation.

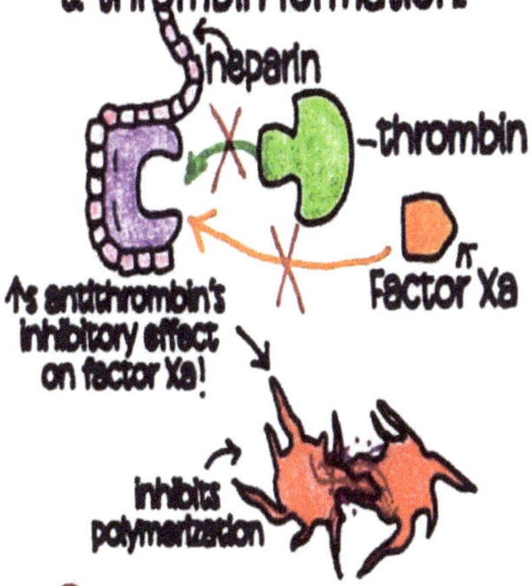

nursing considerations:

- Have protamine sulfate readily available, if needed (this is the antidote/reversal agent for heparin)! Heparin is a high-alert drug; always verify c̄ another RN when initiating a gtt, titrating, hanging a new bag, administering a bolus, &/or restarting the infusion!
- Draw baseline labs: PT/INR, CBC/platelet count, & anti-Xa ā initiating a gtt; titrate according to orders until anti-Xa or aPTT levels are therapeutic (the order should specify whether anti-Xa or aPTT).
- Monitor for bleeding & S/S of heparin-induced thrombocytopenia (HIT).
- Know heparin's contraindications: hypersensitivity, severe thrombocytopenia, uncontrolled bleeding (exception to this is DIC).
- Ensure that any pre-existing orders for SQ heparin/enoxaparin are D/C'd, if the patient is on a heparin gtt.
- IV heparin is weight-based, so make sure the patient's weight is up-to-date & accurate.
- In patients c̄ impaired renal function, the clearance of heparin may be ↓, increasing the risk of bleeding.

IBUTILIDE

(Corvert)

WHAT IT IS

A short-acting IV class III antiarrhythmic (K+ channel blocker) that is used to convert atrial fibrillation/flutter to normal sinus rhythm.

@icunursingnotesbycaitlyn

HOW IT WORKS

It works by prolonging cardiac action potential duration in cardiac muscle cells, and it increases both atrial & ventricular refractoriness.

NURSING IMPLICATIONS

- Consider giving 2 grams of IV magnesium prior to administering ibutilide to ↓ the risk of torsades.
- Ensure that your patient's K+ & magnesium levels are within the normal range, & replete PRN before giving ibutilide.
- It can be given to patients c̄ pre-excited A-Fib in the setting of Wolff-Parkinson White Syndrome.
- Put defibrillation pads on the patient & have a code cart nearby.
- Typical dose is 1 mg IV over 10 minutes. Dilute one vial (1 mg) in a 50 mL bag of NS).
- Know your patient's baseline QTc before giving ibutilide.
- Avoid giving other drugs that prolong the QT interval (i.e. Zofran, other antiarrhythmics, etc).
- If the patient converts to NSR, then stop the infusion.
- Ibutilide is more effective for converting A-flutter than A-Fib.
- It generally doesn't affect the patient's hemodynamics.
- If A-flutter or A-Fib persists 10 min after completing the first dose, a second dose of 1 mg can be given over 10 min.
- A patient must be on continuous ECG monitoring for a minimum of 4 hours after the infusion or until the QTc has returned to baseline.

USES:

- EP study/cardiac ablation
- postoperative bradycardia s/p heart transplant
- heart block (not first-line)

CLASS:

beta-1 & beta-2 agonist

HEMODYNAMIC EFFECTS

↑ heart rate
↑ or ↓ BP
↑ ♥ contractility
↑ cardiac output
↓ SVR (afterload)

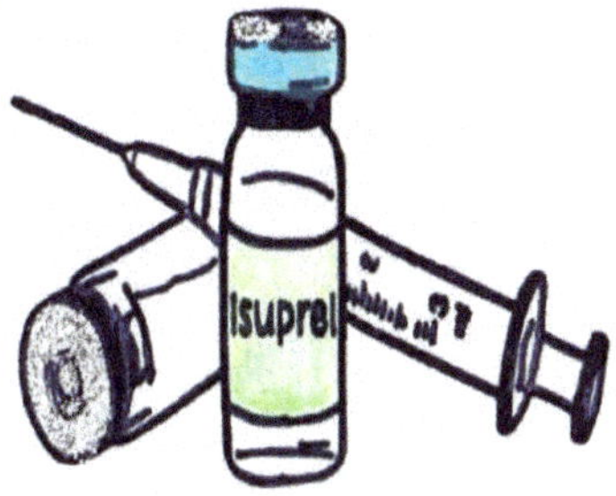

isoproterenol (ISUPREL)

NURSING CONSIDERATIONS

- Isuprel may be used to increase HR in patients c̄ a denervated heart s/p cardiac transplant; these patients will not respond to atropine!
- Other medications (i.e. atropine) & interventions (i.e. pacing) are ideally used before Isuprel is considered.
- It increases myocardial oxygen demand (MvO2) & limits coronary filling and perfusion (secondary to tachycardia), thereby increasing the risk of cardiac ischemia - this is why it's important to know your patient's history!
- Monitor for side effects (tachycardia, arrhythmias, hypotension, & S/S of cardiac ischemia).
- Monitor for changes in HR, BP, UOP, cardiac output (if the patient has a Swan).
- Titrate accordingly (check your orders, always).
- Administer an Isuprel gtt centrally, if possible.

@icunursingnotesbycaitlyn

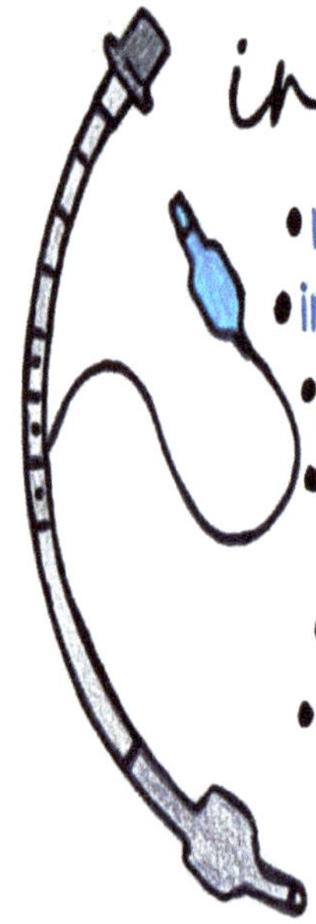

indications

- multimodal analgesia
- induction agent for RSI
- procedural sedation
- acute/chronic pain management
- status epilepticus
- treatment-resistant depression, PTSD, & eating disorders

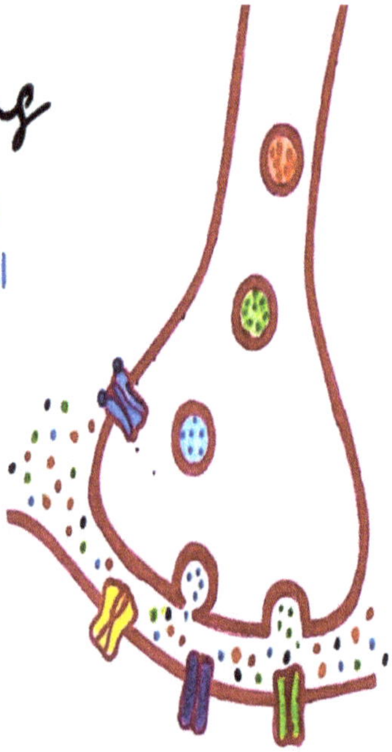

how it works

Ketamine's mechanism of action is complex but, in general, it's a NMDA receptor antagonist & a dissociative anesthetic. It blocks glutamate, an excitatory neurotransmitter, from binding to NMDA receptors within the CNS; this mechanism is thought to be responsible for ketamine's dissociative & analgesic effects. It also interacts c̄ many other binding sites including opioid, cholinergic, nicotinic & muscarinic receptors.

Ketamine

general nursing considerations:

- Know your state's board of nursing guidelines/hospital policy for the RN administration of ketamine.
- Ketamine ↑s sympathetic tone & inhibits catecholamine reuptake channels, so anticipate an ↑ in your patient's BP & HR. Use c̄ caution in patients who have uncontrolled HTN &/or CAD (it ↑s myocardial O2 demand).
- Unlike other sedatives, ketamine typically preserves airway reflexes, ventilation, & hemodynamics, making it valuable in many clinical situations; it can be useful in cases where we want to avoid intubation (i.e. cardiac tamponade, asthma, etc) unless it's absolutely necessary!
- Use ketamine c̄ caution in catecholamine-depleted states (common in ICU patients) – it can cause a paradoxical ↓ in BP & HR and act as a myocardial depressant (negative inotropic effect) in these patients!
- Ketamine can be given IV, IO, IM, or IN c̄ dosing ranges based on the desired effect; its effects are dose-dependent.
- There's no strong evidence to support that ketamine ↑s ICP in head injuries (a previously-thought contraindication).
- Remember that ketamine's effects are synergistic (rather than just additive).
- Emergence delirium can occur when higher/dissociative doses of ketamine are administered & start to wear off; consider the coadministration of a PRN benzodiazepine, like midazolam (Versed), to help minimize this risk.

labetalol

Drug Class & Use:

Labetalol is a combined alpha- & beta-adrenergic blocking agent that is used to ↓ blood pressure in the setting of:

- refractory hypertension
- hypertensive crises
- preeclampsia/eclampsia
- catecholamine crises (pheochromocytoma)

How It Works:

By blocking epi & norepi from binding to alpha-1, beta-1, & beta-2 receptors in the body, labetalol reduces systemic vascular resistance (SVR) and, in turn, ↓ arterial blood pressure with minimal effect on the heart rate, stroke volume, & cardiac output.

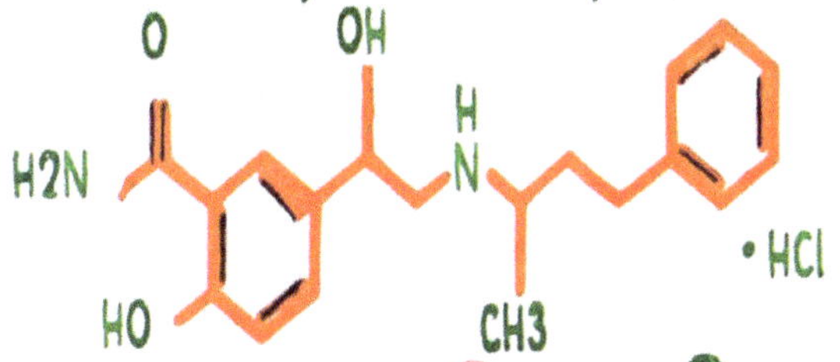

Nursing Considerations:

- Labetalol is a non-cardioselective beta blocker. Because it blocks beta-2 receptors in the lungs, it should not be given to patients c̄ asthma or COPD 2/2 bronchoconstriction.
- It decreases afterload (SVR) without a reflex tachycardia (a compensatory ↑ in the heart rate when the blood pressure drops). It has little to no effect on the heart rate.
- Because of its alpha-1 effects, labetalol is more effective at lowering arterial blood pressure than pure beta-blockers (i.e. metoprolol).
- Don't give labetalol to patients c̄ acute decompensated heart failure (ADHF)/HFrEF; it ↓s cardiac contractility & can exacerbate CHF.
- It can be administered IV or PO. An initial IV bolus of 20 mg is typically given &, if needed, it's repeated q 10 minutes c̄ escalating doses of 20-80 mg up to a cumulative dose of 300 mg in 24 hours.
- Orthostatic hypotension can occur for up to 3 hours after IV administration.
- It can mask the S/S of hypoglycemia in patients c̄ diabetes.
- When very tight blood pressure control is needed (i.e. aortic dissection), easily titratable agents like nicardipine or sodium nitroprusside are better options. Labetalol has a long half-life (2-6 hours depending on the dose), so it's not easy to titrate as a continuous IV infusion.

Magnesium sulfate

Indications:

- hypomagnesemia
- torsades de pointes
- prolonged QT interval
- refractory A-Fib c̄ RVR
- acute asthma exacerbation
- preterm labor (works as a tocolytic)
- preeclampsia/ecclampsia & HELLP Syndrome
- adjunct to multimodal anesthesia

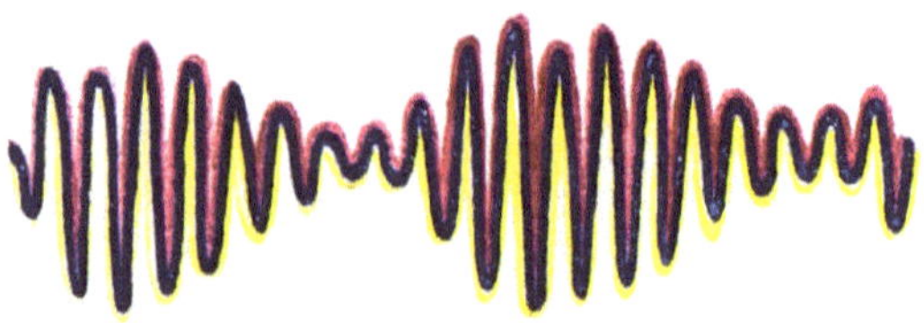

The Pharmacology:

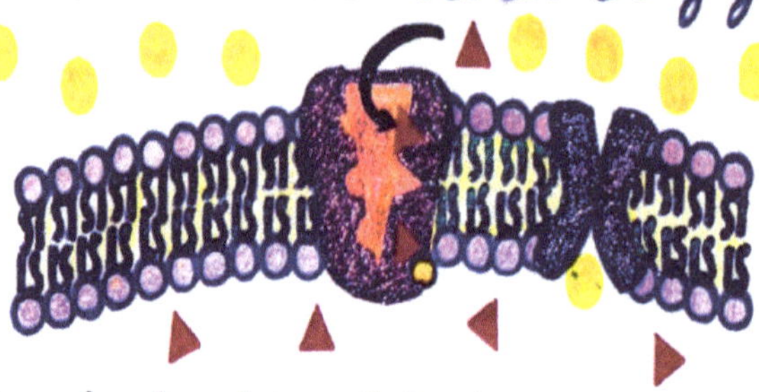

Magnesium is an intracellular electrolyte & cation that regulates neuronal conduction, vascular tone, myocardial excitation, & muscular contraction. It acts as a coenzyme (a needed substance for the function of enzymes) in a variety of ion channels & pumps in the heart. It works like a calcium channel blocker, but c̄ minimal negative inotropic effects (doesn't weaken cardiac contraction)!

Nursing Considerations:

- Know the normal level: 1.5 to 2.2 mEq/L.
- If you're taking care of a post-cardiac arrest patient undergoing targeted temperature management (TTM), keep a close eye on the magnesium level & anticipate repleting the Mg^{2+} especially during the cooling & rewarming phases 2/2 intracellular shifts in electrolytes.
- If you're having trouble correcting a low potassium or calcium, then consider checking the patient's mag level; correcting the magnesium first will allow the K^+ & Ca^{2+} to be corrected. The body will not hang on to K^+ if the magnesium level is low!
- Hypomagnesemia ↑s the risk of torsades de pointes - a type of polymorphic VT associated c̄ a prolonged QT interval. The treatment for this is IV magnesium, IV isoproterenol/Isuprel & overdrive pacing (if refractory), defibrillation/CPR (pulseless) or cardioversion (unstable c̄ a pulse).
- The routine use of magnesium for cardiac arrest isn't recommended unless torsades is present.
- Use c̄ caution in your patients c̄ renal failure. Monitor UOP!
- If given too quickly, IV mag can cause transient hypotension & a warm, flushed feeling 2/2 vasodilation.
- Calcium gluconate is the antidote for magnesium toxicity. S/S include hyporeflexia & hypotension; if your patient still has DTRs, then magnesium toxicity is unlikely! @icunursingnotesbycaitlyn

USES

- myocardial infarction
- A-Fib/flutter & SVT
- stable heart failure
- hypertension

CLASS

cardioselective beta blocker

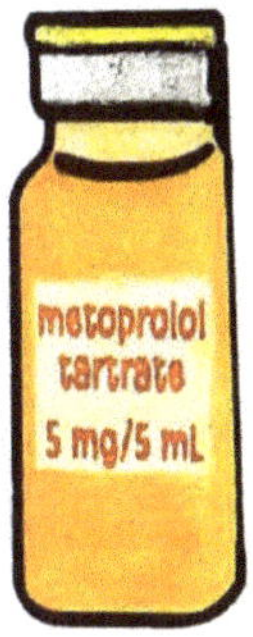

HEMODYNAMIC EFFECTS

↓ heart rate
↓ blood pressure
↓ cardiac output
↓ contractility

metoprolol (Lopressor)

NURSING CONSIDERATIONS:

- Metoprolol is cardioselective (it's ok for patients c̄ asthma or COPD).
- Do not give a beta blocker to a patient in acute decompensated HF (CHF exacerbation) - remember that beta blockers are negative inotropes (↓cardiac contractility) & ↓cardiac output.
- Monitor for bradycardia, hypotension, & S/S of worsening heart failure.
- Always check your patient's BP & HR before giving a beta blocker; in general, hold it for a HR < 60 bpm &/or a SBP < 90 mmHg (your order should have HR & BP parameters).
- Beta blockers can mask the typical signs & symptoms of hypoglycemia.
- *The oral dose of Lopressor should be increased gradually until an adequate maintenance dose is reached.*

DRUG CLASS & USES:

A short-acting benzodiazepine & central nervous system (CNS) depressant c̄ sedative, hypnotic & amnestic properties that is used for:

- the induction of anesthesia
- sedation in the ICU
- conscious sedation
- seizures

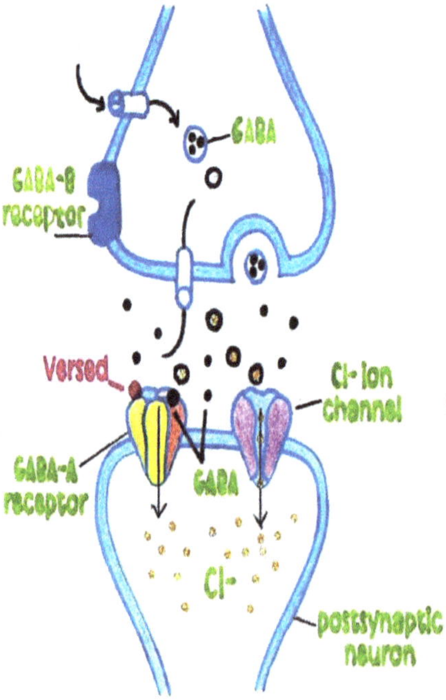

HOW IT WORKS:

Versed enhances the effects of gamma-aminobutyric acid (GABA), the primary inhibitory neurotransmitter for the central nervous system (CNS), at the GABA-A receptor. Activation of GABA-A ↑s the flow of chloride (Cl-) anions into the cell by ↑ the frequency of Cl-channel opening: this ↓s the neurons' ability to fire an action potential (hyperpolarization) & thereby inhibits neural transmission, resulting in sedation, anxiolysis & amnesia!

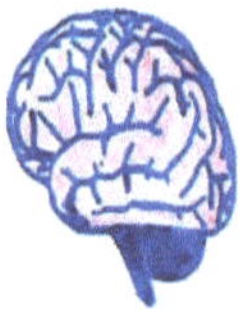

MIDAZOLAM (VERSED)

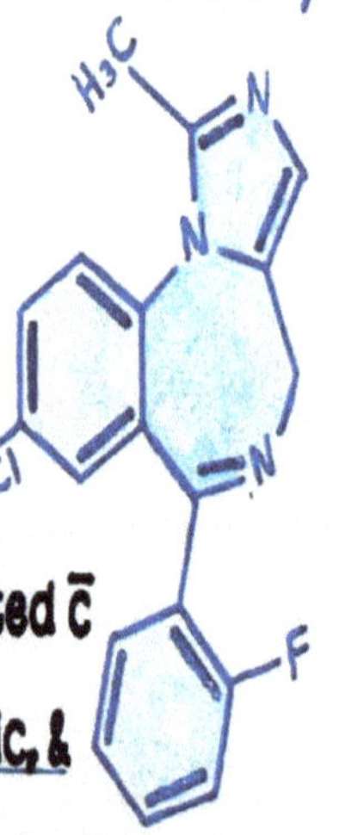

NURSING CONSIDERATIONS:

- It can be administered via several routes: IV, IM, PO, SL, IN & PR.
- Monitor for side effects: oversedation, Δs in HR & BP, respiratory depression, & N/V.
- Know that the reversal agent (antidote) for Versed is flumazenil (Romazicon).
- Versed can ↑ the risk of confusion & agitation in older adults (paradoxical reaction), so use cautiously & at a reduced dose.
- Patients c̄ COPD are extremely sensitive to the respiratory depressant effects associated c̄ Versed. Ensure that you assess the patient's respiratory status before giving Versed!
- Sedation & pain control are not synonomous! Although Versed has sedating, anxiolytic, & amnestic effects, it does nothing for pain!
- Concomitant opioid administration can potentiate the respiratory depressant & sedative effects of Versed. Consider using a ↓ dose of Versed in this instance. A good rule of thumb: start low & go slow!
- Always have your rescue equipment readily available (code cart, BVM, & suction).
- Continuous IV midazolam infusions for sedation have fallen out of favor in the ICU 2/2 the drug's ↑ context-sensitive half-time, risk for benzo tolerance/withdrawal & ↑ risk of ICU delirium.

@icunursingnotesbycaitlyn

INDICATIONS:

angina
decompensated ♥ failure
cardiac catheterization
NSTEMI/STEMI

exception: anterior MI/
RV infarction

PHARMACOLOGY:

The body converts NTG into nitric oxide - a potent vasodilator. The dilation of the venous system ↓s the amount of blood returning to the ♥ c̄ each beat and, consequently, reduces myocardial workload & ventricular wall tension. These Δs ↓ myocardial oxygen demand (MvO2), which helps balance oxygen supply & demand - the classic problem in cardiac ischemia & infarction. It also dilates the coronary arteries & ↑s blood flow to ischemic regions of the heart muscle.

nitroglycerin

nursing considerations

- Nitro can be administered via several routes (SL, PO, transdermal, IV, intra-arterial & intracoronary)
- Sublingual 0.4 mg (1 SL tab) q 5 min x 3, then consider advocating for a nitro gtt for unrelieved c/p.
- Monitor for side effects - hypotension & reflex tachycardia.
- A nitro-induced H/A is common (Tylenol usually helps).
- It's easily titratable when used as a gtt (short half-life & rapid onset).
- Nitro ↓s preload at lower doses, & ↓s afterload at higher doses because it dilates the veins more than the arteries.
- Know your patient's history! You wouldn't want to give NTG to a patient c̄ severe aortic stenosis (AS), hypertrophic obstructive cardiomyopathy (HOCM), or in the setting of an anterior MI/RV infarction (remember that these patients are preload-dependent)..Use caution in an inferior MI (risk of RV involvement)!
- Know your patient's medications! Don't give NTG to a patient who has recently taken a PDE5 inhibitor like sildenafil or Cialis (≤24 hrs).
- Monitor BP & HR and for ongoing c/p. Don't give NTG if the patient's BP can't tolerate it.
- Use special IV tubing for a nitro gtt & make sure that the glass bottle isn't directly exposed to light.

norepinephrine (LEVOPHED)

@cnursingnotesbycaitlyn

Indications:

- severe hypotension
- cardiogenic shock
- distributive shock (septic & neurogenic)
- hypotension s/p ROSC
- cardiothoracic surgery (intra-op & post-op)

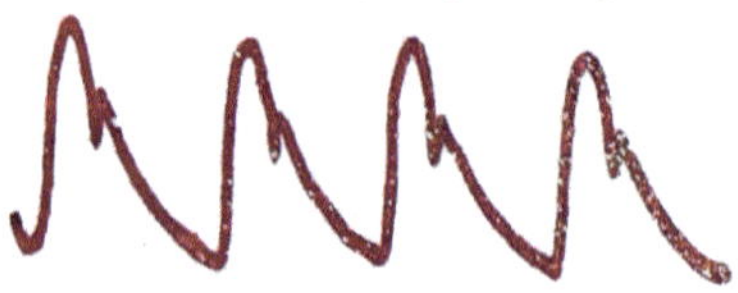

73/50
(58)

How it Works:

Levophed is a vasopressor that acts on alpha-1, alpha-2, & beta-1 receptors. Activation of alpha receptors on smooth muscle cells causes vasoconstriction, thereby ↑ systemic vascular resistance (SVR) c̄ a subsequent ↑ in BP & mean arterial pressure (MAP). Activation of beta-1 receptors on the heart muscle ↑ s the HR & enhances contractility, thereby ↑ cardiac output!

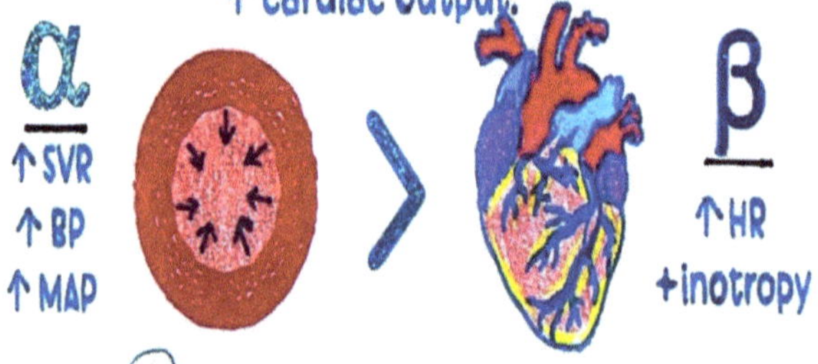

Nursing Considerations:

- Avoid using Levophed as the first-line pressor for patients c̄ hypertrophic obstructive cardiomyopathy (HOCM), as it can worsen the left ventricular outflow obstruction. Phenylephrine (Neo) is first-line for these patients!
- Know its effects on hemodynamics: ↑ CO, ↑ SVR, ↑ PVR, & ↑ MAP.
- Clinically, Levophed's alpha effects (vasoconstriction) are greater than its beta effects (↑ HR & ↑ contractility).
- Titrate according to the ordered BP or MAP goal. An invasive ABP reading from an arterial line is ideal.
- Acidosis will ↓ its effectiveness, so check your patient's pH if the patient isn't responding to Levo.
- Ensure that your patient receives adequate volume resuscitation in addition to initiating vasopressors (the exception here is cardiogenic shock)!
- Levophed often slightly ↑ s the heart rate, but it can also cause a reflex bradycardia in some patients 2/2 the ↑ in afterload (SVR) from alpha-1 receptor stimulation.
- High doses & long-term use ↓ s perfusion to the skin/extremities 2/2 excessive vasoconstriction, which can lead to tissue necrosis, limb loss, & end-organ damage. Assess your patient regularly for S/S of ↓ perfusion (cyanosis, ↓ capillary refill time, diminished/absent peripheral pulses, ↓ UOP, etc).
- Ideally, Levophed should be infused through a central line to prevent extravasation (treat c̄ phentolamine).
- It can be administered as a weight-based (mcg/kg/min) or non-weight based (mcg/min) IV infusion.

indications

- hypotension c̄↓SVR
- push-dose pressor for transient hypotension ("Neo sticks")
- hypotension in the setting of severe aortic stenosis (AS) & hypertrophic obstructive cardiomyopathy (HOCM)
- Tetralogy of Fallot (tet spell)

pharmacology

Phenylephrine ("Neo") is primarily an alpha-1 agonist that↑s arterial blood pressure via vasoconstriction by acting on alpha receptors located in vascular smooth muscle. Because it's purely alpha, Neo↑s afterload (SVR) s̄ a subsequent↑in contractility. In a critically ill patient c̄ already impaired ♥ function, the↑in afterload will only make the work harder & further↓the cardiac output & ↑MvO2.

↑afterload = reduced contraction (↓stroke volume)!

phenylephrine ("Neo")

Nursing Considerations

- It can be given as a bolus dose (push-dose pressor) or as a continuous IV infusion.
- Neo is generally used as a last resort for refractory hypotension (the patient will likely be already maxed on 2 or more pressors when Neo is considered).
- Monitor for reflex bradycardia & arrhythmias.
- Monitor arterial BP, HR & rhythm, UOP (strict I&O), Δs in skin color/temp, hemodynamics (CO/CI & SVR), & labs (Cr, ScVO2 or SvO2, lactate, etc).
- Neo will↑the BP without ↑ the HR & force of contractility.
- It can be useful if a patient is both hypotensive & tachycardic!
- If a patient is hypotensive & has severe aortic stenosis (AS) or hypertrophic obstructive cardiomyopathy (HOCM), Neo is useful because it ↑s BP s̄↑contractility (which could worsen the outflow obstruction).
- Administer through a central line!

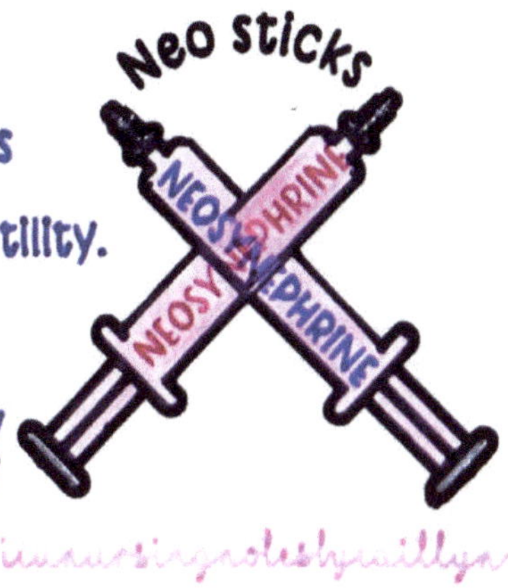

Indications

- induction & maintenance of general anesthesia
- sedation for intubated patients in the ICU.
- procedural sedation

Pharmacology

Propofol potentiates GABA (one of the primary inhibitory neurotransmitters in the central nervous system) & alters chloride ion channels, leading to hyperpolarization of neurons. Propofol causes a direct reduction in myocardial contractility, SVR, & preload, making it a poor choice in the setting of shock.

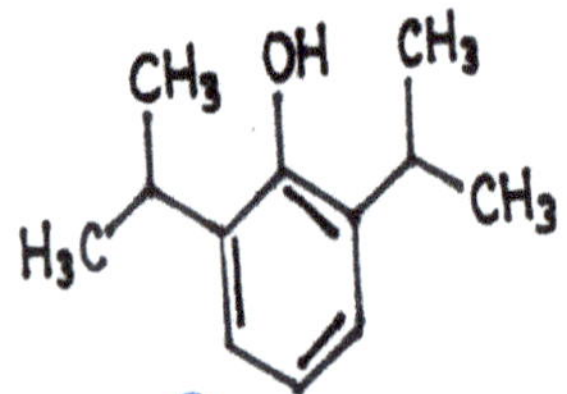

DIPRIVAN

(Propofol)

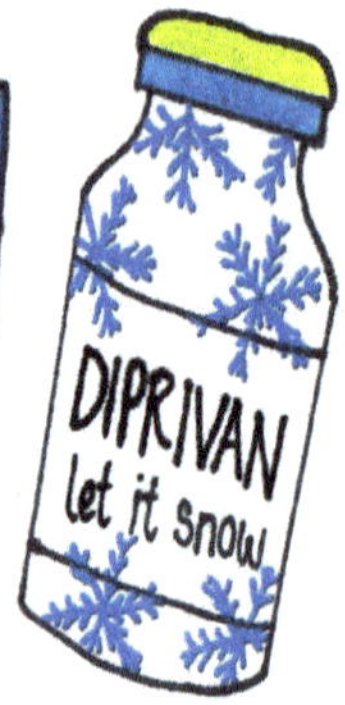

Nursing Care

- Easily titratable and allows for earlier extubation.
- Weight-based medication; titratable gtt with a range of 10 to 100 mcg/kg/min
- Titrate according to RASS score (usually to -2)
- Remember that propofol does not have analgesic effects; treat pain!
- Use caution in hypovolemic &/or catecholamine-depleted patients (common in the ICU).
- It can run peripherally or centrally; change IV tubing q 12 hours & use disinfectant caps on ports.
- Lowers blood pressure & suppresses respiratory drive.
- Monitor for propofol-infusion syndrome (PRIS) with high dose, long-duration infusions.

Side Effects

- bradycardia
- hypotension
- ↓ afterload
- respiratory depression
- ↑ triglycerides
- propofol-infusion syndrome
- green discoloration of urine (due to phenolic metabolites)
- amnesia
- pain at the injection site
- myoclonic movements
- antiemetic & anticonvulsant properties

@icunursingnotesbycaitlyn

@icunursingnotesbycaitlyn

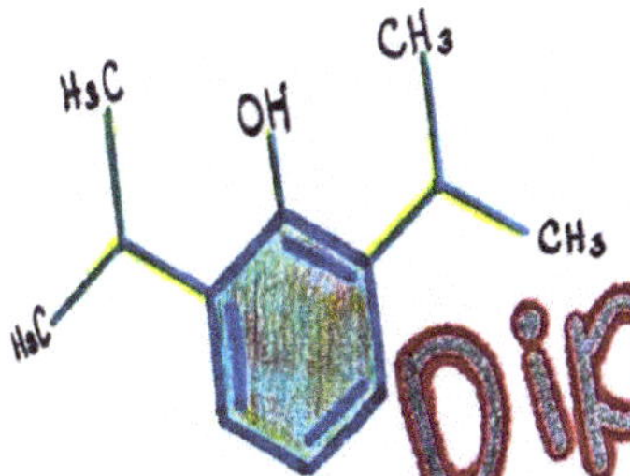

Diprivan | Precedex

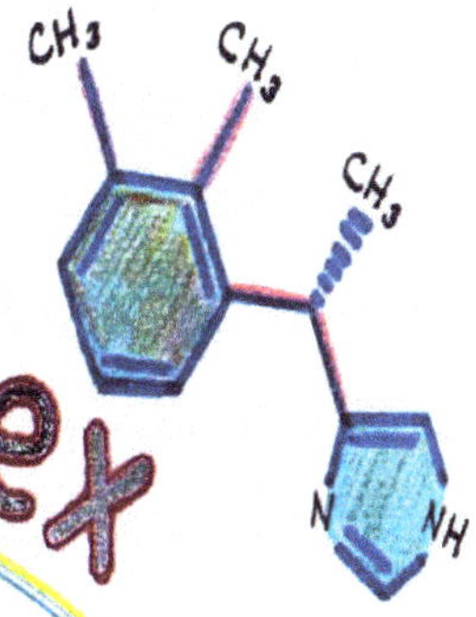

Diprivan

- Greater effect on BP (hypotension)
- causes respiratory depression
- provides no analgesia
- works on GABA-A receptors in the CNS
- can ↑ triglyceride levels c̄ prolonged use
- propofol-related infusion syndrome (PRIS) is a rare complication of its use
- provides deep sedation
- can cause green discoloration of urine
- quicker onset of action

Both

- titratable
- IV sedatives
- associated c̄ a ↓ in BP & HR
- both cross the blood-brain barrier
- weight-based dosing

Precedex

- Greater effect on HR (bradycardia)
- doesn't cause respiratory depression
- has some analgesic effects
- works on alpha-2 receptors
- doesn't accumulate in the body c̄ prolonged infusions
- provides light to moderate sedation (arousable)
- can be used to facilitate extubation
- can cause a transient initial ↑ in BP
- slower onset of action

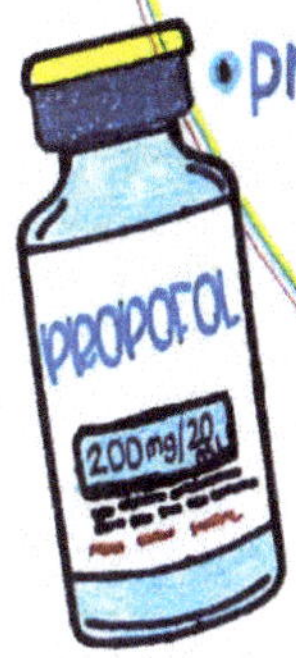

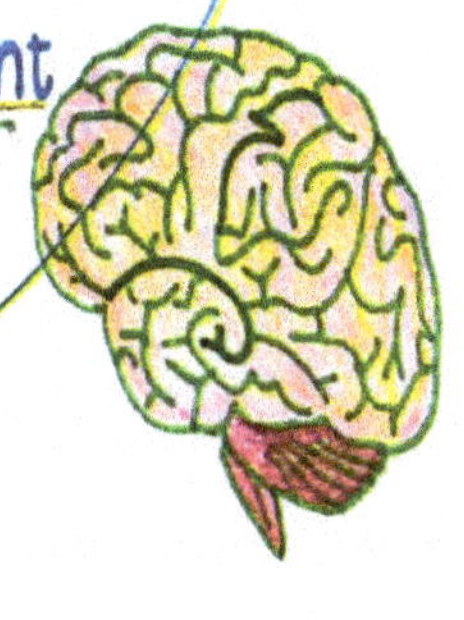

protamine sulfate

what it is:

It's an IV protein used to reverse heparin anticoagulation in the setting of:

- severe heparin-associated bleeding
- cardiothoracic & vascular surgeries
- heparin overdose

@icunursingnotesbycaitlyn

how it works:

Protamine is a strong base that neutralizes the anticoagulant effect of heparin, which is a strong acid. It binds to heparin molecules to form a stable, neutral salt that has no active anticoagulation effect.

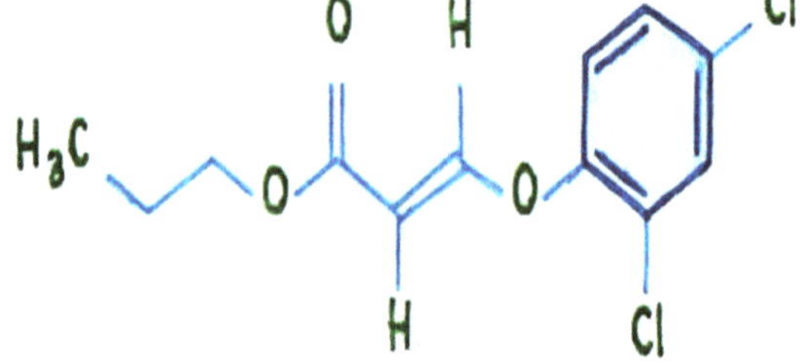

nursing considerations

- Always administer a "test dose" (usually 5-10 mg IV) before giving the full dose to assess for a reaction (anaphylaxis, hypotension, bradycardia, pulmonary hypertension, & pulmonary edema).
- Administer it SLOWLY! Usually over 15-20 min in a 50 cc bag of NS. Rapid IV administration can cause hypotension 2/2 histamine release. Monitor the patient closely during & after giving protamine.
- Dosing depends on the amount of heparin given & the time that it's administered but, in general, 1 mg of protamine can reverse the effects of 100 units of heparin.
- No more than 50 mg of protamine should be given in any one dose.
- Check an ACT or aPTT 15 minutes after giving the full dose of protamine.
- Protamine hypersensitivity reactions are more common in patients taking NPH insulin, those c̄ fish allergies, & those who have had vasectomies.
- Monitor for spontaneous bleeding, as "heparin rebound" can occur 2-3 hours after protamine administration; this happens because the half-life of protamine is significantly shorter than heparin. It's treated c̄ additional protamine administration.
- Protamine fully reverses unfractionated heparin, but it only partially reverses the anticoagulant effect of low-molecular weight heparin (LMWH).

CLASS & USE

a short-acting opioid & mu (μ)-receptor agonist used as an adjunct to anesthetic agents during the induction &/or maintenance of general anesthesia!

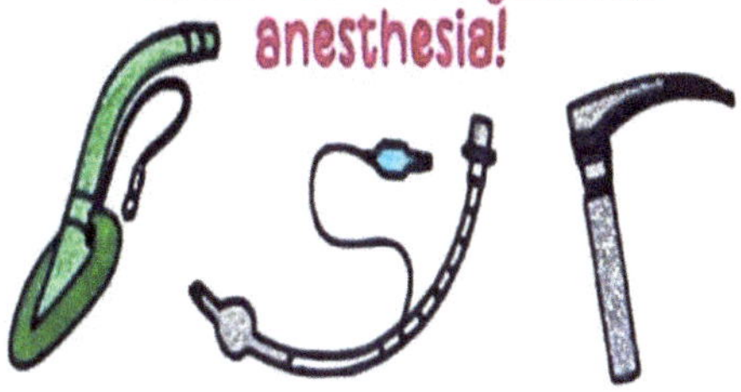

HOW IT WORKS

It binds to mu (μ)-opioid receptors at many sites in the central nervous system (CNS), ↑ pain threshold, altering pain reception, & inhibiting ascending pain pathways.

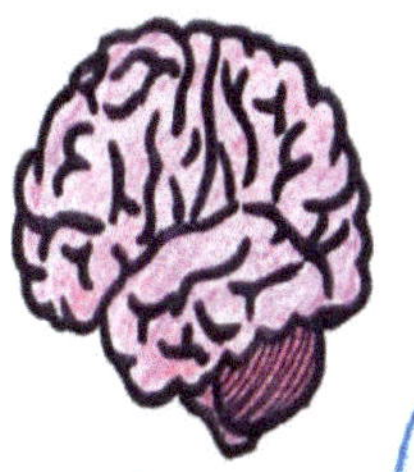

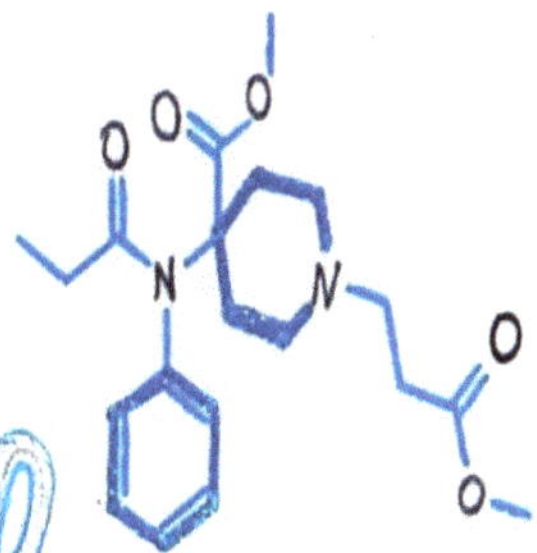

remifentanil

@icunursingnotesbycaitlyn

CLINICAL PEARLS:

- Remifentanil is typically administered via continuous IV infusion by an anesthesiologist or CRNA, and it's 200-300x more potent than morphine!
- It has an extremely short half-life (5 minutes) because it doesn't rely on an organ (liver) for metabolism; its metabolized by enzymes in the bloodstream.
- Allows for a more rapid recovery from anesthesia.
- Its clearance is relatively unaffected by Δs in liver &/or kidney function, making it ideal for patients c̄ liver &/or kidney failure.
- It can cause bradycardia & hypotension, respiratory depression, nausea & muscle rigidity
- Its analgesic effects will quickly subside 2/2 its short half-life, so remifentanil, alone, is not used for post-operative pain (a multimodal approach c̄ longer-acting narcotics, ketamine, etc is best).

INDICATIONS

- normal-anion-gap metabolic acidosis (NAGMA) 2/2 HCO_3^- loss (RTA, fistula losses, etc)
- Na^+ channel blocker, TCA, & salicylate toxicity
- chronic kidney disease (CKD)
- indigestion
- hyperkalemia (controversial)
- high-dose methotrexate administration
- Impella (Abiomed) purge solution

PHARMACOLOGY

Sodium bicarb ($NaHCO_3^-$) is an alkalizing agent that reacts c̄ hydrogen ions (H^+) to ultimately form H_2O & CO_2 which, in turn, is exhaled by the lungs. $NaHCO_3^-$, in the presence of metabolic acidosis & tissue hypoxia, can ↑ lactate production, & cause worsening acidosis. If the metabolic acidosis isn't associated c̄ tissue hypoxia (i.e. renal or GI loss of HCO_3^- as in renal tubular acidosis), then $NaHCO_3^-$ may raise the blood's pH & actually be beneficial.

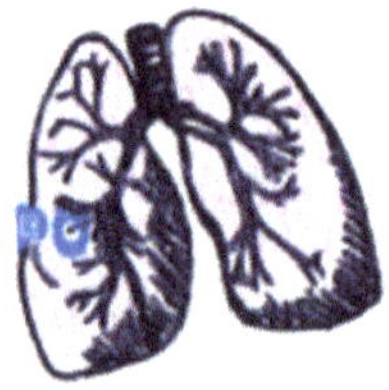

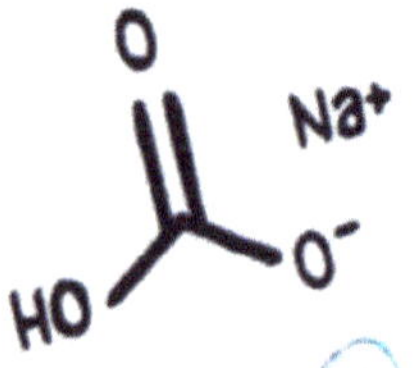

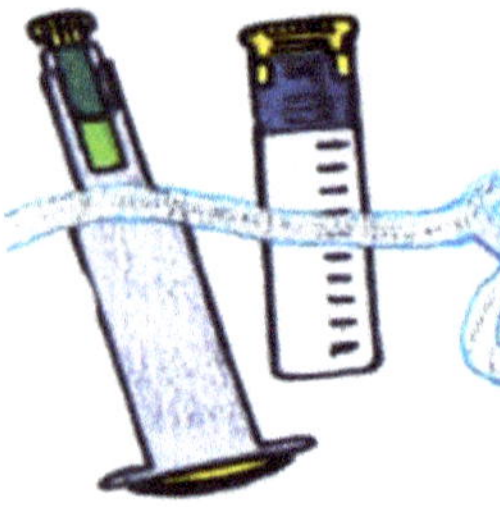

sodium bicarb

@icunursingnotesbycaitlyn

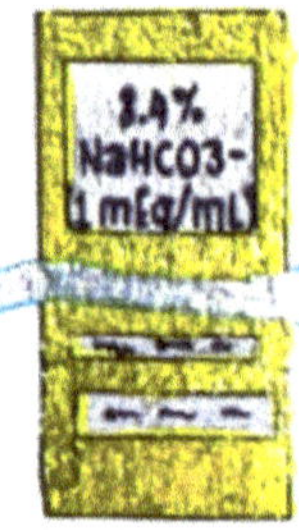

NURSING CONSIDERATIONS

- $NaHCO_3^-$ is a band-aid, not a solution, for severe metabolic acidosis. Although it can buy valuable time for other interventions to kick in, it doesn't fix the patient's underlying problem.
- The American Heart Association (AHA) discourages its routine use in cardiac arrest management (unless the cause of the arrest is hyperkalemia or Na^+ channel blocker/TCA toxicity).
- Monitor for fluid overload, ↑ Na^+, ↓ Ca^{2+} (ionized), hypoperfusion, neuro changes, hypercapnia, & trend labs (ABG/VBG, lactate, & electrolytes).
- Because acidosis often ↓ s the efficacy of many interventions (i.e. vasopressors, pacing, etc), $NaHCO_3^-$ is often used to transiently ↑ the blood pH to, essentially, "buy time" to identify & treat the underlying cause.
- Question the empiric use of $NaHCO_3^-$. The literature suggests that it results in more harm than good/poor outcomes in patients c̄ respiratory acidosis, lactic acidosis, diabetic ketoacidosis, & undifferentiated cardiac arrest.
- Anticipate a normal ↑ in the patient's $EtCO_2$ after giving an amp of $NaHCO_3^-$, & understand it doesn't reflect ROSC.

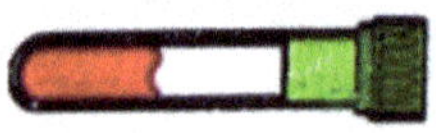

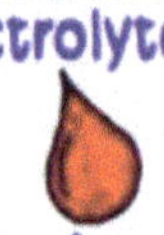

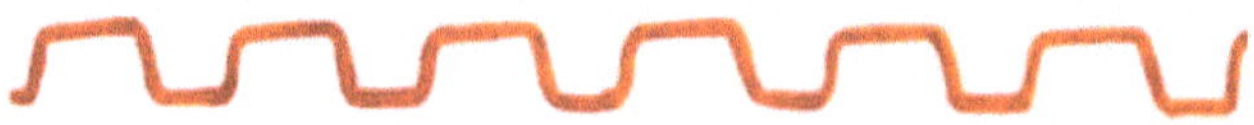

- Ventilation is important, & patients need to be able to handle the ↑ CO_2 load from $NaHCO_3^-$ administration. $NaHCO_3^-$ can exacerbate acidosis, especially in patients who are already tachypneic & maximally compensating (i.e. DKA).

sodium nitroprusside (NIPRIDE)

INDICATIONS

Nipride is a potent arterial & venous vasodilator that is used in the management of:

- hypertensive crisis
- acute aortic dissection
- acute decompensated heart failure (ADHF)
- no-reflow s/p PCI

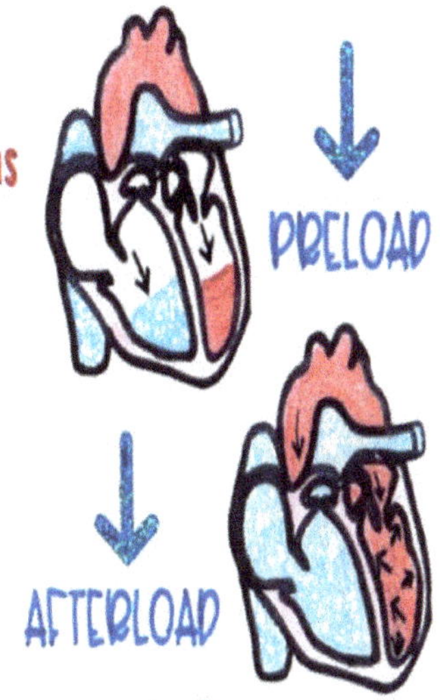

HOW IT WORKS

Nipride is metabolized into nitric oxide (NO), causing arterial & venous dilation c̄ a subsequent ↓ vascular resistance (systemic & pulmonary). This, in turn, reduces arterial blood pressure & ↓ intracardiac filling pressures. Although Nipride ↓ preload, it has a greater effect on afterload reduction!

NURSING CONSIDERATIONS

- These patients should have an arterial line for continuous blood pressure monitoring. Make sure that you level your transducer! Accurate & precise pressure readings are imperative!
- The dose range for a continuous IV infusion is 0.5 to 10 mcg/kg/min. Titrate the infusion according to the ordered hemodynamic parameters. 10 mcg/kg/min is the maximum infusion rate! Monitor heart rate, as Nipride can cause a reflex tachycardia 2/2 to a ↓ in SVR.
- Nipride has an immediate onset & a short half-life. Expect to see a ↓ in BP within 2 min of initiating the infusion or ↑ the infusion rate.
- Once mixed, Nipride is only stable for 24 hours. Protect the IV bag and tubing from light.
- If you're caring for a patient on a Nipride infusion for a hypertensive crisis, avoid ↓ the BP too quickly (general rule: MAP should be reduced by no more than 25% over the first hour)! Monitor for cyanide toxicity! Impaired renal function & prolonged infusions (≥ 48 hours) ↑ this risk.
- Early signs of cyanide toxicity are metabolic acidosis, confusion, & tinnitus. Sodium thiosulfate is used to treat cyanide toxicity!
- Nipride can cause intra-pulmonary shunting, so consider this in the setting of a sudden ↓ in SpO_2 & a ↓ in SaO_2 and PaO_2 on ABGs.
- It's used in conjunction with a beta blocker (esmolol) to manage a type B acute aortic dissection.

indications

- vasodilatory shock states
- post-cardiac surgery vasoplegia
- hepatorenal syndrome (HRS)
- diabetes insipidus (DI)
- esophageal variceal bleeding

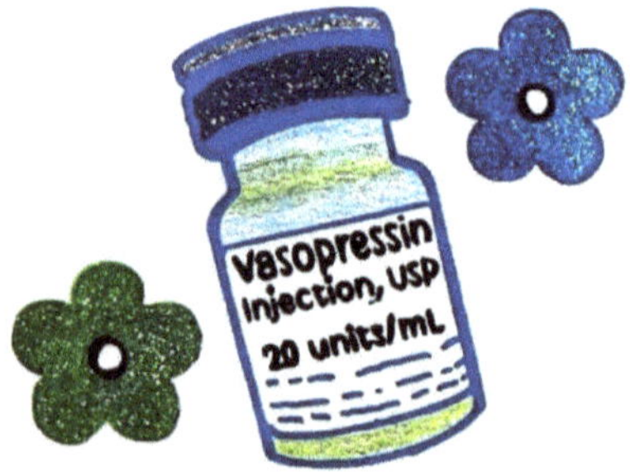

pharmacology

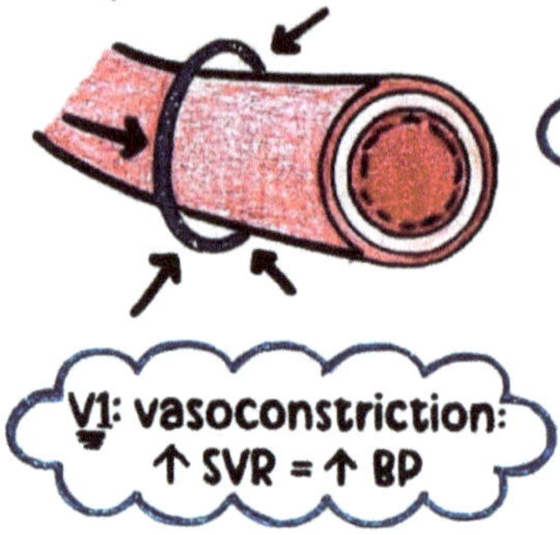

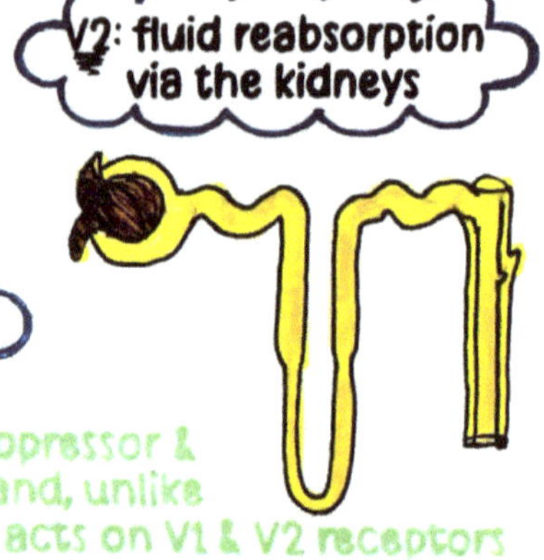

Vasopressin is a pure vasopressor & a potent vasoconstrictor and, unlike traditional vasopressors, it acts on V1 & V2 receptors rather than alpha & beta (catecholamine) receptors. These receptors are found in vascular smooth muscle (V1) & in the kidneys (V2). Vasopressin ↑ s the MAP by ↑ the SVR (afterload) & intravascular volume, but it does so without directly augmenting cardiac contractility.

VASOPRESSIN

nursing considerations:

- Its half-life is ≈ 15 to 20 min, so don't anticipate an immediate ↑ in the BP; this is important to consider when starting or titrating a vaso infusion.
- It may be a better alternative to norepinephrine (Levophed) for ↑ MAP in patients c̄ pulmonary HTN, RV failure, or a massive PE because it will ↑ the SVR without having any significant effect on the pulmonary vascular resistance (PVR).
- It's generally not used alone (risk of reflex bradycardia); it's used as an adjunct to the catecholamine vasopressors (i.e. norepi & epi); monitor for signs of coronary/mesenteric/tissue ischemia 2/2 extreme vasoconstriction.
- Unlike the catecholamine vasopressors, vasopressin still works in acidotic states & potentiates other vasoactive drugs because of its unique mechanism of action.
- Vasopressin is a pure vasoconstrictor c̄ little to no effect on HR (chronotropy) or cardiac contractility (inotropy), so it will ↑ the afterload on the heart & potentially ↓ cardiac output (depending on the heart's ability to tolerate the ↑ in afterload).
- It's associated c̄ a lower risk of new-onset arrhythmias (NOAs) because it primarily acts on vascular smooth muscle, causing less direct stimulation of the heart's conduction system.
- Consider using it earlier in vasopressin deficient states (i.e. liver failure/cirrhosis, septic shock, etc). Vasopressin deficiency potentiates hypotension!
- Compared to traditional vasopressor infusions which are routinely titrated, vasopressin may or may not be titrated (varies according to institution & provider preference) – check your orders!

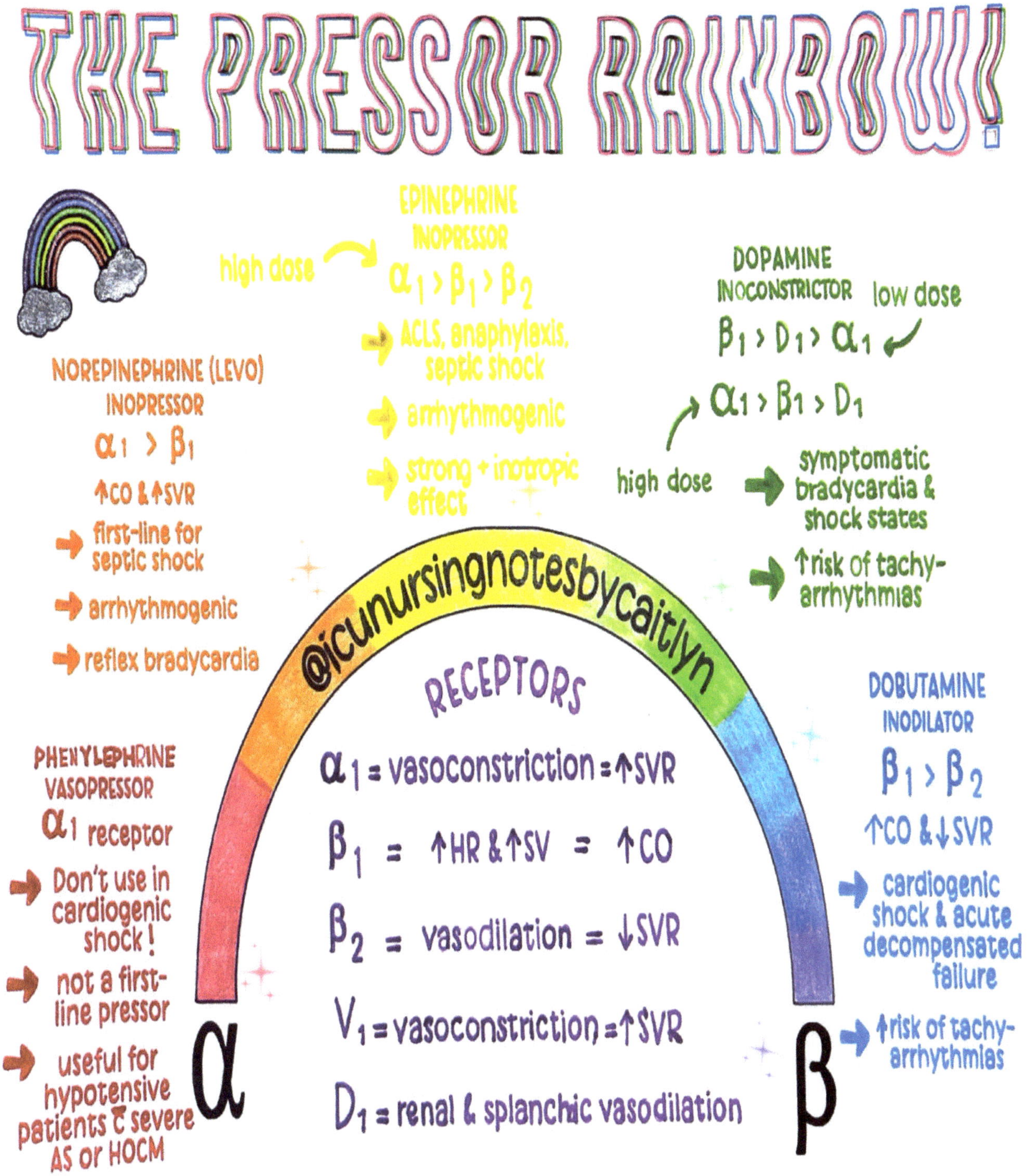

Drawing inspired by the work of Maxwell Coll, MD.

Topic Index

Citations

Abbott, J.D., Vallabhajosyula, S., & Kapur, N.K. (2024). The need to define high-dose pharmacological circulatory support in cardiogenic shock. *Mayo Clinic Proceedings,* 99(7), 1035–1037.

Abdildin, Y., Tapinova, K., Nemerenova, A., & Viderman, D. (2024). The impact of ketamine on outcomes in critically ill patients: a systematic review with meta-analysis and trial sequential analysis of randomized controlled trials. *Acute and Critical Care*, 39(1), 34–46.

Abiomed. (2021). Automated Impella controller™ overview. HeartRecovery.

Abiomed. (2020). Impella CP® with SmartAssist instructions or use & clinical reference manual.

Abiomed. (2024). Impella RP® with SmartAssist® instructions for use & clinical reference manual. Heart Recovery.\

Abiomed. (2024). Impella RP® with SmartAssist® patient management. Abiomed Academy.

Ackerman, M.J., Priori, S.G., Dubin A.M, et al. (2017). Beta-blocker therapy for long QT syndrome and catecholaminergic polymorphic ventricular tachycardia: are all beta-blockers equivalent? Heart Rhythm.

Adlam, D., Cuculi, F., Lim, C., & Banning, A. (2010). Management of spontaneous coronary artery dissection in the primary percutaneous coronary intervention era. *Journal of Invasive Cardiology*. 22(11): 549–553.

Aehlert, B.J. (2022). ECGs made easy (7th ed.). Elsevier.

Aggarwal, B. & Raymond, C.E. (2015). Therapeutic goals in patients with acute aortic dissection: management before surgery. *Journal of the American College of Cardiology* (JACC), 65(15): 1599–1600.

Agrawal, N., Kumar, A., Aggarwal, P., & Jamshed, N. (2016). Sympathetic crashing acute pulmonary edema. *Critical Care Medicine*, 20(12): 719-723.

Ahmed, T, Nautiyal, A., Kapadia, S., & Nissen, S. (2020). Delayed presentation of STEMI complicated by ventricular septal rupture in the era of the COVID-19 pandemic. *JACC Case Reports*, 2(10z), 1599-1602.

Ahn, S., Kim, Y.J., Sohn, C.H, et al. (2018). Sodium bicarbonate on severe metabolic acidosis during prolonged cardiopulmonary resuscitation: a double-blind, randomized, placebo-controlled pilot study. *Journal of Thoracic Disease*, 10(4), 2295–2302.

Al-Saady, N.M., Obel, O.A., & Camm, A.J. (1999). Left atrial appendage: structure, function, and role in thromboembolism. *Heart*, 82(5).

Alajaji, W.A., Akl, E.A., Farha, A., Jaber, W.A, et al. (2015). Surgical versus medical management of patients with acute ischemic mitral regurgitation: a systematic review. *BMC Research Notes*, 8, 712.

Alerhand, S., Adrian, R.J., Long, B, et al. (2022). Pericardial tamponade: a comprehensive emergency medicine and echocardiography review. *Am J Emerg Med*. 58: 159-74.

Alexander, J. & Rizzolo, D. (2023). Wellens' syndrome: an important consideration in patients with chest pain. *Journal of the American College of Cardiology (JACC)*, 36(2): 25-29.

Alfonso, F., Byrne, R.A., Rivero, F., Kastrati, A. (2014). Current treatment of in-stent restenosis. *Journal of the American College of Cardiology (JACC)*, 63: 2659-2673.

Alkhunaizi, F.A., Smith, N., Brusca, S.B., & Furfaro, D. (2024). The management of cardiogenic shock from diagnosis to devices: a narrative review. *CHEST Critical Care*, 2(2).

Almarzooq, Z.I., Song, Y., Dahabreh, I.J., Kochar, A, et al (2023). Comparative effectiveness of percutaneous microaxial left ventricular assist device vs intra-aortic balloon pump or no mechanical circulatory support in patients with cardiogenic shock. *JAMA Cardiology*, 8(8), 744-754.

American Association of Critical-Care Nurses & Johnson, K. (2023). AACN procedure manual for acute and critical care (8th ed). Saunders/Elsevier.

Amit, G., Cafri., C, et al. (2006). Intracoronary nitroprusside for the prevention of the no-reflow phenomenon after primary percutaneous coronary intervention in acute myocardial infarction: a randomized, double-blind, placebo-controlled clinical trial. *The American Heart Journal*, 152(5), 887.e9-887e14.

Anozie, O. (2021). The vitals: pulsus paradoxus. *Critical Care Now*.

Antunes, M.J. (2021). Left ventricular free wall rupture: a real nightmare. *Journal of Cardiac Surgery*, 36(9), 3334-3336.

Argulian, E. & Messerli, F. (2013). Misconceptions and facts about pericardial effusion and tamponade. *The American Journal of Medicine*, 126(10): 858-861.

Arif, A.W., Khan, M.S., Masri, A. et al. (2020). BRASH syndrome with hyperkalemia: an under-recognized clinical condition. *Methodist Debakey Cardiovascular Journal*, 16(3): 241-244.

Arvanitaki, A., Gatzoulis, M.A., Opotowsky, A.R, et al. (2022). Eisenmenger syndrome: JACC state-of-the-art review. *Journal of the American College of Cardiology*, 79(12): 1183-1198.

Ashraf, F. (2017). Wellens' syndrome: a predictor of critical left anterior descending artery stenosis. *Postgraduate Medical Journal,* 93, 53-53.

Atchley, E., Tesoro, E., Meyer, R., Bauer, A., Pulver, M., & Benken, S. (2022). Hemodynamic effects of ketamine compared with propofol or dexmedetomidine as continuous ICU sedation. *The Annals of Pharmacotherapy*, 56(7), 764–772.

Aten, K., Raney, K., & Alomar, A. (2022). Dressler's syndrome: not just a relic of the past. Cureus, 14(10).

Atkinson, T.M., Ohman, E.M., O'Neill, W.W., Rab, T., & Cigarroa J.E. (2016). A practical approach to mechanical circulatory support in patients undergoing percutaneous coronary intervention: an interventional perspective. *JACC: Cardiovascular Interventions*, 9(9), 871-883.

Bacich, A., Bernard, S., Churchill, T.W., Namasivayam, M., & Bertrand, P.B. (2020). Agitated saline contrast echocardiography in the identification of intra- and extracardiac shunts: connecting the dots. *Journal of the American Society of Echocardiography.*

Baran D.A., Grines C.L., Bailey S, et al. (2019). SCAI clinical expert consensus statement on the classification of cardiogenic shock. *Catheterization & Cardiovascular Interventions*, 94(1): 29-37.

Barash, P.G., Cullen, B.F., & Stoelting, R.K. et al. (2017). Clinical anesthesia. (8th ed.). Lippincott Williams & Wilkins.

Barison, A., Del, A., & Todiere G. (2016). Hemodynamic findings in obstructive hypertrophic cardiomyopathy: pulsus bisferiens & Brockenbrough-Braunwald-Morrow sign. *Journal of Cardiovascular Medicine.*

Barlow, B., Landolf, K., LaPlante, R., Cercone, J, et al. (2023). Electrolyte considerations in targeted temperature management. *American Journal of Health-System Pharmacy*, 80(3), 102–110.

Barrett, W., Buxhoeveden, M., & Dhillon, S. (2020). Ketamine: a versatile tool for anesthesia and analgesia. *Current Opinion in Anesthesiology*, 33(5), 633–638.

Basir, M.B., Lemor, A., Gorgis, S, et al. (2022). Vasopressors independently associated with mortality in acute myocardial infarction and cardiogenic shock. *Catheterization & Cardiovascular Interventions*, 99(3): 650–65.

Bauer, S.R., Sacha, G.L., Siuba, M.T., Lam, S.W., Reddy, A.J., Duggal, A., & Vachharajani, V. (2022). Association of arterial pH with hemodynamic response to vasopressin in patients with septic shock: an observational cohort study. *Critical Care Explorations.*

Beigel, R., Wunderlich, N.C., Ho, S.Y, et al. (2014). The left atrial appendage: anatomy, function, and noninvasive evaluation. *Journal of the American College of Cardiology,* 7(12): 1251-65.

Bellezzo, J. (2016). Archimedes' screw: is Impella® the future of mechanical circulatory support? Resuscionist-Initiated Extracorporeal Life Support & Enhanced CPR.

Bertini, P. & Guarracino, F. (2021). Pathophysiology of cardiogenic shock. *Current Opinion in Critical Care*, 27(4): 409-415.

Bhandari, R., Ekladious, A., & Javaid, M.M. (2024). Demystifying normal-anion-gap metabolic acidosis (NAGMA): pathophysiology, etiology, evaluation and diagnosis. *Internal Medicine Journal*, 54(7), 1056-1065.

Bilchick, K.C. & Wise, R.A. Paradoxical physical findings described by Kussmaul: pulsus paradoxus and Kussmaul's sign.

Bishop, R.L. & Weisfeldt, M.L. Sodium bicarbonate administration during cardiac arrest: effect on arterial pH, pCO2, and osmolality. *Journal of the American Medical Association*, 235(5): 506–509.

Block, P. C. (2018). DAPT, our genome and clopidogrel resistance: are we near an answer to "which drug and when?" *A*merican College of Cardiology.

Bloom, J.E., Chan, W., Kaye, D.M., & Stub, D. (2023). State of shock: contemporary vasopressor and inotrope use in cardiogenic shock. *Journal of the American Heart Association,* 12(15).

Boivin-Proulx, L.A., Haddad, K., Lombardi, M, et al. (2023). Pathophysiology of myocardial infarction with nonobstructive coronary artery disease: a contemporary systematic review. *CJC Open*, 380-390.

Borlaug, B.A. (2019). Pulsus paradoxus. UpToDate.

Boston Scientific. (2024). Agent™ drug-coated balloon.

Brener, M.I., Rosenblum, H.R., & Burkhoff, D. (2020). Pathophysiology and advanced hemodynamic assessment of cardiogenic shock. *Methodist DeBakey Cardiovascular Journal*, 16(1), 7–15.

Briggs, L. (2024). Stealthy enemy: ischemic nonobstructive coronary artery disease.

Brown, D. L. (2022). Manual of cardiac intensive care. Elsevier.

Brown, K. & Tucker, C. (2020). Ketamine for acute pain management and sedation. *Critical Care Nurse,* 40(5): 26–32.

Bruno, R.R., Wolff, G., Kelm, M., & Jung, C, et al. (2022). Pharmacological treatment of cardiogenic shock - a state of the art review. *Pharmacology & Therapeutics*. Elsevier.

Buckley,, M. S., Smithburger, P. L., Wong, A, et al. (2021). Dexmedetomidine for facilitating mechanical ventilation extubation in difficult-to-wean ICU patients: systematic review and meta-analysis of clinical trials. *Journal of Intensive Care Medicine,* 36(8). 925-936.

Buller, C. (2022). Langston® dual lumen catheter reintroduction. *Cath Lab Digest.*

Burchum, J., & Rosenthal, L. (2018). Lehne's pharmacology for nursing care (10th ed). Saunders.

Butterworth, J.F., Mackey, D.C.,Wasnick, J.D, et al. (2018). Morgan & mikhail's clinical anesthesiology (6th ed.). McGraw-Hill Education.

Camaj, A., Fuster, V., Giustino, G, et al. (2022). Left ventricular thrombus following acute myocardial infarction: JACC state-of-the-art review. *Journal of the American College of Cardiology (JACC)*, 79: 1010–22.

Carey, M.G., Salah, S., Al-Zaiti, T.M., & Kozik, M.P. (2014). Holiday heart syndrome. *The American Journal of Critical Care,* 23(2): 171–172.

Carmen, M, et al. (2019). Opioid and benzodiazepine iatrogenic withdrawal syndrome in patients in the intensive care unit. *AACN Adv Crit Care*, 30(4): 353–364.

Casassus, F., et al. (2015). The use of Impella 2.5® in severe refractory cardiogenic shock complicating an acute myocardial infarction. *Journal of Interventional Cardiology*. 28 (1), 41-50.

Case B.C. & Satler L.F. (2021). The challenges of coronary no-reflow phenomenon. *Catheterization & Cardiovascular Interventions*, 97: 612–613.

Cattaneo, M. (2010). New P2Y12 inhibitors. *Circulation*, 12(1), 171-179.

Celenk, V. & Celenk, C. (2022). Myocardial bridging in adults with hypertrophic cardiomyopathy: imaging findings with coronary computed tomography angiography. *Radiology Case Reports*, *17*(12), 4627–4631.

Chang, Y. F, et al. (2018). Comparison of dexmedetomidine versus propofol on hemodynamics in surgical critically ill patients. *The Journal of Surgical Research*, 228, 194-200.

Chua, H.R., Schneider, A., & Bellomo, R. (2011). Bicarbonate in diabetic ketoacidosis — a systematic review. *Annals of Intensive Care*, 1(1), 23.

Chung, M. K., Eckhardt, L. L., Chen, L. Y., Ahmed, H. M., Gopinathannair, R, et al. (2020). Lifestyle and risk factor modification for reduction of atrial fibrillation: a scientific statement from the American Heart Association. *Circulation*, 141(16), 750–772.

Conrad, H. (2023). Anomalous left coronary artery from the pulmonary artery (ALCAPA) illustration.

Convissar, D. (2022). Pericardiocentesis. Count Backwards from Ten.

Convissar, D. (2022). Pulsus paradoxus.

Convissar, D. (2023). Master the machines: a clinical course in mechanical circulatory support. www.masterthemachines.com.

Crea, F. & Niccoli, G. (2024). Myocardial infarction or ischemia with no obstructive coronary atherosclerosis. UpToDate. *Critical Care Medicine*, 52(1).

Cullington, D., Goode, K. M., Zhang, J., Cleland, J. G., & Clark, A. L. (2014). Is heart rate important for patients with heart failure in atrial fibrillation? *Journal of the American College of Cardiology (JACC)*, 2(3), 213–220.

Curtis, A.B. (2017). Fundamentals of cardiac pacing. Jones & Bartlett.

Dai, W. (2018). Effect of preoperative loading dose ticagrelor and clopidogrel on no-reflow phenomenon during intervention in patients with ST-segment elevation myocardial infarction undergoing primary percutaneous coronary intervention: a systematic review and meta-analysis. *Drug Design, Development, & Therapy*, 12, 2039-2049.

Dalia, T., Lahan, S., Ranka, S. et al. (2021). Warfarin versus direct oral anticoagulants for treating left ventricular thrombus: a systematic review and meta-analysis. *Thrombosis Journal*, 19(1), 7.

Damani, S.B. & Topol, E.J. (2010). The case for routine genotyping in dual-antiplatelet therapy. *Journal of the American College of Cardiology (AJCC),* 56(2): 109–11.

Damluji, A.A., Van Diepen, S., Katz, J.N., et al. (2021). Mechanical complications of acute myocardial infarction: a scientific statement from the AHA. *Circulation*, 144(2), 16-35.

Dangas, G.D., Claessen, B.E., Caixeta, A, et al. (2010). In-stent restenosis in the drug-eluting stent era. *Journal of the American College of Cardiology*, 56: 1897-1907.

Davidson, L., Cleveland, J., Welt, F. et al. (2022). A practical approach to left main coronary artery disease: JACC state-of-the-art review. *Journal of the American College of Cardiology (JACC),* 80(22), 2119-2134.

De Zwaan, C., Bar, F.W., & Wellens, H.J. (1982). Characteristic electrocardiographic pattern indicating a critical stenosis high in left anterior descending coronary artery in patients admitted because of impending myocardial infarction. *American Heart Journal,* 103, 730–736.

De, Ferrari., G.M., Dusi, V., Spazzolini, C, et al. (2015). Clinical management of catecholaminergic polymorphic ventricular tachycardia: the role of left cardiac sympathetic denervation. *Circulation*, 131(25): 2185-2193.

Deglin, J. H. & Vallerand, A.H. (2022). Davis's drug guide for nurses. (14th ed). F.A. Davis.

Dennison, R.D. (2018). Pass CCRN® (5th ed.). Mosby.

Desai, S.R., & Hwang, N.C. (2020). Strategies for left ventricular decompression during venoarterial extracorporeal membrane oxygenation - a narrative review. *Journal of Cardiothoracic Vascular Anesthesia*, 34(1): 208–218.

Devlin, J.W. & Roberts, R.J. (2009). Pharmacology of commonly used analgesics and sedatives in the ICU: benzodiazepines, propofol, and opioids. *Crit Care Clin*, 25(3), 431–449.

Devlin, J.W., Skrobik, Y., Gélinas, C, et al. (2018). Clinical practice guidelines for the prevention and management of pain, agitation/sedation, delirium, immobility, and sleep disruption in adult patients in the ICU. *Crit Care Med*, 46(9): 825-873.

Di Biase, L., Santangeli, P., Anselmino, M, et al. (2012). Does the left atrial appendage morphology correlate with the risk of stroke in patients with atrial fibrillation? Results from a multicenter study. *Journal of the American College of Cardiology*, 60(6): 531-8.

DiNicolantonio, J.J., Liu, J., & O'Keefe, J.H. (2018). Magnesium for the prevention and treatment of cardiovascular disease. *Open Heart*, 5(2).

Dukkipati S.R., Kar, S., Holmes D.R., et al. (2018). Device-related thrombus after left atrial appendage closure: incidence, predictors, and outcomes. *Circulation*, 138(9): 874-885.

Ekenback, C., Tornvall, P., & Agewall, S. (2022). MINOCA from A to Z. The American College of Cardiology.

Elliott, A.D., Middeldorp, M.E., Van Gelder, I.C, et al. (2023). Epidemiology and modifiable risk factors for atrial fibrillation. *Nature Reviews Cardiology*, 20(6), 404-417.

Ellis, M.F. (2015). Use of bicarbonate in patients with metabolic acidosis. *Critical Care Nurse*, 35(5), 73–75.

Eraky, A.M., Yerramalla,Y., Khan, A., Mokhtar, Y., Wright, A, et al. (2024). Complexities, benefits, risks, and clinical implications of sodium bicarbonate administration in critically ill patients: a state-of-the-art review. *Journal of Clinical Medicine*, 13(24), 7822.

Ettinger, P.O., Wu, C.F., Weisse, A.B, et al. (1978). Arrhythmias and the "holiday heart": alcohol-associated cardiac rhythm disorders. *The American Heart Journal*, 95(5): 555–562.

Fang, J.C. & Jones, T.L. (2020). Can a pulmonary artery catheter improve outcomes in cardiogenic shock? *The Journal of the American College of Cardiology (JACC)*, 8(11): 914–916.

Farkas, J.D., Long, B., Koyfman, A., & Menson, K. (2020). BRASH syndrome: bradycardia, renal failure, atrioventricular nodal blockade, shock, and hyperkalemia. *Journal of Emergency Medicine,* 59(2), 216-223.

Fefer, P., Bogdan, A., Grossman, Y., Berkovitch, A., Brodov, Y., et al. (2018). Impact of rapid ventricular pacing on outcome after transcatheter aortic valve replacement. *Journal of the American Heart Association*, 7(14).

Ferri, L.A., Beneduce, A., Ancona, M.B, et al. (2022). A systematic transoesophageal echocardiography study of suture-mediated percutaneous patent foramen ovale closure.

Fincke, R., Hochman, J.S., Lowe, A.M., Menon, V., Slater, J.N., Webb, J.G, et al. (2004). Cardiac power is the strongest hemodynamic correlate of mortality in cardiogenic shock: A report from the SHOCK trial registry. *Journal of American College of Cardiology*, 44(2), 340-348.

Flood, P., Rathmell, J. P., & Shafer, S. (2014). Stoelting's pharmacology & physiology in anesthetic practice (5th ed.). Lippincott Williams and Wilkins.

Flower, L., Arrowsmith, J.E., Bewley, J, et al. (2023). Management of acute aortic dissection in critical care. *Journal of the Intensive Care Society,* 24(4), 409-418.

Fragen, R.J. (1997). Pharmacokinetics and pharmacodynamics of midazolam given via continuous intravenous infusion in intensive care units. *Clin Ther*, 19(3): 405-419.

Frazier, S.K. (2014). 20 things you didn't know about measurement of cardiac output. The Journal of Cardiovascular Nursing, 29(2): 155-157.

Galbraith, E.M., McDaniel, M.C., Jeroudi, A.M., Kashlan, O.R, (2010). Comparison of location of "culprit lesions" in left anterior descending coronary artery among patients with anterior wall ST-segment elevation myocardial infarction having ramus intermedius coronary arteries versus patients not having such arteries. *The American Journal of Cardiology*, 106(2), 162–166.

Gallagher, C., Hendriks, J.M.L, Elliott, A.D., Wong, C.X., Rangnekar, G, et al. (2017). Alcohol and incident atrial fibrillation - a systematic review and meta-analysis. *International Journal of Cardiology*, 246, 46-52.

Gallo M., Blitzer D., Laforgia P.L., et al. (2022). Percutaneous coronary intervention versus coronary artery bypass graft for left main coronary artery disease: a meta-analysis. *The Journal of Thoracic & Cardiovascular Surgery*, 163(1), 94-105.

Garan, A.R., Kanwar, M., Thayer, K.L., Whitehead, E., Zweck, E, et al. (2020). Complete hemodynamic profiling with pulmonary artery catheters in cardiogenic shock is associated with lower in-hospital mortality. *The Journal of the American College of Cardiology (JACC)*, 8(11), 903–913.

Garber, J. S., Gross, M., Slonim, A. D., Allbee, B. H., & Marcucci, L. (2017). Avoiding common nursing errors. Lippincott Williams & Wilkins.

Garcia, T. (2015). 12-lead ECG: the art of interpretation (2nd ed). Jones & Bartlett Learning.

Gaubert, M., Laine, M., Resseguier, N., Aissaoui, N, et al. (2020). Hemodynamic profiles of cardiogenic shock depending on their etiology. *Journal of Clinical Medicine*, 9(11):1.

Gaudino M., Antoniades C., Benedetto U., et al. (2017). Mechanisms, consequences, & prevention of coronary graft failure.

Circulation, 136(18): 1749–1764.

George, R., Condrey, J., & Wilson, S. (2018). Magnesium: a powerful tool in the perioperative setting. American Society of Regional Anesthesia & Pain Medicine.

Gerlach, A., Blais, D., Jones, G, et al. (2016). Predictors of dexmedetomidine-associated hypotension in critically ill patients. *International Journal of Critical Illness and Injury Science*, 6(3): 109-114.

Gianstefani, S., Douri, A., Delithanasis, I, et al. (2014). Incidence and predictors of early left ventricular thrombus after ST-elevation myocardial infarction in the contemporary era of primary percutaneous coronary intervention. *The American Journal of Cardiology*, 113(7), 111-1116. .

Gibson, A.J. (2014). Keeping pace: Understanding temporary transvenous cardiac pacing. *Nursing Critical Care*, 9(5): 20-7.

Giustino, G., Colombo, A., Camaj, A, et al. (2022). Coronary in-stent restenosis: JACC state-of-the-art review. *Journal of the American College of Cardiology*, 80(4): 348–372.

Glazier J J. & Kaki, A. (2018). Improving survival in cardiogenic shock: is Impella® the answer? *American Journal of Medicine*, 131(10): 403–404.

Glazier, J. J. & Kaki, A. (2019). The Impella® device: historical background, clinical applications & future directions. *The International Journal of Angiology*, 28(2), 118–123.

Glineur, D. & Hanet, C. (2012). Competitive flow in coronary bypass surgery: is it a problem? *Current Opinion in Cardiology*, 27(6): 620-628.

Gordon, A.C., Mason, A.J., Thirunavukkarasu, N., Perkins, G.D, et al. (2016). Effect of early vasopressin vs norepinephrine on kidney failure in patients with septic shock: the VANISH randomized clinical trial. *Journal of the American Medical Association*, 316(5): 509-18.

Gori, A.M., Marcucci, R., Migliorini, A, et al. (2008). Incidence and clinical impact of dual nonresponsiveness to aspirin and clopidogrel in patients with drug-eluting stents. *Journal of the American College of Cardiology (AJCC)*, 52(9), 734–739.

Grandin, E., Nunez, J., Willar, B., et al. (2022). Mechanical left ventricular unloading in patients undergoing venoarterial extracorporeal membrane oxygenation. *Journal of the American College of Cardiology*, 79(13), 1239-1250.

Grant A.O. (2009). Cardiac ion channels. *Circulation: Arrhythmia Electrophysiology*, 2(2), 185-194.

Gray, A., Goodacre, S., Newby, D. E., Masson, M., Sampson, F, et al. Noninvasive ventilation in acute cardiogenic pulmonary edema. *The New England Journal of Medicine*, 359(2), 142–151.

Guigui, S. A., Torres, C., Escolar, E., & Mihos, C.G. (2022). Systolic anterior motion of the mitral valve in hypertrophic cardiomyopathy. *Journal of Thoracic Disease*, 14(6), 2309-2325.

Guntheroth, W.G., Morgan, B.C., & Mullins, G.L. Effect of respiration on venous return and stroke volume in cardiac tamponade. *Circulation Research*, 20(4): 381-90.

Gutierrez, E. (2021). Bicarbonate for respiratory acidosis: not so fast.

Gutierrez, E. (2023). The vasopressor & inotrope handbook: a practical guide for healthcare professionals. Kindle Direct Publishing.

Gutierrez, E.J. (2019). Replace/correct the magnesium deficiency before potassium (hypokalemia)!

Guy, C., Holmes, N.E., Kishore, K, et al. (2023). Decompensated metabolic acidosis in the emergency department: epidemiology, sodium bicarbonate therapy, & clinical outcomes. *Critical Care Resuscitation*, 25(2), 71–77.

Hagahmed, M. (2022). Catecholaminergic polymorphic ventricular tachycardia: recognize & treat it early. *Critical Care Now.*

Hajjar L.A. & Teboul, J. (2019). Mechanical circulatory support devices for cardiogenic shock: state of the art. *Critical Care*, 23(76).

Hamada, M., Ikeda., & Shigematsu, Y. (2014). Advances in medical treatment of hypertrophic cardiomyopathy. *The American Journal of Cardiology*, 64(1): 1–10.

Harari, R., Bansal, P., Yatskar, L., Rubinstein, D, et al. (2017). Papillary muscle rupture following acute myocardial infarction: anatomic, echocardiographic, and surgical insights. *Echocardiography*, 34(11): 1702-1707.

Hardin, S. R., & Kaplow, R. (2016). Cardiac surgery essentials for critical care nursing. Jones & Bartlett Learning.

Hartjes, T. M. & American Association of Critical Care Nurses. (2018). Core curriculum for high acuity progressive and critical care nursing (7th ed). Elsevier.

Hartmann, S., Farris, R.W., & Di Gennaro, J.L. (2015). Systematic review and meta-analysis of end-tidal carbon dioxide values associated with return of spontaneous circulation during cardiopulmonary resuscitation. *Journal of Intensive Care Medicine*, 30(7) :426-435.

Hayashi, H., Abe, Y., Morita, Y., Yamaji, Y., Nakane, E., Haruna, Y., Haruna, T., & Inoko, M. (2019). Impact of stroke volume on prognostic outcome in patients with atrial fibrillation and concomitant heart failure with preserved ejection fraction. *Journal of Cardiology*, 73(4), 307–312.

Hayes S.N., Kim E.S., Saw, J, et al. (2018). Spontaneous coronary artery dissection: current state of the science: a scientific statement from the American Heart Association. *Circulation*, 137(19): 523–557.

Heldman, A.W. Drug-eluting stent solutions: examining the antiproliferative drug paclitaxel. *Cath Lab Digest.*

Helgestad, O., Josiassen, J., Hassager, C, et al. (2020). Contemporary trends in use of mechanical circulatory support in patients with acute myocardial infarction and cardiogenic shock. *Open Heart,* 7(1).

Hess, A.S. & Long, M.T. (2023). Bicarbonate: from physiology to clinical practice. *Anesthesiology*, 139(4), 549.

Hodge, T. (2020). Fast facts for the cardiac surgery nurse. Springer.

Holmes, C.L., Landry, D.W. & Granton, J.T. (2004). Vasopressin and the cardiovascular system part II – clinical physiology. *Critical Care,* 8(1), 15-23.

Holmes, D.R., Doshi, S.K., Kar, S., et al. (2015). Left atrial appendage closure as an alternative to warfarin for stroke prevention in atrial fibrillation: a patient-level meta-analysis. *Journal of the American College of Cardiology (JACC)*, 65: 2614-2623.

Huang, C.L. & Kuo, E. (2007). Mechanism of hypokalemia in magnesium deficiency. *Journal of the American Society of Nephrology*, 18(10): 2649-52.

Imazio, M., & Hoit, B.D. (2013). Post-cardiac injury syndromes: an emerging cause of pericardial diseases. *International Journal of Cardiology*, 168(2): 648-52.

Imazio, M., Gaita, F., & LeWinter, M. (2015). Evaluation and treatment of pericarditis: a systematic review. *The Journal of the American Medical Association (JAMA)*, 314(14), 1498-1506.

Imberti, J.F., Underwood, K., Mazzanti, A., & Priori, S.G. (2016). Clinical challenges in catecholaminergic polymorphic ventricular tachycardia. *Heart Lung Circ*, 25: 777-83.

Interpreting intra-aortic balloon pump waveforms. (2015). *Critical Care Challenges*, 39(2): 9-10.

Ireland, S. & Christifulli, T. (2023). Coronary dominance. www.foamfrat.com.

Jaber, S., Paugam, C., Futier, E, et al. (2018). Sodium bicarbonate therapy for patients with severe metabolic acidaemia in the intensive care unit (BICAR-ICU): a multicentre, open-label, randomised controlled, phase III trial. *Lancet*, 392(10141), 31-40.

Jaffe, R., Charron, T., Puley, G., Dick, A., & Strauss, B.H. (2008). Microvascular obstruction and the no-reflow phenomenon after percutaneous coronary intervention. *Circulation*, 117(24), 3152–3156.

Jakob, S.M, et al. (2012). Dexmedetomidine vs midazolam or propofol for sedation during prolonged mechanical ventilation: two randomized controlled trials. *Journal of the American Medical Association,* 307(11): 1151-1160.

Jakowenko, N.D., Murata, J., Kopp, B.J., & Erstad, B.L. (2022). Influence of timing and catecholamine requirements on vasopressin responsiveness in critically ill patients with septic shock. *Journal of Intensive Care Medicine*, 37(11), 1512-1519.

Jasti, J.R., Jasty, T.N., Gudiwada, M.C., & Jitta, S.R. (2023). Bradycardia, renal failure, atrioventricular nodal blockade, shock and hyperkalemia (BRASH) syndrome: a clinical case study. *Cureus*, 15(2).

Jayne, J.E., Catherwood, E., Niles, N.W., & Friedman, B.J. Double-lumen catheter assessment of aortic stenosis: comparison with separate catheter technique. *Catheterization and Cardiovascular Diagnosis*, 29(2): 157–160.

Jazayeri, M.A., Vuddanda, V., Parikh, V., & Lakkireddy, D.R. (2017). Percutaneous left atrial appendage closure: current state of the art. *Current Opinion in Cardiology*, 32(1): 27–38.

Jeboda, J. Aortic arch anatomy coloring page. JennMedArt.

Jentzer, J.C., Van Diepen, S., Barsness, G.W, et al. (2019). Cardiogenic shock classification to predict mortality in the cardiac intensive care unit. *The Journal of the American College of Cardiology (JACC),* 74: 2117–2128.

Joyce, D. L., Joyce, L. D., & Loebe, M. (2021). Mechanical circulatory support: principles and applications. McGraw-Hill Professional.

Juarez, P. (2022). Barron's test prep: adult CCRN exam. Kaplan.

Kang, G., Ha, R., & Banerjee, D. (2016). Pulmonary artery pulsatility index predicts right ventricular failure after left ventricular assist device implantation. *The Journal of Heart and Lung Transplantation,* 35(1), 67–73.

Kapur, N.K., Esposito, M.L., Bader, Y., Morine, K.J., Kiernan, M.S, et al. (2017). Mechanical circulatory support devices for acute right ventricular failure. *Circulation*, 136(3): 314-326.

Karami, M., Hemradj, V.V., Ouweneel, D.M, et al. (2020). Vasopressors and inotropes in acute myocardial infarction related cardiogenic shock: a systematic review and meta-analysis. *The Journal of Clinical Medicine,* 9(7): 2051.

Karbach, S. (2023). Coronary arteries & ECG regions. Nurse Dose Podcast.

Kassimis, G., Karagiannidis, E., Triantafyllou, K, et al. (2020). Fatal post-infarction late left ventricular free wall rupture in the era of COVID-19. Journal of the American College of Cardiology (JACC), 13(16), 157-158.

Katzung B.G., & Vanderah T.W. (2021). Basic & clinical pharmacology. McGraw Hill.

Kaul, S., & Ito, H. (2004). Microvasculature in acute myocardial ischemia: evolving concepts in pathophysiology, diagnosis, and treatment. *Circulation*, 109(2), 146-149.

Kaur, G., et al. (2021). Pathophysiology, diagnosis, and management of coronary no-reflow phenomenon. *The International Journal of Angiology*, 30(1), 15-21.

Kaur, M., & Singh, P. M. (2011). Current role of dexmedetomidine in clinical anesthesia and intensive care. *Anesthesia Essays & Researches*, 5(2), 128-133.

Kawano, T., Grunau, B., Scheuermeyer, F.X, et al. (2017). Prehospital sodium bicarbonate use could worsen long-term survival with favorable neurological recovery among patients with out-of-hospital cardiac arrest. *Resuscitation*, 119, 63–69.

Kawata, H., Ohno, S., Aiba, T, et al. (2016). Catecholaminergic polymorphic ventricular tachycardia (CPVT) associated with ryanodine receptor (RyR2) gene mutations - long-term prognosis after initiation of medical treatment. *Circulation*, 80(9), 1907-1915.

Keech, B.M. & Laterza, R.D. (2020). Anesthesia secrets (6th ed.). Elsevier.

Kennon, T. (2024). What to know about mechanical circulatory support in the treatment of cardiogenic shock. American Association of Critical Care Nurses.

Kern, M. (2014). Measurement of cardiac output in the cath lab: how accurate is it? *Cath Lab Digest.*

Khachatryan, A., Srivastava, M.C., Cinar, T, et al. (2024). The ramus intermedius: a bridge to survival in the setting of triple-vessel total occlusion, *Cureus*, 16(5).

Khalid, S., Seepana, J., Sundhu, M, et al. (2017). Left ventricular free wall rupture in transmural myocardial infarction. *Cureus*, 9(8): 1610.

Kibos, A., Campeanu, A., & Tintoiu, I. (2007). Pathophysiology of coronary artery in-stent restenosis. *Acute Cardiac Care*, 9(2), 111–119.

Kini, A. & Sharma, S.K. (2021). Practical manual of interventional cardiology. Springer.

Klabunde, R.E. (2020). Cardiovascular physiology concepts. Lippincott Williams & Wilkins/Wolters Kluwer.

Knapp, R. (2020). Hemodynamic monitoring made incredibly visual. Wolters Kluwer.

Kodama, S., Saito, K., Tanaka, S, et al. (2017). Alcohol consumption and risk of atrial fibrillation: a meta analysis. *Journal of the American College of Cardiology (JACC)*, 57(4): 427–436.

Komatsu, R., Turan, A.M., Orhan-Sungur, M, et al. Remifentanil for general anesthesia: a systematic review.

Kovacevic, M, et al. (2021). Left main trifurcation and its percutaneous treatment. *Circulation: Cardiovascular Interventions*, 14(3).

Krishna, M., & Zacharowski, K. (2018). Principles of intra-aortic balloon pump counterpulsation. *Continuing Education in Anesthesia Critical Care*, 9(1): 24-28.

Krittanawong C, Kumar A, Johnson KW, et al. (2019). Conditions and factors associated with spontaneous coronary artery dissection. *American Journal of Cardiology*, 123(2), 249-253.

Kucia, A.M. & Horowitz, J.D. (2023). Pathogenesis of acute coronary syndromes. Cardiac Care.

Kucia A. M. & Quinn, T. (2010). Acute cardiac care: a practical guide for nurses.

Kufner, S., Cassese, S., Valeskini, M., et al (2015). Long-term efficacy and safety of paclitaxel-eluting balloon for the treatment of drug-eluting stent restenosis: 3-year results of a randomized controlled trial. *Journal of the American College of Cardiology Cardiovascular Interventions*, 8(7): 877-884.

Kumar, R. (2018). Bicarbonate. RK.MD.

Kumar, R. (2017). Combining vasoactive/inotropic agents. RK.MD.

Kumar, R. (2020). Overview of temporary pacemakers. RK.MD.

Kumar, R. (2017). Pulmonary artery catheter/Swan-Ganz structure and waveforms. RK.MD.

Kundu, A. & Moliterno, D.J. (2024). Drug-coated balloons for in-stent restenosis—finally leaving nothing behind for patients. *Journal of the American Medical Association*, 331(12), 1011-1012.

Kupchik, N. L. (2020). Ace the CCRN®!: you can do it: study guide.

Kupchik, N. L. (2023). Critical care survival guide. Nicole Kupchik Consulting.

Kupchik, N.L. (2022). Facing pacing: emergent pacing essentials for nurses.

Labrada, L., Patil, A., Kumar, J, et al. (2020). Papillary muscle rupture complicating acute myocardial infarction: a tale of teamwork. *Journal of the American College of Cardiology*, 2(15): 2283–2288.

Lange, R.L, et al. Diagnostic signs in compressive cardiac disorders: constrictive pericarditis, pericardial effusion, and tamponade. *Circulation*, 33(5): 763-777.

Lau, W.C., Gurbel, P.A., Watkins, P.B, et al. (2004). Contribution of hepatic cytochrome P450 3A4 metabolic activity to the phenomenon of clopidogrel resistance. *Circulation*, 109(2), 166-171.

Lauten, A., et al. (2013). Percutaneous left-ventricular support with the Impella-2.5-assist device® in acute cardiogenic shock.

Circulation: Heart Failure, 6(1), 23-30.

Layon, J., Gabrielli, A., Yu, M., & Wood, K.E. (2018). Civetta, Taylor, & Kirby's critical care.

Leather, H.A., Segers, P., Berends, N., Vandermeersch, E., & Wouters, P.F. (2002). Effects of vasopressin on right ventricular function in an experimental model of acute pulmonary hypertension. *Critical Care Medicine*, 30(11), 2548–2552.

Lemaire, A., Anderson, M.B., Lee, L.Y., Scholz, P., Prendergast, T., Goodman, A., Lozano, A.M., Spotnitz, A, & Batsides, G. (2014). The Impella device for acute mechanical circulatory support in patients in cardiogenic shock. Ann Thorac Surg. 97(1): 133-8.

Levine, G., McEvoy, J., Fang, J., Ibeh, C, et al. (2022). Management of patients at risk for and with left ventricular thrombus: a scientific statement from the American Heart Association. *Circulation*, 146(15), 205–223.

Levine, G.N. (2022). Cardiology secrets (6th ed.). Elsevier.

Levy, B., Buzon, J., & Kimmoun, A. (2019). Inotropes and vasopressors use in cardiogenic shock: when, which and how much? *Current Opinion in Critical Care*, 25(4), 384–390.

Lewis, T.C., Aberle, C., Altshuler, D., Piper, G.L., & Papadopoulos, J. (2019). Comparative effectiveness and safety between milrinone or dobutamine as initial inotrope therapy in cardiogenic shock. *Journal of Cardiovascular Pharmacology and Therapeutics*, 24(2): 130-138.

Li, J., Cooper, M., Shults, C. et al. (2023). Post-myocardial infarction free-wall rupture: rapid diagnosis and management. *Journal of the American College of Cardiology (JACC) Case Reports,* 18, 101915..

Li, J., Patel, S.M., Parikh, M.A., Parikh, S.A. (2016). Unprotected left main disease: indications and optimal strategies for percutaneous intervention. *Curr Treat Options Cardiovasc Med*, 18(3), 19.

Li, K.H., Lee, S., Yin, C., Liu, T., et al (2020). Brugada syndrome: a comprehensive review of pathophysiological mechanisms and risk stratification strategies. *International Journal of Cardiology,* 26, 100468.

Lim, H.S. (2016). Cardiogenic shock: failure of oxygen delivery and oxygen utilization. *Clinical Cardiology*, 39(8): 477–483.

Link, M.S. (2012). Commotio cordis: ventricular fibrillation triggered by chest impact-induced abnormalities in repolarization. *Circulation: Arrhythmia & Electrophysiology*, 5(2): 425-432.

Link, M.S. & Estes, N.A. (2010). Athletes and arrhythmias. *Journal of Cardiovascular Electrophysiology*, 21(10): 1184-1189.

Lo, K.B., Garvia, V., Stempel, J.M., Ram, P., & Rangaswami, J. (2020). Bicarbonate use and mortality outcome among critically ill patients with metabolic acidosis: a meta analysis. *Heart & Lung: The Journal of Acute and Critical Care*, 49(2), 167–174.

Lowenstein, S.R., Gabow, P.A., Cramer, J., Oliva, P.B., & Ratner, K. (1983). The role of alcohol in new-onset atrial fibrillation. *Archives of Internal Medicine*, 143(10), 1882-1885.

Madhavan, M.V., Kirtane, A.J., Redfors, B, et al. (2020). Stent-related adverse events > 1 year after percutaneous coronary intervention. *Journal of the American College of Cardiology*, 75(6): 590-604.

Madias, C., Maron BJ, Weinstock J, et al. (2007). Commotio cordis: sudden cardiac death with chest wall impact. *Journal of Cardiovascular Electrophysiology,* 18(1), 115-122.

Majeed, H., Khan, A., Khalid, S. et al. (2023). Brash syndrome: a systematic review of reported cases. *Current Problems in Cardiology,* 48(6), 101663.

Manabe, S., Kasegawa, H., Arai, H., Takanashi, S. (2018). Management of systolic anterior motion of the mitral valve: a mechanism-based approach. *Gen Thorac Cardiovasc Surg*, 66(7): 379-389.

Manning, W. & Black, J. (2018). Overview of acute aortic dissection and other acute aortic syndromes. UpToDate.

Marchena, E. & Gomez, C. (2023). Mastering structural heart disease. John Wiley & Sons.

Marian, A. J., & Braunwald, E. (2017). Hypertrophic cardiomyopathy: genetics, pathogenesis, clinical manifestations, diagnosis, & therapy. *Circulation Research*, 121(7), 749-770.

Maron, B., Desai, M., Nishimura, R, et al. (2022), Management of hypertrophic cardiomyopathy. *Journal of the American College of Cardiology (JACC)*, 79(4), 390-414.

Martinez, L.G. (2012). Spontaneous coronary artery dissection: a rare threat to young women. *Critical Care Nurse*, 32(4): 19-26.

Mathew, A., Berry, E., Tirou, M., & Kumar, P. (2020). Left ventricular rupture: a rare complication and an unusual presentation. *BMJ Case Reports*, 13(2).

Mathew, R., Di Santo, P., Jung, R.G, et al. (2021). Milrinone as compared with dobutamine in the treatment of cardiogenic shock. *The New England Journal of Medicine*, 385(6): 516-525.

Mathew, R., Visintini, S.M., Ramirez, F.D, et al. (2019). Efficacy of milrinone and dobutamine in low cardiac output states: a systematic review and meta-analysis. *Clinical & Investigative Medicine,* 42(2): 26-32.

Mathieu, D., Neviere, R., Billard, V., Fleyfel, M., & Wattel, F. Effects of bicarbonate therapy on hemodynamics & tissue oxygenation in patients with lactic acidosis: a prospective, controlled clinical study. *Critical Care Medicine,* 19(11): 1352-1356.

Mattu, A., Tabas, J.A., & Brady, W.J. (2019). Electrocardiography in emergency, acute & critical care.

McCarthy C.P., Vaduganathan, M., McCarthy K, et al. (2018). Left ventricular thrombus after acute myocardial infarction: screening, prevention, and treatment. *Journal of the American Medical Association*, 3(7): 642-649.

McCulloch, B.K. (2022). Fast facts for the cath lab nurse. Springer.

McGee, W.T., Headley, J.M., Frazier, J.A. (2015). Quick guide to cardiopulmonary care. Edwards Lifesciences.

Mclean, H., Wells, L., & Marler, J. (2021). The effect of pre-arrest acid-base status on response to sodium bicarbonate and achievement of return of spontaneous circulation. *Annals of Pharmacotherapy.*

Mead, N.E. & O'Keefe, K.P. (2009). Wellens' syndrome: an ominous ECG pattern. *Journal of Emergencies, Trauma & Shock,* 2(3), 206-208.

Meani, P., Lorusso, R., & Pappalardo, F. (2022). ECPella: concept, physiology and clinical applications. *Journal of Cardiothoracic Vascular Anesthesia*, 36: 557–566.

Medtronic Corp. (2020). Model 5392 dual chamber temporary pacemaker technical manual.

Medtronic. (2022). Transvenous pacing: basic pacing concepts. Medtronic Academy.

Merelman, A.H., Perlmutter, M.C, & Strayer, R.J. (2019). Alternatives to rapid sequence intubation: contemporary airway management with ketamine. *The Western Journal of Emergency Medicine,* 20(3): 466-471.

Mileva, N., Nagumo, S., Mizukami, T., Sonck, J, et al. (2022). Prevalence of coronary microvascular disease and coronary vasospasm in patients with nonobstructive coronary artery disease: systematic review and meta-analysis. *Journal of the American Heart Association*, 11(7).

Mind the Graph. Atrial appendage closure device Watchman™ illustration & icon. www.mindthegraph.com.

Mind the Graph. Shockwave intravascular lithotripsy coronary balloon illustration & icon. www.mindthegraph.com.

Mind the Graph. Heart left atrial appendage cut illustration & icon. www.mindthegraph.com.

Mind the Graph. Transcatheter aortic valve replacement illustration & icon. www.mindthegraph.com.

Minor, J. & George, E. Critical care: using mixed venous oxygen saturation to improve patient assessments. Wolters Kluwer.

Mobrien, K.M., Jones, G.M., MacDermott, J.R., & Murphy, C.V. (2014). Remifentanil, ketamine, and fospropofol: a review of alternative continuous infusion agents for sedation in the critically ill. *Critical Care Nurse*, 37(2): 137-151.

Mohr, F.W., Morice, M.C., Kappetein, A.P., et al.(2013). Coronary artery bypass graft surgery versus percutaneous coronary intervention in patients with three-vessel disease and left main coronary disease: 5-year follow-up of the randomized, clinical SYNTAX trial. *Lancet*, 381(9867), 629-638.

Mohsin, I., Namburu, L., Sadiq, Z., Newberry, B., & Ahmed, H.M. (2021). Competitive flow: closure of internal thoracic artery graft after successful coronary artery bypass graft surgery. Elsevier.

Mojadidi, M.K., Zaman, M.O., Elgendy, I.Y, et al. (2018). Cryptogenic stroke and patent foramen ovale. *Journal of the American College of Cardiology*, *71*(9), 1035–1043.

Morrow, D.A. (2019). The changing face of cardiogenic shock: a challenge in cardiac critical care. *The Journal of the American College of Cardiology (JACC),* 73(14): 1792–1794.

Moulakakis, K.G, et al. (2014). Management of complicated and uncomplicated acute type B dissection: a systematic review and meta-analysis. *Annals of Cardiothoracic Surgery,* 3(3), 234-246.

Nagarakanti, R, & Ezekowitz, M. (2008). Diastolic dysfunction and atrial fibrillation. *Journal of Interventional Cardiac Electrophysiology*, 22(2): 111–118.

Nagelhout, J.J. & Elisha, S. (2018). Nurse anesthesia (6th ed.). Elsevier.

Naidu, S.S. (2015). Diagnosis and management of hypertrophic cardiomyopathy: expert analysis. The American College of Cardiology.

Namana, V., Gupta, S.S., Sabharwal, N., & Hollander, G. (2018). Clinical significance of atrial kick. *Quarterly Journal of Medicine*, 111(8): 569-570.

Ndrepepa, G., Tiroch, K, et al. (2010). Predictive factors and impact of no-reflow after primary percutaneous coronary intervention in patients with acute myocardial infarction. *Circulation: Cardiovascular Interventions,* 3(1), 27-33.

Netter, F. (2019). Atlas of human anatomy (7th ed.). Philadelphia, PA: Saunders.

Nienaber, C.A. & Clough, R.E. (2015). Management of acute aortic dissection. *Lancet*, 385(9970), 800–811.

Nishimura, R.A., Seggewiss, H., & Schaff, H.V. (2018). Hypertrophic obstructive cardiomyopathy: surgical myectomy and septal ablation. *Circulation Research,* 121(7), 771-783.

Noessler, N., Schweintzger, S., & Kurath-Koller, S. (2021). Holiday heart syndrome: an upcoming tachyarrhythmia in today's youth? *Cardiology in the Young*, 31(6): 1054-1056.

Nogic, J., MacPherson, M., Roberts, L, et al. (2022). Magnesium in the management of atrial fibrillation with rapid ventricular response. *Journal of the American College of Cardiology (JACC),* 8(6), 800-802.

O'Neil, J., Mazumder, S., Sanborn, D.Y., & Wu, S. (2021). A case of spontaneous coronary artery dissection in patients with severe anorexia nervosa. *Case Reports in Cardiology*.

Opotowsky, A. R., Hess, E., Maron, B. A., et al. (2017). Thermodilution vs estimated fick cardiac output measurement in clinical practice. *Journal of the American Medical Association.*

Osmancik, P., Herman, D., Neuzil P., et al. (2020). Left atrial appendage closure versus direct oral anticoagulants in high-risk patients with atrial fibrillation. *Journal of the American College of Cardiology (JACC),* 75(25): 3122-3135.

Ouellette, R.G., & Joyce, J.A. (2010). Pharmacology for nurse anesthesiology. Jones and Bartlett.

Ouweneel, D.M., Eriksen, E., Seyfarth, M., & Henriques, J.P. (2017). Percutaneous mechanical circulatory support versus intra-aortic balloon pump for treating cardiogenic shock: a meta-analysis. *Journal of the American College of Cardiology*, 69(3): 358–360.

Ouweneel, D.M., Eriksen, E., Sjauw, K.D, et al. (2017). Impella CP versus intra-aortic balloon pump support in acute myocardial infarction complicated by cardiogenic shock. The Journal of the American College of Cardiology (JACC), 69: 278–287.

Overbay, D. & Criddle, L. Mastering temporary invasive cardiac pacing. *Critical Care Nurse*, 24(3): 25–32.

Overgaard, C.B., & Dzavík, V. Inotropes and vasopressors: a review of physiology and clinical use in cardiovascular disease. *Circulation*, 118(10): 1047-1056.

Pahuja, M., Chitturi, K.R., Tuli, A., Saxena, A, et al. (2025). Impact of pulmonary artery catheterization in patients with acute myocardial infarction cardiogenic shock. Cardiovascular Revascularization Medicine.

Paola, M., Wilde, A., & Hanno, T.L. (2005). Pathophysiological mechanisms of Brugada syndrome: depolarization disorder, repolarization disorder, or more? *Cardiovascular Research*, 67(3), 367-378.

Paone, S, Clarkson, L, Sin, B., & Punnapuzha, S. (2018). Recognition of sympathetic crashing acute pulmonary edema (SCAPE) and use of high-dose nitroglycerin infusion. *Am J Emerg Med*, 36(8).

Pape, L.A., Awais, M., Woznicki, E.M, et al. (2015). Presentation, diagnosis, and outcomes of acute aortic dissection: 17-year trends from the international registry of acute aortic dissection. *Journal of the American College of Cardiology (JACC),* 66(4): 350-358.

Pappalardo, F., Schulte, C., Pieri, M., et al. (2017). Concomitant implantation of Impella® on top of veno-arterial extracorporeal membrane oxygenation may improve survival of patients with cardiogenic shock. *Journal of Heart Failure,* 19(3), 404-412.

Parikh, K.S., Agarwal, R., Mehrotra, A.K, et al. (2012). Wellens' syndrome: a life-saving diagnosis. American Journal of Emergency Medicine, 30(1).

Parissis V., Graham S., et al. (2016). IABP: history, evolution, pathophysiology, & indications: what we need to know. *Journal of Cardiothoracic Surgery,* 11(1), 122.

Parsons P. E., Wiener-Kronish, J. P., Stapleton R. D., & Berra L. (2019). Critical care secrets. Elsevier.

Pasupathy, S., Air, T., Dreyer, R.P., Tavella, R., & Beltrame, J.F. (2015). Systematic review of patients presenting with suspected myocardial infarction and nonobstructive coronary arteries. *Circulation*, 131(10): 861-870.

Pasupathy, S., Tavella, R., & Beltrame, J. (2017). Unraveling the enigma of MI with nonobstructive coronary arteries. *The American College of Cardiology*, 10(2), 79-82.

Patel, S.M., Lipinski, J., Al-Kindi, S.G, et al. (2019). Simultaneous venoarterial extracorporeal membrane oxygenation and percutaneous left ventricular decompression therapy with Impella® is associated with improved outcomes in refractory cardiogenic shock. *ASAIO Journal*, 65: 21–28.

Peacock, W.F., Hilleman, D.E., Levy, P.D., Rhoney D.H., & Varon, J. A systematic review of nicardipine vs. labetalol for the management of hypertensive crises. *The American Journal of Emergency Medicine*, 30(6), 981-993.

Peck, T. E., & Hill, S. A. (2014). Pharmacology for anesthesia and intensive care. *Cambridge University Press.*

Pelliccia, F. & Camici, P.G. (2023). Updates on MINOCA and INOCA through the 2022 publications in the international journal of cardiology. *International Journal of Cardiology,* 374, 8-11.

Peltenberg, P.J., Kallas, D., Bos, J.M, et al. (2021). An international multi-center cohort study on beta-blockers for the treatment of symptomatic children with CPVT. *Circulation*, 145(5), 333-344.

Pelter, M., Carey, M., & Salah, A. (2011). Coronary artery dominance. *American Journal of Critical Care,* 20(5), 401-402.

Perel, A. (2017). The value of dynamic preload variables during spontaneous ventilation. *Current Opinion in Critical Care,* 23(4): 310-317.

Perman, S.M., Elmer, J., Maciel, C.B., Uzendu, A., & American Heart Association (2024). 2023 american heart association focused update on adult advanced cardiovascular life support: an update to the american heart association guidelines for cardiopulmonary resuscitation and emergency cardiovascular care. *Circulation*, 149(5), 254–273.

Pepin, J. (2021). Sodium bicarbonate for cardiac arrest: time to put it away. *Critical Care Now.*

Pflaumer, A, & Davis, A.M. (2012). Guidelines for the diagnosis and management of catecholaminergic polymorphic ventricular tachycardia. *Heart Lung Circ*, 21(2): 96-100.
Pourafkari, L., Kinninger, A., Fazlalizadeh, H, et al. (2023). Presence of ramus intermedius artery is associated with higher atherosclerotic plaque burden in the left main stem in coronary ct angiography. *Circulation*.
Price M.J., Slotwiner, D., Du, C., et al. (2022). Clinical outcomes at 1 year following transcatheter left atrial appendage occlusion in the United States. *JACC Cardiovascular Interventions*, 15(7): 741-750.
Price, M.J. (2014). Left atrial appendage occlusion with the WATCHMAN™ for stroke prevention in atrial fibrillation. *Rev Cardiovasc Med*, 15(2): 142-5.
Prichard, B.N. & Richards, D.A. (1981). The pharmacological basis for the use of labetalol in the treatment of hypertension. *Journal of Cardiovascular Pharmacology*.
Pritts, W. (2023). Case studies in BRASH syndrome: bradycardia, renal failure, AV blocker, shock, & hyperkalemia.
Privitera, D., Capsoni, N., Vailati, P., Terranova, G., & Aseni, P. (2022). Standardized nursing approach to the acute aortic dissection patient: a practice update. *Sage Open Nursing*.
Prondzinsky, R., Lemm, H., Swyter, M, et al. (2010). Intra-aortic balloon counterpulsation in patients with acute myocardial infarction complicated by cardiogenic shock - the prospective, randomized IABP SHOCK Trial for attenuation of multi-organ dysfunction syndrome. *Critical Care Medicine*, 38(1): 152–160.
Propper, S. (2023). The cath lab visual orientation manual. Propper Consulting, LLC.
Propper, S. (2023). The RCIS study guide. Propper Consulting, LLC.
Puckett, S.D. & Andrews, J.J. Update for nurse anesthetists: a comprehensive review of remifentanil: the next generation opioid. *American Association of Nurse Anesthesiology Journal*, 66(3): 220.
Purves, P. D., Klein, G.J., Leong-Sit, P., Yee, R., Skanes, A.C., & Gula, L.J. (2012). Cardiac electrophysiology: a visual guide for nurses, techs and fellows.
Quaal, S.J. (2001). Interpreting the arterial pressure waveform in the intra-aortic balloon-pump patient. *Progress in Cardiovascular Nursing*, 16(3), 116-125.
Quick reference guide: IABP insertion. (2022). Maquet.
Ragnhildstveit, A., Slayton, M., Jackson, L. K, et al. (2022). Ketamine as a novel psychopharmacotherapy for eating disorders: evidence and future directions. *Brain Sciences*, 12(3), 382.
Ragoonanan, D. & Friedman, L. (2021). Clinical update on vasopressors and titration strategies. *AACN Advanced Critical Care*, 32(4), 369–374.
Ragosta M. (2015). Left main coronary artery disease: importance, diagnosis, assessment, and management. *Current Problems in Cardiology*, 40(3), 93-126.
Ragosta M. (2017). Textbook of clinical hemodynamics. Elsevier.
Ragosta, M. (2010). Cases in interventional cardiology. Saunders.
Ramadan, R., Boden, W.E., & Kinlay S. (2018). Management of left main coronary artery disease. *Journal of the American Heart Association*, 7(7).
Ramesh, T., Lee, P.Y., Mitta, M, et al. (2021). Intravenous magnesium in the management of rapid atrial fibrillation: a systematic review and meta-analysis. *Journal of Cardiology*, 78(5), 375-381.
Rao, B.N. (2023). Clinical examination in cardiology (3rd edition). Elsevier.
Reynolds, H.R., Srichai, M.B., Iqbal, S.N., Slater, J.N, et al. (2011). Mechanisms of myocardial infarction in women without angiographically obstructive coronary artery disease. *Circulation*, 124(13): 1414–1425.
Rezkalla, S.H., Dharmashankar, K.C, et al. (2010). No-reflow phenomenon following percutaneous coronary intervention for acute myocardial infarction: incidence, outcome, and effect of pharmacologic therapy. *Journal of Interventional Cardiology*, 23(5), 429-436.
Riker, R.R., Shehabi, Y., Bokesch, P.M. et al. (2009). Dexmedetomidine vs midazolam for sedation of critically ill patients: a randomized trial. *Journal of the American Medical Association*, 301(5), 489-499.
Rishi, K. (2024). The left atrial appendage. RK.MD.
Rizik, D.G., Klassen, K.J., Burke, R.F., Hodgson, J.M., & Stone, G.W. (2015). Interventional management of unprotected left main coronary artery disease: patient selection and technique optimization. *Journal of Interventional Cardiology*, 28(4), 326-338.
Robinson, A., Jain, A., Gentry, M., & McNamara, R. (2016). Left ventricular thrombi after STEMI in the primary PCI era: a systematic review and meta-analysis. *Int. J. Cardiol*, 221, 554–559.
Rodés-Cabau, J., Philippon, F., & Farjat-Pasos, J. (2024). Rapid pacing in TAVR procedures: going minimalist. *Journal of American College of Cardiology Cardiovascular Interventions*, 17(8), 1029–1031.
Rosani, N.S., Zamin, R.M., Zulkafli, I.S, et al. (2021). Presence of ramus intermedius increases the risk of atherosclerotic plaque

formation at the left main bifurcation's region: a retrospective study from CT coronary angiography in UMMC. *International Journal of Cardiology*, 345, 19–19.

Russell, J.A. (2019). Vasopressor therapy in critically ill patients with shock. *Intensive Care Medicine*, 45(11): 1503-1517.

Sabik, J.F. & Blackstone, E.H. (2008). Coronary artery bypass graft patency and competitive flow. *Journal of the American College of Cardiology*, 51(2): 126-8.

Sabik, J.F., Olivares, G., Raza, S., Lytle, B.W., & et al. (2016). Does grafting coronary arteries with only moderate stenosis affect long-term mortality? *J Thorac Cardiovasc Surg*, 151(3), 806-811.

Sahinovic, M., M, Struys., & Absalom, A.R. (2018). Clinical pharmacokinetics and pharmacodynamics of propofol. *Clinical Pharmacokinetics*, 57(12), 1539-1558.

Saldivar, L., Beasley, S., Romesser, C. et al. (2023). Bradycardia, renal failure, atrioventricular nodal blocking agents, shock and hyperkalemia: a rare syndrome threatening cardiovascular collapse. *Journal of the American College of Cardiology (JACC).*

Sammour Y., Krishnaswamy A., Kumar A, et al. (2021). Incidence, predictors, and implications of permanent pacemaker requirement after transcatheter aortic valve replacement. *Journal of American College of Cardiology Cardiovascular Interventions*, 14(2): 115–134.

Samsky, M.D., Morrow, D.A., Hochman, J.S, et al. (2021). Cardiogenic shock after acute myocardial infarction: a review. *The Journal of the American Medical Association (JAMA)*, 326(18), 1840–1850.

Sardana, M., Shaikh, A., & Smith, C. (2018). The atrial kick: atrioventricular dyssynchrony causing paroxysms of hypotension in the setting of acute left ventricular dysfunction. *Journal of the American College of Cardiology (JACC).*

Sasse, T., & Eriksson, U. (2017). Post-cardiac injury syndrome: etiology, diagnosis, and treatment. *e-Journal of Cardiology Practice*, 15(21).

Saw, J., Humphries, K., Aymong, E, et al. (2017). Spontaneous coronary artery dissection: clinical outcomes and risk of recurrence. *Journal of the American College of Cardiology (JACC).* 70(9), 1148–1158.

Scalone, G., Niccoli, G., & Crea, F. (2019). The pathophysiology, diagnosis and management of MINOCA: an update. *Journal of Acute Cardiovascular Care*, 8(1): 54–62.

Scanlon, T. (2021). Basic cardiac rhythms: the visual nurse's guide. www.thevisualnurse.com.

Scanlon, T. (2021). Ejection fraction. www.thevisualnurse.com.

Scheeren, T.W.L., Bakker, J., Kaufmann, T, et al. (2021). Current use of inotropes in circulatory shock. *Annals of Intensive Care*, 11(1), 21.

Scheller, B., Hehrlein, C., Bocksch, W., et al. (2006). Treatment of coronary in-stent restenosis with a paclitaxel-coated balloon catheter. *The New England Journal of Medicine*, 355(20), 2113-2124.

Schnur, M. (2022). Alpha adrenergic blockers - how do they work? Lippincott Nursing Center.

Schnur, M.B. (2021). Understanding pulsus paradoxus. Lippincott Nursing Center.

Schrage, B., Becher, P.M., Bernhardt, A, et al.(2020). Left ventricular unloading is associated with lower mortality in patients with cardiogenic shock treated with venoarterial extracorporeal membrane oxygenation: results from an international, multicenter cohort study. *Circulation*, 142: 2095–2106.

Serafini, G., Howland, R.H., Rovedi, F., Girardi, P., & Amore, M. (2014). The role of ketamine in treatment-resistant depression: a systematic review. *Current Neuropharmacology*, 12(5), 444–461.

Shamloo, B.K., Chintala, R.S., Nasur, A., et al. (2010). Spontaneous coronary artery dissection: aggressive vs. conservative therapy. *Journal of Invasive Cardiology*, 22(5): 222–228.

Shankar, A., Gurumurthy, G., Vallabhajosyula, S, et al. (2022). A clinical update on vasoactive medication in the management of cardiogenic shock. *Clinical Medicine Insights.*

Shehabi, Y., Howe, B.D., Bellomo, R., Arabi, Y, et al. (2019). Early sedation with dexmedetomidine in critically ill patients. *The New England Journal of Medicine*, 380(26), 2506–2517.

Sheikh, A. S., & Ranjan, K. (2014). Brugada syndrome: a review of the literature. *Clinical Medicine*, 14(5), 482–489.

Sheng X.Y., An H.J., et al. (2022). High-dose clopidogrel versus ticagrelor in CYP2C19 intermediate or poor metabolizers after percutaneous coronary intervention: a meta-analysis of randomized control trials. *Journal of Clinical Pharmacy.* 47(8):1112–1121.

Sherrid, M.V., Pearle, G., & Gunsburg, D.Z. (1998). Mechanism of benefit of negative inotropes in obstructive hypertrophic cardiomyopathy. *Circulation*, 97(1), 41-47.

Sherrid, M.V., Balaram, S., Kim, B, et al. (2016). The mitral valve in obstructive hypertrophic cardiomyopathy. *Journal of the American College of Cardiology*, 67(15), 1846-1858.

Sherrid, M.V., Shetty, A., Winson, G, et al. (2013). Treatment of obstructive hypertrophic cardiomyopathy symptoms and

gradient resistant to first-line therapy with β-blockade or verapamil. *Circulation: Heart Failure*, 6(4), 694-702.
Shishehbor, M.H., Moazami, N., Tong, M.Z, et al. (2017). Cardiogenic shock: from ECMO to Impella and beyond. *Cleveland Clinic Journal of Medicine*, 84(4), 287–295.
Shiyovich, A., & Nesher, L. (2012). Contained left ventricular free wall rupture following myocardial infarction. *Case Reports in Critical Care*.
Simmons, J. & Ventetuolo, C.E. (2017). Cardiopulmonary monitoring of shock. *Current Opinion in Critical Care*, 23(3), 223–231.
Simmons, T. & Blazar, E. (2019). Synergistic bradycardia from beta blockers, hyperkalemia, and renal failure. *Journal of Emergency Medicine*, 57(2).
Simon, T., Verstuyft, C., Mary-Krause, M., et al. (2009). Genetic determinants of response to clopidogrel and cardiovascular events. *New England Journal of Medicine*, 360(4): 363–75.
Singh, S., Wann, L.S., Schuchard, G.H., Klopfenstein, H.S, et al. Right ventricular and right atrial collapse in patients with cardiac tamponade - a combined echocardiographic and hemodynamic study. *Circulation*, 70(6): 966-71.
Siopi, S.A.,Tagarakis, G., Voucharas, C, et al. (2024). Cardiac failure and cardiogenic shock: insights into pathophysiology, classification, and hemodynamic assessment. *Cureus*, 16(10).
Skelding, K.A., Goldstein, J.A, et al. (2002). Resolution of refractory no-reflow with intracoronary epinephrine. *Catheterization & Cardiovascular Interventions*, 57(3), 305-309.
Slama, M., Tribouilloy, C., Maizel, J. (2016). Left ventricular outflow tract obstruction in ICU patients. *Curr Opin Crit Care*, 22(3): 260-266.
Snoep, J.D., Hovens, M.M., Eikenboom, J.C., et al. Clopidogrel nonresponsiveness in patients undergoing percutaneous coronary intervention with stenting: a systematic review and meta-analysis. *American Heart Journal*. 154(2): 221–231.
Soda, T., Brunetti, V., Berra-Romani, R., & Moccia, F. (2023). The emerging role of N-methyl-D-aspartate (NMDA) receptors in the cardiovascular system: physiological implications, pathological consequences, and therapeutic perspectives. *International Journal of Molecular Sciences*, 24(4), 3914.
Sole, M. L., Klein, D. G., & Moseley, M.J. (2016). Introduction to critical care nursing. Saunders.
Sorajja, P., Lim, M.J., & Kern, M.J. (2020). Kern's cardiac catheterization handbook (7th ed.). Elsevier.
Spontaneous coronary artery dissection. (2022). BioRender.
Standring, S. (2016) Gray's anatomy: the anatomical basis of clinical practice. Elsevier.
Stemple, K, DeWitt, K.M., Porter, B.A., Sheeser, M., Blohm, E., & Bisanzo, M. (2021). High-dose nitroglycerin infusion for the management of sympathetic crashing acute pulmonary edema (SCAPE): a case series. *Am J Emerg Med*, 44, 262-266.
Stoltenberg, E., & Joffe, A. (2020). Analgesia, sedation, and neuromuscular blockade. *Critical Care*. McGraw-Hill Education.
Sullivan, B.L., Bartels, K., & Hamilton, N. (2015). Insertion and management of a temporary pacemaker. Seminars in *CardioThoracic Vascular Anesthesia*. 20(1): 52–62.
Swami, A. & Spodick, D.H. Pulsus paradoxus in cardiac tamponade: a pathophysiologic continuum. *Clinical Cardiology*, 26(5): 215-7.
Swan-Ganz catheter. (2023). BioRender.
Swan-Ganz thermodilution catheters. (2017). Edwards Lifesciences.
Tamis-Holland, J.E., Jneid, H., Reynolds, H.R, et al. (2019). Contemporary diagnosis and management of patients with myocardial infarction in the absence of obstructive coronary artery disease: a scientific statement from the American Heart Association. *Circulation*, 1399(18): 891–908.
Tehrani, B.N., Truesdell, A.G., Psotka, M.A, et al. (2020). A standardized and comprehensive approach to the management of cardiogenic shock. *Journal of the American College of Cardiology: Heart Failure*, 8(11), 879–891.
Tepper, S., Masood, M.F., Baltazar, G., et al. (2017). Left ventricular unloading by Impella device versus surgical vent during extracorporeal life support. *Ann Thorac Surg*, 104(3), 861–867.
Thiele, H., Ohman, M., & Desch, S. (2015). Management of cardiogenic shock. American Association of Critical Care Nurses. 278-297.
Thomas, M.R. & Storey, R.F. (2017). Clinical significance of residual platelet reactivity in patients treated with platelet P2Y12 inhibitors. *Vascular Pharmacology*, 84, 25-27.
Timothy, P.R. & Rodeman, B.J. Temporary pacemakers in critically ill patients: assessment and management strategies. *AACN Clinical Issues*, 15(3): 305–325.
Tweet, M.S., Best, P., & Hayes, S.N. (2017). Unique presentations and etiologies of myocardial infarction in women. *Current Treatment Options in Cardiovascular Medicine*, 19(9), 66.
Tweet, M.S., Hayes, S.N., Codsi, E., et al. (2017). Spontaneous coronary artery dissection associated with pregnancy. *Journal of the American College of Cardiology (JACC)*, 70(4), 426–435.

Vahdatpour, C., Collins, D., & Goldberg, S. (2019). Cardiogenic shock. *The Journal of the American Heart Association,* 8(8).

Vallabhajosyula, S., Shankar, A., Patlolla, S.H., Prasad, A, et al. (2020). Pulmonary artery catheter use in acute myocardial infarction-cardiogenic shock. *ESC Heart Failure,* 7(3), 1234–1245.

Van Diepen, S., Katz, J.N., Albert, N.M, et al. Contemporary management of cardiogenic shock: a scientific statement from the American Heart Association. *Circulation,* 136(16): 232–268.

VanDyck, T.J., Pinsky, M.R. (2021). Hemodynamic monitoring in cardiogenic shock. *Current Opinion in Critical Care,* 27(4): 454-459.

Vargas, K.G., Jäger, B., Kaufmann, C.C., Biagioli, A., Watremez, S., Gatto, F., Özbek, C., Razouk, A., Geppert, A., & Huber, K. (2020). Impella in cardiogenic shock following acute myocardial infarction: a systematic review and meta-analysis.

Velissaris, D., Karamouzos, V., Ktenopoulos, N, et al. (2015). The use of sodium bicarbonate in the treatment of acidosis in sepsis: a literature update on a long term debate. *Critical Care Research and Practice.*

Velissaris, D., Karamouzos, V., Pierrakos, C, et al. (2016). Use of sodium bicarbonate in cardiac arrest: current guidelines and literature review. *Journal of Clinical Medicine Research,* 8(4), 277–283.

Ventetuolo, C.E., & Klinger, J.R. (2014). Management of acute right ventricular failure in the intensive care unit. *Annals of the American Thoracic Society,* 11(5), 811–822.

Vilacosta, I., San Román, J, et al. Acute aortic syndrome revisited: JACC state-of-the-art review. *Journal of the American College of Cardiology (JACC),* 78(21), 2106–2125.

Voskoboinik, A., Prabhu, S., Ling, L.H, et al. (2016). Alcohol and atrial fibrillation: a sobering review. *Journal of the American College of Cardiology (JACC),* 68(23): 2567–2576.

Waksman, R. & Chitturi, K. (2024). Myths and truths in the management of drug-eluting stent in-stent restenosis. *Journal of the American College of Cardiology,* 17(1), 14–16.

Waksman, R., Pahuja, M., Van Diepen, S, et al. (2023). Standardized definitions for cardiogenic shock research and mechanical circulatory support devices: scientific expert panel from the shock Academic research consortium. *Circulation,* 148(14): 1113–1126.

Wang L, Yuan S, Borgquist R, Hoijer CJ, Brandt J. (2014). Coronary sinus cannulation with a steerable catheter during biventricular device implantation.

Wang, K. & Samai, K. (2020). Role of high-dose intravenous nitrates in hypertensive acute heart failure. *Am J Emerg Med,* 39(1):132-137.

Wardi, G., Holgren, S., Gupta, A., Sobel, J, et al. (2023). A review of bicarbonate use in common clinical scenarios. *The Journal of Emergency Medicine,* 65(2), 71-80.

Watson, S., & Gorski, K.A. (2023). Invasive cardiology: a manual for cath lab personnel. Jones & Bartlett Learning.

Webb, A.J., Seisa, M.O., Nayfeh, T., Wieruszewski, P.M., Nei, S.D., & Smischney, N.J. (2020). Vasopressin in vasoplegic shock: a systematic review. *World Journal of Critical Care Medicine,* 9(5): 88-98.

Weerink, M., Struys M., Hannivoort, L, et al. (2017). Clinical pharmacokinetics and pharmacodynamics of dexmedetomidine. *Clinical Pharmacokinetics,* 56(8), 893-913.

Weinstein, S., Hagle, M., Magee, S., Fischer, A., Saltzber, D., & Druding, S. (2014). Plumer's principles & practice of infusion therapy. Lippincott Williams & Wilkins.

Werner, G.S., Lang, K., Kuehnert H, et al. (2002). Intracoronary verapamil for reversal of no-reflow during coronary angioplasty for acute myocardial infarction. *Catheter Cardiovasc Interv,* 57(4), 444-451.

White, K. (2016). Fast facts for critical care – the original critical care pocket reference.

Willis, L. M. (2023). Fluids & electrolytes made incredibly easy! Wolters Kluwer.

Wilson, S.S.,, Kwiatkowski, G.M., Millis, S.R., Purakal, J.D., Mahajan, A.P., & Levy, P.D. (2017). Use of nitroglycerin by bolus prevents intensive care unit admission in patients with acute hypertensive heart failure. *Am J Emerg Med,* 35(1): 126-131.

Wiviott, S.D., Braunwald, E., McCabe, C.H, et al. (2007). Prasugrel versus clopidogrel in patients with acute coronary syndromes. *The New England Journal of Medicine,* 357(20), 2001-2015.

Woodruff, D. (2020). Critical care nursing made incredibly easy! (4th ed.). Wolters Kluwer

Wu, K.H., Chang, C.Y, et al. (2020). Effectiveness of sodium bicarbonate administration on mortality in cardiac arrest patients: a systematic review and meta-analysis. *Journal of Emergency Medicine,* 59(6), 856-864.

Yang, D., Park, B., Kang, S., & An, W.S. (2024). Sodium bicarbonate supplementation may be harmful in septic patients with severe lactic acidosis: a retrospective analysis. *Journal of the American Society of Nephrology.*

Yang, L., Zhang, X., Jin, Q., et al. (2021). Pericardial effusion during the perioperative period for left atrial appendage closure.

Yasuhiro, O., Masanobu, I., So, I, et al. (2024). Current overview of myocardial infarction with nonobstructive coronary arteries, *Journal of Coronary Artery Disease.*

Yeh, R.W., Shlofmitz, R., & Moses, J., et al. (2024). Paclitaxel-coated balloon vs uncoated balloon for coronary in-stent restenosis: the AGENT IDE randomized clinical trial. *Journal of the American Medical Association*, 331(12), 1015-1024.

Yildiz, O., Gamze, A., Zumrut, D.T., Yenigun, C.D., & Yazicioglu, N. (2017). Evaluation of resting cardiac power output as a prognostic factor in patients with advanced heart failure. *The American Journal of Cardiology*, 120(6), 973-979.

Zhou, Y., Wang, Y., et al. (2017). Individualized dual antiplatelet therapy based on platelet function testing in patients undergoing percutaneous coronary intervention: a meta-analysis of randomized controlled trials. *BMC Cardiovascular Disorders*.

Zipes, D., Libby, P., Bonow, R., et al. (2021). Braunwald's heart disease: a textbook of cardiovascular medicine Elsevier/Saunders.

Zipes, D.P., Jalife, J., & Stevenson, W.G. (2021). Cardiac electrophysiology: from cell to bedside. Saunders/Elsevier.

About Me

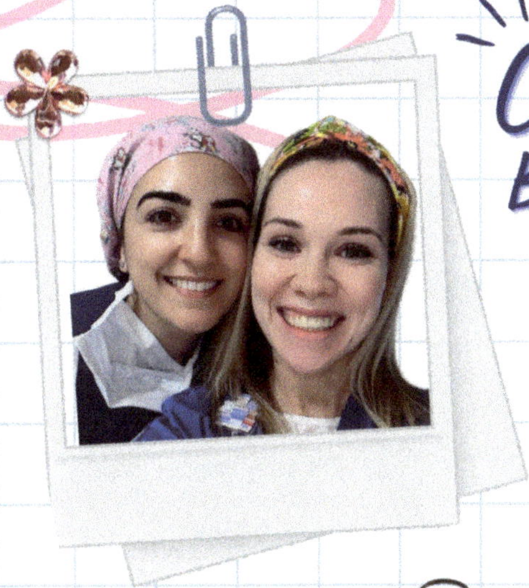

Caitlyn Nichols
BSN, RN, CCRN-CMC

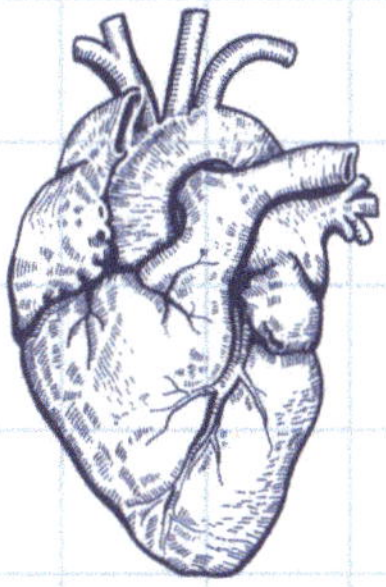

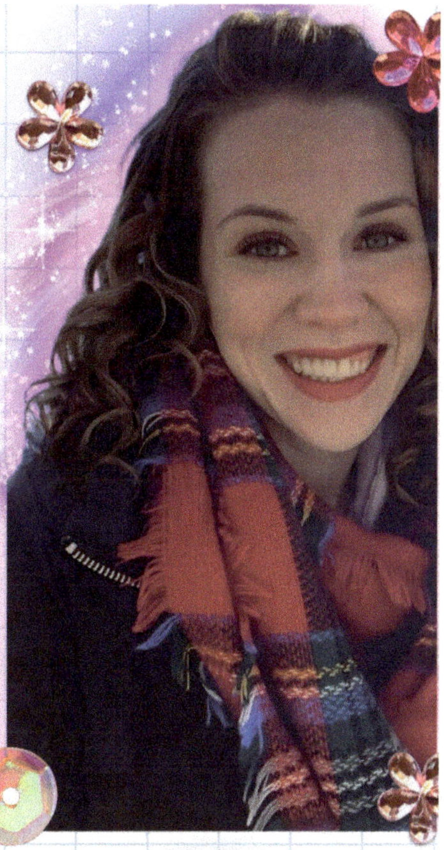

- I graduated from Fairfield University in 2021.
- I've been artistic for as long as I can remember.
- I'm a dog lover.
- I've been skydiving 7 times.
- I'm an old soul at heart!
- My favorite band is the 1975.
- I love learning new things!

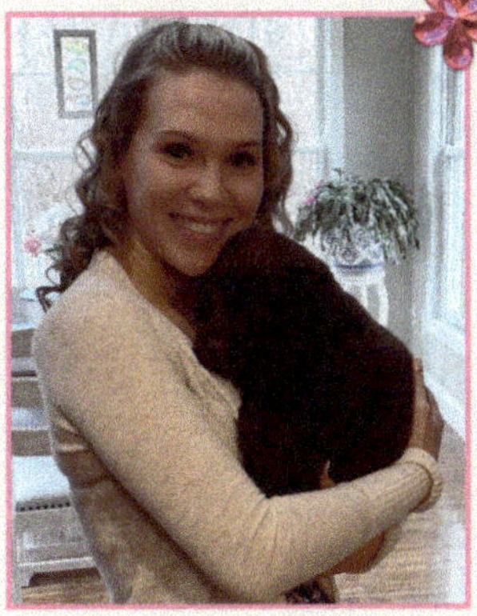

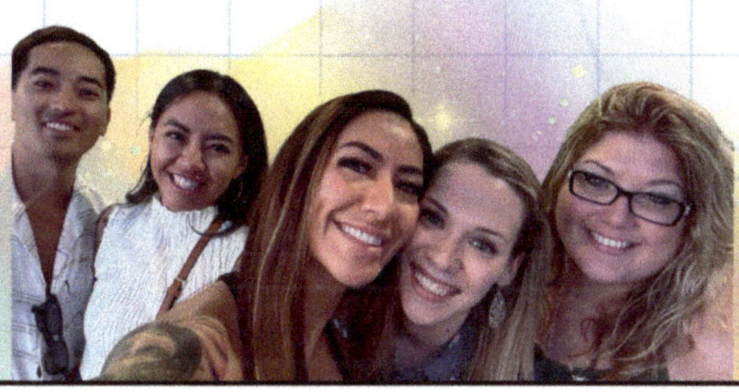

icunursingnotesbycaitlyn

Caitlyn Nichols | BSN, RN, CCRN-CMC

348 posts · 72.3K followers · 282 following

Education
Just a critical care cath lab RN simplifying & sharing my love + passion for critical care nursing & education!

@icunursingnotesbycaitlyn

Etsy www.Etsy.com/shop/icunursingnotes

JEBWizard Publishing

Books with Character

www.ingramcontent.com/pod-product-compliance
Lightning Source LLC
LaVergne TN
LVHW070850210926
848482LV00016B/903

* 9 7 9 8 9 8 7 7 1 7 4 8 6 *